Update on Acute Severe Respiratory Infections

Update on Acute Severe Respiratory Infections

Guest Editor
Jean-Francois Timsit

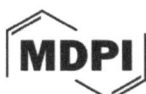

Basel • Beijing • Wuhan • Barcelona • Belgrade • Novi Sad • Cluj • Manchester

Guest Editor
Jean-Francois Timsit
Medical and Infectious
Diseases ICU
APHP Bichat Hospital F
Paris
France

Editorial Office
MDPI AG
Grosspeteranlage 5
4052 Basel, Switzerland

This is a reprint of the Special Issue, published open access by the journal *Journal of Clinical Medicine* (ISSN 2077-0383), freely accessible at: https://www.mdpi.com/journal/jcm/special_issues/9042H9KMCN.

For citation purposes, cite each article independently as indicated on the article page online and as indicated below:

Lastname, A.A.; Lastname, B.B. Article Title. *Journal Name* **Year**, *Volume Number*, Page Range.

ISBN 978-3-7258-4265-0 (Hbk)
ISBN 978-3-7258-4266-7 (PDF)
https://doi.org/10.3390/books978-3-7258-4266-7

© 2025 by the authors. Articles in this book are Open Access and distributed under the Creative Commons Attribution (CC BY) license. The book as a whole is distributed by MDPI under the terms and conditions of the Creative Commons Attribution-NonCommercial-NoDerivs (CC BY-NC-ND) license (https://creativecommons.org/licenses/by-nc-nd/4.0/).

Contents

Giorgia Lüthi-Corridori, Maria Boesing, Andrea Roth, Stéphanie Giezendanner, Anne Barbara Leuppi-Taegtmeyer, Philipp Schuetz and Joerg D. Leuppi
Predictors of Length of Stay, Rehospitalization and Mortality in Community-Acquired Pneumonia Patients: A Retrospective Cohort Study
Reprinted from: *J. Clin. Med.* **2023**, *12*, 5601, https://doi.org/10.3390/jcm12175601 1

Pratima Chowdary, Banwari Agarwal, Maria Rita Peralta, Sanjay Bhagani, Simon Lee, James Goldring, Marc Lipman, Emal Waqif, Mark Phillips, Helen Philippou, et al.
Nebulized Recombinant Tissue Plasminogen Activator (rt-PA) for Acute COVID-19-Induced Respiratory Failure: An Exploratory Proof-of-Concept Trial
Reprinted from: *J. Clin. Med.* **2023**, *12*, 5848, https://doi.org/10.3390/jcm12185848 16

Szymon Białka, Michał Zieliński, Magdalena Latos, Marlena Skurzyńska, Michał Żak, Piotr Palaczyński and Szymon Skoczyński
Severe Bacterial Superinfection of Influenza Pneumonia in Immunocompetent Young Patients: Case Reports
Reprinted from: *J. Clin. Med.* **2024**, *13*, 5665, https://doi.org/10.3390/jcm13195665 33

Maire Röder, Anthony Yong Kheng Cordero Ng and Andrew Conway Morris
Bronchoscopic Diagnosis of Severe Respiratory Infections
Reprinted from: *J. Clin. Med.* **2024**, *13*, 6020, https://doi.org/10.3390/jcm13196020 46

Nadir Ullah, Ludovica Fusco, Luigi Ametrano, Claudia Bartalucci, Daniele Roberto Giacobbe, Antonio Vena, et al.
Diagnostic Approach to Pneumonia in Immunocompromised Hosts
Reprinted from: *J. Clin. Med.* **2025**, *14*, 389, https://doi.org/10.3390/jcm14020389 66

Ágnes Jakab, Andrea Harmath, Zoltán Tóth, László Majoros, József Kónya and Renátó Kovács
Epidemiology and Clinical Relevance of *Pneumocystis jirovecii* in Non-Human Immunodeficiency Virus Patients at a Tertiary Care Center in Central Europe: A 3-Year Retrospective Study
Reprinted from: *J. Clin. Med.* **2025**, *14*, 2820, https://doi.org/10.3390/jcm14082820 91

Maside Ari, Aslı Haykir Solay, Tarkan Ozdemir, Murat Yildiz, Oral Mentes, Omer Faruk Tuten, et al.
Neutrophil Percentage-to-Albumin Ratio as a Prognostic Marker in Pneumonia Patients Aged 80 and Above in Intensive Care
Reprinted from: *J. Clin. Med.* **2025**, *14*, 3033, https://doi.org/10.3390/jcm14093033 100

David Mokrani and Jean-François Timsit
Role of Respiratory Viruses in Severe Acute Respiratory Failure
Reprinted from: *J. Clin. Med.* **2025**, *14*, 3175, https://doi.org/10.3390/jcm14093175 114

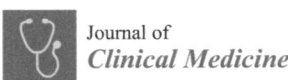

Article

Predictors of Length of Stay, Rehospitalization and Mortality in Community-Acquired Pneumonia Patients: A Retrospective Cohort Study

Giorgia Lüthi-Corridori [1,2], Maria Boesing [1,2], Andrea Roth [1,2], Stéphanie Giezendanner [1,2], Anne Barbara Leuppi-Taegtmeyer [1,2,3], Philipp Schuetz [2,4] and Joerg D. Leuppi [1,2,*]

[1] University Centre of Internal Medicine, Cantonal Hospital Baselland, Rheinstrasse 26, 4410 Liestal, Switzerland; giorgia.luethi-corridori@ksbl.ch (G.L.-C.)
[2] Faculty of Medicine, University of Basel, Klingelbergstrasse 61, 4056 Basel, Switzerland
[3] Department of Patient Safety, University Hospital Basel, Petersgraben 4, 4031 Basel, Switzerland
[4] Cantonal Hospital Aarau, University Department of Medicine, Tellstrasse 25, 5001 Aarau, Switzerland
* Correspondence: joerg.leuppi@ksbl.ch

Abstract: Background: Community-acquired pneumonia (CAP) represents one of the leading causes of hospitalization and has a substantial impact on the financial burden of healthcare. The aim of this study was to identify factors associated with the length of hospital stay (LOHS), rehospitalization and mortality of patients admitted for CAP. Methods: A retrospective cohort study was conducted with patients presenting to a Swiss public hospital between January 2019 and December 2019. Zero-truncated negative binomial and multivariable logistic regression analyses were performed to assess risk factors. Results: A total of 300 patients were analyzed (median 78 years, IQR [67.56, 85.50] and 53% males) with an average LOHS of 7 days (IQR [5.00, 9.00]). Of the 300 patients, 31.6% (97/300) were re-hospitalized within 6 months, 2.7% (8/300) died within 30 days and 11.7% (35/300) died within 1 year. The results showed that sex (IRR = 0.877, 95% CI = 0.776–0.992, p-value = 0.036), age (IRR = 1.007, 95% CI = 1.002–1.012, p-value = 0.003), qSOFA score (IRR = 1.143, 95% CI = 1.049–1.246, p-value = 0.002) and atypical pneumonia (IRR = 1.357, 95% CI = 1.012–1.819, p-value = 0.04) were predictive of LOHS. Diabetes (OR = 2.149, 95% CI = 1.104–4.172, p-value = 0.024), a higher qSOFA score (OR = 1.958, 95% CI = 1.295–3.002, p-value = 0.002) and rehabilitation after discharge (OR = 2.222, 95% CI = 1.017–4.855, p-value = 0.044) were associated with a higher chance of being re-hospitalized within 6 months, whereas mortality within 30 days and within one year were both associated with older age (OR = 1.248, 95% CI = 1.056–1.562, p-value = 0.026 and OR = 1.073, 95% CI = 1.025–1.132, p-value = 0.005, respectively) and the presence of a cancer diagnosis (OR = 32.671, 95% CI = 4.787–369.1, p-value = 0.001 and OR = 4.408, 95% CI = 1.680–11.43, p-value = 0.002, respectively). Conclusion: This study identified routinely available predictors for LOHS, rehospitalization and mortality in patients with CAP, which may further advance our understanding of CAP and thereby improve patient management, discharge planning and hospital costs.

Keywords: community-acquired pneumonia; length of hospital stay; rehospitalization; mortality; prediction; CAP; LOHS

1. Introduction

Community-acquired pneumonia (CAP) is one of the leading causes of hospitalization and is responsible for approximately 2.5 million deaths worldwide every year [1,2]. In Europe, CAP also leads to high hospitalization rates, causing a significant financial burden for the healthcare system [3,4]. The financial impacts of CAP due to prolonged hospitalizations or increased hospitalization rates have been documented in previous studies [5–7]. Current guidelines emphasize the importance of discharging patients as soon as they achieve clinical stability and have access to a safe environment where continuity of care can be ensured [8]. The recommendations particularly underline the importance of increasing outpatient treatment to decrease the cost of hospitalizations and the risk of hospital-acquired complications [8]. However, the length of hospital stay (LOHS) for patients with CAP continues to be variable and for that reason, the development of accurate models to predict the LOHS using patients' baseline profiles from an early stage is needed. Obtaining accurate predictive models upon admission has multiple advantages. First of all, they allow us to identify the profiles of patients at risk of prolonged hospitalization, and whenever possible, to promptly act on modifiable factors. Moreover, discharge strategies can be improved. The implementation of a precise prediction model would additionally permit the evaluation of hospital performance, thereby fostering advancements in hospital management.

The LOHS in patients with CAP can be influenced by a variety of factors, including sociodemographic, health-related and hospital care-related characteristics [9–21]. A number of previous studies investigating factors that influence the LOHS in CAP identified patient-related variables such as advanced age and specific comorbidities, in addition to disease severity, as predictors of a prolonged LOHS [9–13]. Other studies direct their research focus to laboratory values [14–16], while others concentrate on therapies [17–19] or other interventions during hospitalization [20,21]. Due the wide variety of influencing factors, there is no uniform method for predicting the LOHS in CAP patients; moreover, as mentioned above, several studies included factors that are not available at the time of admission, hindering the chance of predicting the LOHS in the first days of hospitalization.

The primary aim of this study was to identify which factors may affect the length of stay of patients admitted for CAP. The identification of patient characteristics influencing the LOHS may help decision makers properly plan hospital management. Particularly, we retrospectively explored whether the primary outcome, the LOHS for CAP, was associated with commonly available sociodemographic and health-related variables that are measurable at the time of admission to the hospital.

Despite advances in therapy, the mortality rate associated with this disease is still high (6–10%). While a shorter LOHS may decrease hospital costs, it may also negatively impact the quality of care [22]. Moreover, research has indicated that rehospitalization and mortality rates are high among patients with CAP who survive the initial admission. This is primarily attributed to factors related to the aging population, like the presence of multiple medical conditions and other health fragilities [23]. Most elderly CAP patients require special attention from health care professionals after discharge to reduce rehospitalization and mortality rates [24]. For this reason, this study analyzed factors associated with rehospitalization within 6 months and all-cause mortality (30-day and one-year mortalities) as secondary outcomes.

2. Materials and Methods

2.1. Design and Setting

Our study was conducted in the cantonal hospital of Baselland (KSBL), a district general hospital covering a stable population of 280,000 in Northwest Switzerland. We undertook a retrospective cohort study extracting all patients older than 18 years of age who were admitted to the hospital between January and December 2019 and categorized them using an International Classification of Disease (ICD) code related to pneumonia (for more details, see the ICD codes list in the Appendix A). A total of 573 patients were identified.

2.2. Inclusion and Exclusion Criteria

Cases were included in this study if newly diagnosed CAP was the main reason for the patient's hospitalization and their diagnosis was confirmed via a chest X-ray or a microbiological test supported by clinical judgment. CAP was defined according to the Infectious Diseases Society of America (IDSA) criteria [8].

The following criteria were applied for exclusion:
- Denied research consent (n = 31);
- Hospital-acquired pneumonia (n = 26);

- Immunocompromised patients (n = 35);
- Patients with prior therapy prescribed by their general practitioner, not newly diagnosed nor newly treated (n = 83);
- Diagnosis not confirmed (n = 38);
- Directly transferred to rehabilitation (n = 27);
- Palliative care (n = 15);
- Other main diagnosis or main reason for hospitalization (n = 11);
- Consecutive (second or third) admission for CAP in the study period (n = 7).

After the application of the eligibility criteria, the data of 300 patients were included in the analysis (Figure 1).

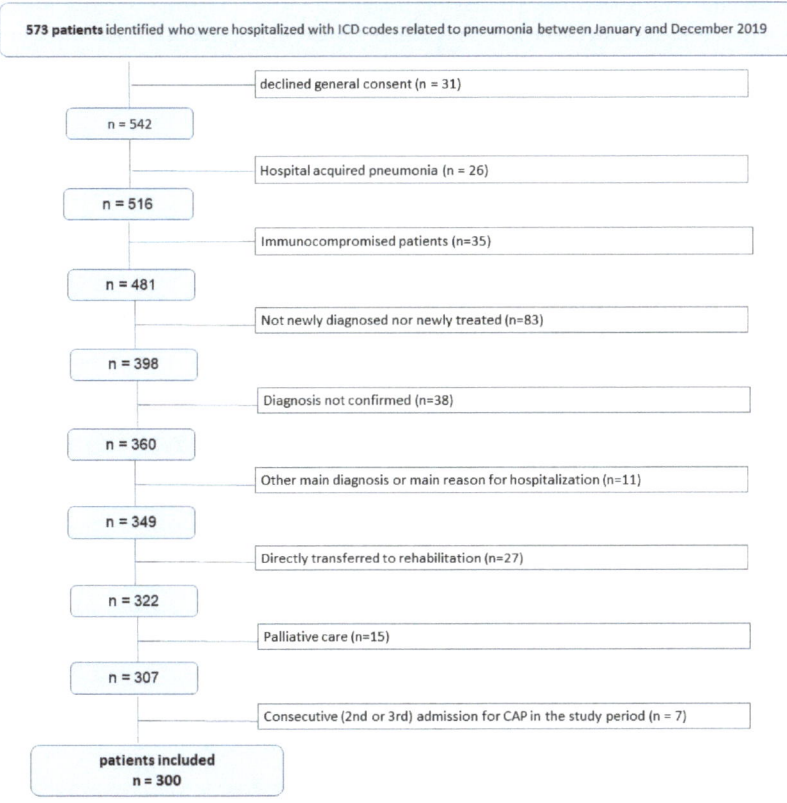

Figure 1. Flowchart diagram for the patient selection process.

2.3. Data Collection

Basic data such as gender, age and the LOHS were automatically extracted from the controlling system. The remaining variables were extracted manually from the electronic patient record by a study physician. To ensure the quality of the data, a subset was reviewed by a health scientist. The primary outcome of interest was the LOHS. Additionally, the secondary outcomes included rehospitalization within six months and all-cause mortality within 30 days and one year. To minimize the risk of bias, optimism and overfitting, we did not perform a data-driven selection of variables. Instead, potential predictors were selected based on the existing literature and clinical knowledge. Two researchers conducted a comprehensive literature review and consulted clinical experts in the field. Predictors for the LOHS included variables available at the time of admission: demographic variables, vital signs, laboratory parameters, comorbidities and risk scores. An "Indication for oxygen supplementation" was defined as the presence of at least one of the following conditions upon admission: oxygen saturation < 90%, oxygen supplementation already in place and respiratory rate ≥ 30. For the analysis of the rehospitalization rate and mortality, events occurring during the hospitalization were also collected, such as oxygen supplementation during hospitalization and rehabilitation after discharge.

2.4. Statistical Analyses

The outcome variables comprised the LOHS (primary outcome), all-cause mortality (at 30 days and 1 year) and rehospitalization within 6 months (secondary outcomes). To minimize the risk of bias, optimism and overfitting, no data-driven selection of variables was conducted. The parameters assessed included age, gender, housing situation before admission, type of pneumonia (atypical pneumonia when an atypical pathogen was identified), medical history and vital signs obtained at the time of admission, laboratory results, therapy and diagnostic work-up score. The analysis of the LOHS was primarily conducted on patients that were discharged alive; since only one patient died in hospital, it was not necessary to perform a sensitivity analysis on the full data set. For the re-hospitalization outcome, we further included the variable LOHS into the model, rehabilitation after discharge and oxygen supplementation during hospitalization. The selection criteria for a multivariate regression of mortality and rehospitalization were tailored to the specific nature of the outcomes under investigation. Distinct from the LOHS analysis, which included admission-time variables like vital signs, the multivariable regression for rehospitalization and mortality focused on long-term outcomes (6 month and 1 year, respectively), retaining factors with minimal temporal variability such as demographics, comorbidities and hospital-related factors (e.g., oxygen during hospitalization, the LOHS and post-discharge rehabilitation) to minimize the risk of susceptibility to temporal fluctuations. We displayed measures of central tendency for descriptive statistics: a median with an interquartile range (IQR) if the distribution was skewed (as determined via a histogram assessment). For categorical variables, we reported absolute and relative frequencies. Variables with missing values of up to 30% were imputed using the k-nearest neighbor algorithm (function knn.impute from the R package "bnstruct") [25,26]. A zero-truncated negative binomial regression was conducted to estimate the LOHS and its association with potential risk factors using the R package "VGAM". Logistic regression models were created to estimate the risk of death and rehospitalization and its association with potential risk factors using the R package "stats". All statistical analyses were performed using R version 4.0.3 statistical software (R Foundation for Statistical Computing). All reported *p*-values were two-sided; statistical significance was defined as $p < 0.05$.

3. Results

3.1. Patient Characteristics

The patient characteristics are presented in Table 1. The median age at the time of hospital admission was 78.5 years, and 53% were males. More than half of the patients had chronic cardiovascular comorbidities (58%); the second most frequent concomitant disease was COPD, followed by diabetes (29.7% and 18.3%, respectively).

Table 1. Patient characteristics.

	All (n = 300)	Missing n (%)
Demographic		
Age at diagnosis, median [IQR]	78.48 [67.56, 85.50]	--
Gender (males), n (%)	160/300 (53.3%)	--
Vital Signs		
Respiratory rate at admission, median [IQR]	21.00 [18.00, 26.00]	77 (25.7%)
Indication for oxygen supplementation, n (%)	102/298 (34.2%)	2 (0.7%)

Table 1. Cont.

	All (n = 300)	Missing n (%)
Oxygen supplementation during hospitalization, n (%)	135/299 (45.2%)	1 (0.3%)
Body temperature at admission, median [IQR]	37.60 [36.95, 38.40]	9 (3.0%)
Fever at admission, n (%)	114/293 (38.9%)	7 (2.3%)
Heart rate at admission, median [IQR])	91.00 [79.00, 104.00]	1 (0.3%)
Systolic blood pressure at admission, median [IQR]	132.00 [112.50, 147.00]	1 (0.3%)
Diastolic blood pressure at admission, median [IQR]	74.00 [65.00, 85.00]	1 (0.3%)
Comorbidities		--
Chronic cardiovascular, n (%)	174/300 (58.0)	--
Hypertension, n (%)	177/300 (59.0%)	--
Cancer, n (%)	32/300 (10.7%)	--
Diabetes, n (%)	55/300 (18.3%)	--
Asthma, n (%)	22/300 (7.3%)	--
COPD, n (%)	59/300 (19.7%)	--
Other chronic respiratory diseases, n (%)	42/300 (14.0%)	--
Risk Scores		
GCS at admission, median [IQR]	15.00 [15.00, 15.00]	7 (2.3%)
qSOFA, median [IQR]	1.00 [0.00, 1.00]	82 (27.3%)
BMI, median [IQR]	26.00 [22.40, 30.25]	137 (45.7%)
Laboratory Values		
Leucocytes at admission, median [IQR]	11.90 [8.97, 15.00]	--
Atypic pneumonia diagnosed, n (%)	19/300 (6.3%)	--
Discharge circumstances		
Rehabilitation, n (%)	51/300 (16.6)	--
Discharged home, n (%)	217/300 (72.3)	--
Discharged to a care facility, n (%)		
Outcomes		
LOHS, median [IQR]	7.00 [5.00, 9.00]	--
Rehospitalization within six months, n (%)	97/300 (31.6%)	--
In-hospital death, n (%)	1/300 (0.3%)	--
30-day mortality, n (%)	8/300 (2.7%)	--
1-year mortality, n (%)	35/300 (11.7%)	--

IQR = interquartile range; COPD = chronic obstructive pulmonary disease; GCS = Glasgow coma scale; qSOFA = quick SOFA; BMI = body mass index; LOHS = length of hospital stay.

3.2. Prediction of the LOHS, Rehospitalization and Mortality

Our primary aim was to examine the factors associated with the LOHS. Table 2 provides coefficient estimates for the predictors of the LOHS in patients who did not die. Regression coefficients are shown as incident risk ratios (IRRs). The median LOHS of the overall cohort was 7 days. The analysis of the prediction model for the LOHS identified four statistically significant predictors: sex, age, qSOFA score and atypical pneumonia. The LOHS prediction at the intercept (7.5 days) is the LOHS when all covariates are at 0 (for categorical covariates) or at their mean (for continuous covariates). The predicted LOHS of the model for each variable is presented for a one-unit increase. A higher increase occurs when the qSOFA score increases the predicted LOHS rise by one unit to 8.5 days. Women tended to stay one night longer than men, while people with atypical pneumonia compared to those without tended to stay three nights longer, assuming all other variables are held constant.

Table 2. Results of multivariable zero-truncated negative binomial regression model for length of hospital stay (LOHS) estimation in CAP patients who survived the first hospital admission (n = 299).

	LOHS Prediction	IRR	(95% CI)	p-Value
(Intercept)	7.458	11.947	1.18–121.0	0.036
Gender (males)	6.562	0.877	0.776–0.992	0.036
Age	7.511	1.007	1.002–1.012	0.003
Chronic cardiovascular	8.217	1.103	0.957–1.273	0.176
COPD	7.126	0.955	0.822–1.108	0.542
Asthma	6.654	0.89	0.708–1.119	0.318
Diabetes	7.148	0.958	0.821–1.118	0.583
Active cancer	8.12	1.09	0.905–1.314	0.364
qSOFA	8.508	1.143	1.049–1.246	0.002
Heart rate at admission	7.472	1.002	0.999–1.005	0.218
Body temperature at admission	7.207	0.966	0.909–1.026	0.26
CRP at admission	7.459	1	1–1.001	0.631
Leucocytes at admission	7.46	1	0.993–1.008	0.936
Atypic pneumonia diagnosed	10.088	1.357	1.012–1.819	0.041

LOHS = length of hospital stay; IRR = incidence rate ratio; CI = confidence interval; COPD = chronic obstructive pulmonary disease; qSOFA = Quick SOFA; CRP = C-reactive Protein.

Our secondary aims included the analyses of factors associated with rehospitalization and mortality. The results for our secondary outcome concerning the rehospitalization rate are reported in Table 3. The odds for rehospitalization within 6 months in the KSBL were also significantly higher for patients with a higher qSOFA score at admission. Moreover, patients with diabetes and those who were admitted to rehabilitation had a higher chance of being rehospitalized within 6 months. No other variable was found to be significantly associated with rehospitalization.

Table 3. Results of multivariable logistic regression model for rehospitalization within 6 months in patients with CAP.

	OR	(95% CI)	p-Value
Gender (males)	0.964	0.549–1.693	0.898
Age	1.016	0.994–1.039	0.164
Chronic cardiovascular	1.123	0.582–2.177	0.73
COPD	1.021	0.504–2.016	0.954
Asthma	1.759	0.622–4.718	0.269
Diabetes	2.149	1.104–4.172	0.024
Active cancer	1.565	0.682–3.557	0.284
qSOFA	1.958	1.295–3.002	0.002
Oxygen during hospitalization	0.636	0.357–1.116	0.118
LOHS	1.055	0.984–1.132	0.134
Rehabilitation after discharge	2.222	1.017–4.855	0.044

OR = odds ratio; CI = confidence interval; COPD = chronic obstructive pulmonary disease; qSOFA = quick SOFA; LOHS = length of hospital stay.

The results of the multivariable logistic regression models for mortality are displayed in Table 4 (30-day mortality) and Table 5 (1-year mortality). In both predictive models, age and an active cancer diagnosis were the only two significant variables associated with mortality. No other variable was found to be significantly associated with mortality.

Table 4. Results of multivariable logistic regression model for 30-day mortality in patients with CAP.

	OR	(95% CI)	p-Value
Gender (males)	13.219	1.235–483.5	0.075
Age	1.248	1.056–1.562	0.026
Chronic cardiovascular	0.953	0.078–25.31	0.972

Table 4. *Cont.*

	OR	(95% CI)	*p*-Value
COPD	0.335	0.012–3.534	0.419
Asthma	0	0–0	0.993
Diabetes	0.956	0.059–9.993	0.971
Active cancer	32.671	4.787–369.1	0.001
qSOFA	0.817	0.198–3.135	0.768
Oxygen during hospitalization	6.787	0.864–101.4	0.103
LOHS	1.144	0.909–1.447	0.246
Rehabilitation after discharge	0.259	0.010–3.353	0.356

OR = odds ratio; CI = confidence interval; COPD = chronic obstructive pulmonary disease; qSOFA = auick SOFA; LOHS = length of hospital stay.

Table 5. Results of multivariable logistic regression model for one-year mortality in patients with CAP.

	OR	(95% CI)	*p*-Value
Gender (males)	1.352	0.594–3.166	0.477
Age	1.073	1.025–1.132	0.005
Chronic cardiovascular	1.53	0.563–4.684	0.425
COPD	0.722	0.247–1.881	0.525
Asthma	0.773	0.106–3.445	0.763
Diabetes	1.847	0.725–4.518	0.185
Active cancer	4.408	1.680–11.43	0.002
qSOFA	1.194	0.665–2.126	0.547
Oxygen during hospitalization	1.6	0.714–3.657	0.256
LOHS	1.025	0.922–1.130	0.63
Rehabilitation after discharge	1.234	0.401–3.541	0.703

OR = odds ratio; CI = confidence interval; COPD = chronic obstructive pulmonary disease; qSOFA = quick SOFA; LOHS = length of hospital stay.

4. Discussion

This retrospective observational cohort study of patients with CAP showed that the LOHS is influenced by demographic factors such as an older age and female gender and by disease-specific factors like the qSOFA score and atypical pneumonia. Other factors, such as other types of comorbidities, vital signs (other than included in the qSOFA) and laboratory values at admission, were not associated with a longer LOHS.

Interestingly, our results show that women had worse outcomes compared to men. Gender differences have been observed in the clinical course, and outcomes of people with CAP and, historically, men have been found to have worse outcomes, particularly in terms of short- and long-term mortality [27,28]. Although little evidence in terms of the LOHS is available, our results are consistent with an international multicenter study by the Community Acquired Pneumonia Organization which followed patients for 10 years. In this study, Arnold and colleagues found that women had significantly longer LOHSs and also worse outcomes in terms of time until clinical stability and mortality within 28 days [29]. Gender differences clearly warrant further confirmation and validation because causal inference cannot be drawn. However, if confirmed in the future, the current concept that female patients have a lower risk than males with CAP may need to be revised and the current scoring system adjusted (for example, the subtraction of 10 points for females in the Pneumonia Severity Index (PSI)).

The quick Sequential (Sepsis-related) Organ Failure Assessment (qSOFA) score is another severity assessment tool and validated prognostic model devised by Seymour et al. [30,31] Originally it was developed to predict sepsis using three main clinical criteria, namely altered mental status, low systolic blood pressure and high respiratory rate. In line with other studies, our results also confirm the prognostic validity of the qSOFA score in predicting the length of hospital stay [30,32–34]. The role of qSOFA in the LOHS was confirmed recently by Koch et al. [35]; however, the impacts of the single items comprising the score were unclear. For this reason, in our study, we also analyzed the items of the qSOFA score separately, and we found that altered mental status (GCS < 15) and blood pressure (Systolic BP $\leq$ 100) were significantly predictive for the LOHS (for more details, see Table A1 in Appendix A). The main advantage of implementing the qSOFA score is that it does not require laboratory tests and allows for rapid and repetitive assessments. In addition to the task force's recommendation to use the qSOFA tool to further investigate potential organ dysfunction or to initiate or escalate appropriate therapy, our results suggest that the qSOFA score can be integrated into predictive models as a risk predictor for an extended LOHS.

Another point worth discussing is the fact that atypical pneumonia was predictive for an extended LOHS. In community-acquired pneumonia, examples of typical pathogens are streptococcus pneumoniae and haemophilus influenzae, and atypical pathogens are mycoplasma pneumoniae, chlamydia pneumoniae and staphylococcus aureus [36]. Atypical pneumonia often expresses more unspecific symptoms such as headache, low fever, dyspnea, dry cough and only slightly elevated inflammatory biomarkers; moreover, the clinical presentation can range from mild symptoms to severe illness with respiratory failure or sepsis [37]. Approximately 7% to 20% of cases of community-acquired pneumonia are believed to be caused by atypical bacterial microorganisms which cannot be detected via Gram staining and pose challenges in terms of culturing [38]. Moreover, the presence of atypical pathogens in some patients with community-acquired pneumonia (CAP) poses a challenge in the selection of empirical antibiotic treatment. These pathogens are inherently resistant to beta-lactam drugs, which are commonly used as an initial antibiotic treatment [39]. This dilemma arises from the fact that adding antibiotic coverage specifically for atypical pathogens might carry the risk of adverse effects and promotes the development of antimicrobial resistance [40]. On the other hand, withholding such coverage may potentially worsen the prognosis if an atypical pathogen is indeed the causative agent of the pneumonia [41,42]. Therefore, in our study, we also considered the presence of atypical pathogens as a potential predictor when examining the length of stay in patients with CAP. We recognized that the use or omission of antibiotic coverage for atypical pathogens could influence the clinical course and outcomes, including the LOHS. Hence, the observed association between atypical pneumonia and an extended length of stay in our study could potentially be attributed to the challenges involved in treatment. Specifically, the addition of antibiotic treatment coverage to address atypical pathogens might inadvertently lead to adverse effects, thereby prolonging the hospitalization period. Alternatively, the diagnostic tests employed to identify atypical pathogens may require additional time, contributing to a longer length of stay.

Our secondary outcomes included rehospitalization in the KSBL within 6 months. We detected that in our study population, rehospitalization within 6 months was significantly associated with factors such as diabetes, qSOFA score and rehabilitation after discharge. The percentage of patients who were rehospitalized within 6 months was 31.6%, which is similar to the ranges of two non-recent studies in which the assessed cumulative readmission rates were 22 and 35.6% [43,44]. In terms of readmission rate, in fact, it is not common to assess long-term outcomes, as stated by Prescott in a systematic review; the majority of published studies in the literature concentrate their focus on the 30-day readmission, and the percentage varies from a minimum of 16.8 to a maximum of 20.1% [45]. The most recent study published in 2021 by Averin et al., which assessed late readmission following hospitalization for pneumonia among American adults, analyzed one-year readmission, and the proportion reached 42.3% of the study population [46]. As previously mentioned the qSOFA score is a validated prognostic tool for sepsis; a recent study investigated the prognostic performance of the qSOFA score for in-hospital mortality and ICU admission [47], but its accuracy in predicting long-term outcome in terms of rehospitalization within 6 months has not been established.

Interestingly, diabetes was the only chronic health condition associated with rehospitalization within 6 months. Previous studies found a relationship between diabetes and the incidence of CAP [48] or hospitalization rate [49] or demonstrated that patients with diabetes have worse discharge outcomes compared to patients without diabetes [50]. A recently published systematic review and meta-analysis by Fang et al. found that diabetes mellitus was significantly associated with the hospital readmission rate among pneumonia patients (pooled OR = 1.18; 95% CI: 1.08–1.28) [24], which is confirmed by our results. So, despite advances in treatment, diabetes is still associated with a higher risk of adverse outcomes, and healthcare providers should take this finding into account. Although CAP patients who also suffer from diabetes are at an elevated risk for adverse events and a complicated clinical course, as explained above, further studies are required in order to clarify the underlying mechanisms and the impact of a disrupted glucose metabolism on the development and clinical outcome of CAP in light of rehospitalization rates.

It is worth mentioning that discharge into rehabilitation was found to be significantly associated with rehospitalization. Patients who were sent to rehabilitation after discharge had a higher chance of being readmitted to the hospital within 6 months compared to those who did not attend rehabilitation. This finding contradicts the initial hypothesis that rehabilitation would reduce the risk of rehospitalization. Possible explanations may include the complexity and severity of the underlying conditions requiring rehabilitation, the intensity or duration of the rehabilitation program, or other unmeasured factors that could influence the outcome. In order to further investigate the underlying reasons for the positive relationship between rehabilitation and rehospitalization, we conducted a post hoc analysis comparing the characteristics of patients who were rehabilitated after hospitalization with those who were not rehabilitated. As displayed in Table A2 in Appendix A, significant differences were detected. The age of patients who received rehabilitation was significantly higher compared to those who did not (medians of 82.73 and 77.35, respectively; p-value = 0.004). Similarly, patients who underwent rehabilitation had a significantly longer LOHS (medians of 11 days and 6 days, respectively 6.00; p-value = 0.001). Other factors, such as chronic cardiovascular disease, COPD, respiratory insufficiency, parapneumonic effusion and cardiovascular complications, also showed significant differences between the two groups. The detected significant differences between the two groups in terms of age, comorbidity burden and hospital complications might explain the positive association between rehabilitation and rehospitalization. Hence, it is necessary to carefully interpret the association between rehabilitation and rehospitalization, considering the confounding effects of these patient characteristics. Moreover, a previous study showed promising results, especially in the short-term, specifically focusing on the 30-day hospital readmission rate [51]. The majority of the studies investigating the positive effects of rehabilitation mainly focused on different outcomes [52–55]. It is important to note that our study differs from these previous investigations as we examined rehospitalization rates within a longer time frame of six months. This extended duration allowed us to capture readmissions that may have occurred beyond the initial 30-day period and provides a more comprehensive understanding of the factors influencing rehospitalization. Further exploration is needed to better understand this unexpected association.

In terms of mortality, we observed that the in-hospital mortality rate was very low: only one patient died during the initial hospitalization, as displayed in Table 1. This can be explained by the fact that all the patients who were transferred for palliative care or directly sent to another hospital were excluded from this study. On the contrary, we noticed that almost one-quarter of the overall mortality within one year happened within thirty days after discharge (22.9%). This trend was also confirmed by Wadhera in a study using population-based data from almost 16300 patients which was conducted in Germany. The research revealed a significant increase in mortality over time, with a 4.7% increase between in-hospital mortality (17.2%) and 30-day mortality (21.9%) [56]. Similarly, a study conducted in the United States with a 10-year cohort of about 3 million CAP patients reported a high 30-day post-discharge mortality of 8.2% [57]. Both multivariable logistic models for 30-day and 1-year mortality revealed that age and a cancer diagnosis were associated with a higher risk of mortality. The findings from our study reinforce prior observations that all-cause mortality during the year subsequent to hospital admission for pneumonia is linked to increasing age and a worsening comorbidity profile [46,58,59]. A recent study concluded that while long-term mortality following CAP was primarily associated with comorbidities, there is potential for early post-discharge complications (within 30 days) to be attributed to CAP-related issues that may benefit from targeted interventions [60]. However, our results did not find different predictors between the two mortality outcomes. Finally, it is important to note that the LOHS was not significantly associated with mortality nor rehospitalization, implying that a shorter LOHS did not show an increased risk of re-admission or post-discharge mortality.

Strengths, Limitations and Further Research

The novelty of our study lies in its comprehensive encompassing of three important quality indicators as research outcomes (the LOHS, rehospitalization and mortality). The prediction models included various factors such as demographic variables, health-related variables and laboratory values available at the time of admission. A further strength of our research was the possibility to investigate long-term outcomes such as mortality within one year, as these data were available for all patients. However, there are certain limitations to consider. As a retrospective study, the quality of the data depended on accurate documentation in the patient files, which may have resulted in incomplete information. It is especially important to note that the presentation of the severity index data, such as the Pneumonia Severity Index (PSI), was hindered by the absence of available data, thereby limiting the depth of the analysis regarding the severity stratification of CAP cases in this study. Furthermore, information on rehospitalization within six months was limited to a specific hospital due to privacy policies, potentially missing readmissions to other healthcare facilities. However, according to a previous study, in Switzerland, most unplanned readmissions occur within the same hospital [61]. The conclusions of this study are limited to the definition of CAP according to the IDSA criteria [8]. The generalizability of other definitions of CAP will have to be assessed. Overall, our study provides a foundation for future research and contributes valuable insights into other aspects of CAP, particularly focusing on the possible predictors of the LOHS, mortality and rehospitalization that are available at the time of admission. The identification of predictors available at the time of admission might help to promptly identify patients who are at a higher risk of adverse outcomes and allow healthcare providers to prioritize their care, allocate appropriate resources and develop personalized management strategies tailored to patients' specific needs. Further studies are needed to investigate the underlying causes contributing to the association between atypical pneumonia and the LOHS. As mentioned before, predictive models could include data regarding antibiotic coverage and time until the diagnosis of atypical pneumonia. By conducting additional research, a more comprehensive understanding can be obtained, and targeted interventions to optimize patient care and reduce the burden associated with prolonged hospital stays can be developed.

5. Conclusions

Understanding the factors that are associated with the LOHS in patients with CAP has clinical implications and may help healthcare providers to deliver efficient care and allocate adequate resources in the management of these patients. In summary, the results of this study showed that female sex, advanced age, a higher qSOFA score and atypical pneumonia were predictive for a longer LOHS. Diabetes, a high qSOFA score and discharge to rehabilitation were associated with a higher chance of rehospitalization within 6 months, whereas mortality rates within 30 days and within one year were both linked to advanced age and the presence of an active cancer diagnosis. However, the potential unfavorable effect of rehabilitation after hospitalization should be interpreted with caution as a post hoc analysis revealed significant disparities in terms of age, LOHS, comorbidities and hospital complications among the studied groups (patients undergoing rehabilitation after hospitalization and those not being rehabilitated). Moreover, our study confirmed the important role of the qSOFA score as a predictive tool not only for sepsis but also for the LOHS and rehospitalization in patients with CAP.

Author Contributions: G.L.-C. and A.R. were responsible for data collection. G.L.-C., S.G. and M.B. were responsible for data analysis. G.L.-C., M.B. and J.D.L. were responsible for designing the study. G.L.-C. drafted the manuscript, A.B.L.-T. and P.S. were responsible for critically assessing data interpretation and revising the manuscript. All authors have read and agreed to the published version of the manuscript.

Funding: The project was financed by the Swiss Personalized Health Network (SPHN Grant #2018DRI08).

Institutional Review Board Statement: The study was conducted in accordance with the Declaration of Helsinki of the World Medical Association. This study protocol was reviewed and approved by the ethics committee of northwest and central Switzerland (Project-ID 2021-00964).

Informed Consent Statement: We included patients whose written informed consent was obtained and patients whose consent exception was permitted by the ethics committee (Art.34 HFG). Patients who denied the hospital general consent were excluded.

Data Availability Statement: All data generated were analyzed during this study and the results are included in this article. The data presented in this study are available upon reasonable request from the corresponding author. The data are not publicly available due to restrictions on data privacy.

Acknowledgments: We thank Philippe Salathé for providing accounting information which helped to design the study.

Conflicts of Interest: Joerg D. Leuppi is supported by grants from the Swiss National Science Foundation (SNF 160072 and 185592), as well as by the Swiss Personalized Health Network (SPHN 2018DR108). He has also received unrestricted grants from AstraZeneca AG Switzerland, Boehringer Ingelheim GmbH Switzerland, GSK AG Switzerland, and OM Pharma AG Switzerland. The authors declare that the research was conducted in the absence of any commercial or financial relationships that could be construed as a potential conflict of interest.

Appendix A

A list of the ICD-10 Codes used for patients' selection, in detail:

- A 48.1 Pneumonic legionnaires disease;
- J 10.0 Influenza due to other identified influenza virus with unspecified type of pneumonia;
- J 12.0 Adenoviral pneumonia;
- J 12.1 Respiratory syncytial virus pneumonia;
- J 12.2 Parainfluenza virus pneumonia;
- J 12.3 Human metapneumovirus pneumonia;
- J 12.8 Other viral pneumonia;
- J 12.9 Viral pneumonia, unspecified;
- J 13 Pneumonia due to Streptococcus pneumoniae;
- J 14 Pneumonia due to Hemophilus influenzae;
- J. 15.1 Pneumonia due to Pseudomonas;
- J 15.2 Pneumonia due to Staphylococcus;
- J 15.3 Pneumonia due to streptococcus, group B;
- J 15.4 Pneumonia due to other streptococci;
- J 15.5 Pneumonia due to Escherichia coli;
- J 15.6 Pneumonia due to other aerobic Gram-negative bacteria;
- J 15.7 Pneumonia due to Mycoplasma pneumoniae;
- J 15.8 Other bacterial pneumonia;
- J 15.9 Unspecified bacterial pneumonia;
- J 16.0 Chlamydial pneumonia;
- J 16.8 Pneumonia due to other specified infectious organisms;
- J 18.0-Bronchopneumonia, unspecified organism;

- J 18.1 Lobar pneumonia, unspecified organism;
- J 18.8 Other pneumonia, unspecified organism;
- J 18.9 Pneumonia, unspecified organism;
- J 85.1 Abscess of lung with pneumonia.

Table A1. Multivariable zero-truncated negative binomial regression model for LOHS estimation in CAP survivors; qSOFA items separately assessed (n = 299).

	LOHS Prediction	IRR	(95% CI)	p-Value
(Intercept)	6.693			
Gender (males)	5.883	0.875	0.775–0.989	0.032
Age	6.738	1.007	1.002–1.012	0.005
Chronic cardiovascular	7.455	1.117	0.970–1.285	0.124
COPD	6.455	0.964	0.831–1.117	0.623
Asthma	5.96	0.887	0.708–1.112	0.299
Diabetes	6.49	0.969	0.830–1.131	0.689
Active cancer	7.463	1.118	0.928–1.347	0.241
Altered mental status (GCS < 15)	8.234	1.235	1.079–1.414	0.002
Systolic BP $\leq$ 100	8.646	1.297	1.064–1.582	0.010
Respiratory rate $\geq$ 22	7.142	1.069	0.947–1.206	0.282
Heart rate at admission	6.708	1.002	0.999–1.006	0.131
Body temperature at admission	6.478	0.967	0.911–1.027	0.274
CRP at admission	6.694	1	1–1.001	0.458
Leucocytes at admission	6.696	1.001	0.993–1.008	0.877
Atypic pneumonia diagnosed	9.251	1.389	1.039–1.856	0.026

LOHS = length of hospital stay, IRR = incidence rate ratio; CI = confidence interval; COPD = chronic obstructive pulmonary disease; GCS = Glasgow coma scale; BP = blood pressure, CRP = C-reactive protein.

Table A2. Post hoc analysis. Comparison between patients undergoing rehabilitation after hospitalization and those not being rehabilitated.

Variables	Overall (n = 300)	Rehabilitation (No) n = 253	Rehabilitation (Yes) n = 47	p-Value	Missing
Age, median [IQR]	78.48 [67.6, 85.5]	77.35 [66.2, 84.6]	82.73 [78.0, 88.5]	0.004	0
LOHS, median [IQR]	7.00 [5.00, 9.00]	6.00 [5.00, 8.00]	11.00 [7.5, 14.5]	<0.001	0
BMI (median [IQR])	26.00 [22.4, 30.2]	26.50 [22.8, 30.4]	25.00 [21.0, 27.3]	0.085	45.7
Oxygen during hospitalization, in days, median [IQR]	1.00 [0.0, 3.0]	1.00 [0.0, 3.0]	3.50 [1.0, 6.7]	0.001	26.3
qSOFA, median [IQR]	1.00 [0.00, 1.00]	1.00 [0.0, 1.0]	1.00 [0.0, 1.0]	0.265	27.3
Gender (male), n (%)	160 (53.3)	138 (54.5)	22 (46.8)	0.414	0
Atypic pneumonia, n (%)	12 (4.0)	10 (4.0)	2 (4.3)	1	0
Chronic cardiovascular disease, n (%)	174 (58.0)	140 (55.3)	34 (72.3)	0.045	0
Diabetes, n (%)	55 (18.3)	49 (19.4)	6 (12.8)	0.385	0
COPD, n (%)	59 (19.7)	44 (17.4)	15 (31.9)	0.036	0
Asthma, n (%)	22 (7.3)	21 (8.3)	1 (2.1)	0.236	0
Other chronic respiratory disease, n (%)	42 (14.0)	31 (12.3)	11 (23.4)	0.073	0
Active cancer, n (%)	32 (10.7)	24 (9.5)	8 (17.0)	0.201	0
Severe immunosuppression, n (%)	2 (0.7)	1 (0.4)	1 (2.1)	0.716	0
Care facility resident, n (%)	50 (16.7)	46 (18.2)	4 (8.5)	0.155	0
Oxygen during hospitalization, n (%)	135 (45.2)	106 (42.1)	29 (61.7)	0.02	0.3
Admission to ICU, n (%)	27 (9.0)	20 (7.9)	7 (14.9)	0.208	0
ARDS, n (%)	300 (100.0)	253 (100.0)	47 (100.0)	NA	0
Sepsis, n (%)	6 (2.0)	4 (1.6)	2 (4.3)	0.525	0
Respiratory insufficiency, n (%)	25 (8.3)	15 (5.9)	10 (21.3)	0.001	0
Cardiovascular complications, n (%)	42 (14.0)	29 (11.5)	13 (27.7)	0.007	0
Acute kidney injury, n (%)	54 (18.0)	45 (17.8)	9 (19.1)	0.987	0
Anemia, n (%)	19 (6.4)	19 (7.6)	0 (0.0)	0.109	1

Table A2. *Cont.*

Variables	Overall (n = 300)	Rehabilitation (No) n = 253	Rehabilitation (Yes) n = 47	p-Value	Missing
Parapneumonic effusion, n (%)	34 (11.3)	22 (8.7)	12 (25.5)	0.002	0
Syncope, n (%)	3 (1.0)	3 (1.2)	0 (0.0)	1	0
In-hospital fall, n (%)	22 (7.4)	16 (6.3)	6 (12.8)	0.214	0.3
Elevated liver parameters, n (%)	23 (7.7)	21 (8.3)	2 (4.3)	0.51	0
Neurological complications, n (%)	14 (4.7)	9 (3.6)	5 (10.6)	0.082	0
Gastrointestinal complications, n (%)	14 (4.7)	12 (4.7)	2 (4.3)	1	0
Electrolyte disorder, n (%)	53 (17.7)	44 (17.4)	9 (19.1)	0.935	0

IQR = interquartile range; LOHS = length of hospital stay; BMI = body mass index; qSOFA = quick SOFA; COPD = chronic obstructive pulmonary disease; ICU = Intensive care unit; ARDS = acute respiratory distress syndrome.

References

1. World Health Organization. *Global Health Estimates 2016: Deaths by Cause, Age, Sex, by Country and by Region, 2000–2016*; World Health Organization: Geneva, Switzerland, 2018. Available online: https://www.who.int/data/gho/data/themes/mortality-and-global-health-estimates (accessed on 1 June 2023).
2. Troeger, C.; Blacker, B.; Khalil, I.A.; Rao, P.C.; Cao, J.; Zimsen, S.R.; Albertson, S.B.; Deshpande, A.; Farag, T.; Abebe, Z.; et al. Estimates of the global, regional, and national morbidity, mortality, and aetiologies of lower respiratory infections in 195 countries, 1990-2016: A systematic analysis for the Global Burden of Disease Study 2016. *Lancet Infect. Dis.* 2018, *18*, 1191–1210. [CrossRef] [PubMed]
3. Torres, A.; Cillóniz, C.; Blasi, F.; Chalmers, J.D.; Gaillat, J.; Dartois, N.; Schmitt, H.-J.; Welte, T. Burden of pneumococcal community-acquired pneumonia in adults across Europe: A literature review. *Respir. Med.* 2018, *137*, 6–13. [CrossRef] [PubMed]
4. Welte, T.; Torres, A.; Nathwani, D. Clinical and economic burden of community-acquired pneumonia among adults in Europe. *Thorax* 2012, *67*, 71–79. [CrossRef] [PubMed]
5. Brown, J.D.; Harnett, J.; Chambers, R.; Sato, R. The relative burden of community-acquired pneumonia hospitalizations in older adults: A retrospective observational study in the United States. *BMC Geriatr.* 2018, *18*, 92. [CrossRef]
6. Vissink, C.E.; Huijts, S.M.; de Wit, G.A.; Bonten, M.J.M.; Mangen, M.-J.J. Hospitalization costs for community-acquired pneumonia in Dutch elderly: An observational study. *BMC Infect. Dis.* 2016, *16*, 466. [CrossRef]
7. Reyes, S.; Martinez, R.; Vallés, J.M.; Cases, E.; Menendez, R. Determinants of hospital costs in community-acquired pneumonia. *Eur. Respir. J.* 2008, *31*, 1061–1067. [CrossRef]
8. Metlay, J.P.; Waterer, G.W.; Long, A.C.; Anzueto, A.; Brozek, J.; Crothers, K.; Cooley, L.A.; Dean, N.C.; Fine, M.J.; Flanders, S.A.; et al. Diagnosis and Treatment of Adults with Community-acquired Pneumonia. An Official Clinical Practice Guideline of the American Thoracic Society and Infectious Diseases Society of America. *Am. J. Respir. Crit. Care Med.* 2019, *200*, e45–e67. [CrossRef]
9. Harrison, G.W.; Escobar, G.J. Length of stay and imminent discharge probability distributions from multistage models: Variation by diagnosis, severity of illness, and hospital. *Health Care Manag. Sci.* 2010, *13*, 268–279. [CrossRef]
10. Suter-Widmer, I.; Christ-Crain, M.; Zimmerli, W.; Albrich, W.; Mueller, B.; Schuetz, P. Predictors for length of hospital stay in patients with community-acquired pneumonia: Results from a Swiss multicenter study. *BMC Pulm. Med.* 2012, *12*, 21. [CrossRef]
11. Iroezindu, M.O.; Isiguzo, G.C.; Chima, E.I.; Mbata, G.C.; Onyedibe, K.I.; Onyedum, C.C.; John-Maduagwu, O.J.; Okoli, L.E.; Young, E.E. Predictors of in-hospital mortality and length of stay in community-acquired pneumonia: A 5-year multi-centre case control study of adults in a developing country. *Trans. R. Soc. Trop. Med. Hyg.* 2016, *110*, 445–455. [CrossRef]
12. Kutz, A.; Gut, L.; Ebrahimi, F.; Wagner, U.; Schuetz, P.; Mueller, B. Association of the Swiss Diagnosis-Related Group Reimbursement System With Length of Stay, Mortality, and Readmission Rates in Hospitalized Adult Patients. *JAMA Netw. Open* 2019, *2*, e188332. [CrossRef] [PubMed]
13. Uematsu, H.; Yamashita, K.; Kunisawa, S.; Imanaka, Y. Prediction model for prolonged length of stay in patients with community-acquired pneumonia based on Japanese administrative data. *Respir. Investig.* 2021, *59*, 194–203. [CrossRef] [PubMed]
14. Farah, R.; Khamisy-Farah, R.; Makhoul, N. Consecutive Measures of CRP Correlate with Length of Hospital Stay in Patients with Community-Acquired Pneumonia. *Isr. Med. Assoc. J.* 2018, *20*, 345–348. [PubMed]
15. Travlos, A.; Bakakos, A.; Vlachos, K.F.; Rovina, N.; Koulouris, N.; Bakakos, P. C-Reactive Protein as a Predictor of Survival and Length of Hospital Stay in Community-Acquired Pneumonia. *J. Pers. Med.* 2022, *12*, 1710. [CrossRef]
16. Rivera-Saldivar, G.; Zamudio-Osorio, H.; Vega-Castro, S. Laboratories as predictors of length of hospital stay in patients with pneumonia. *Rev. Med. Inst. Mex. Seguro Soc.* 2023, *61*, 82–87.
17. Gómez Gómez, J.; Gómez Torres, J.L.; Hernández Torres, A.; García Córdoba, J.A.; Canteras Jordana, M. Influence of initial protocolized treatment with steroids in length of stay and costs of community acquired pneumonia. *Rev. Esp. Quimioter.* 2017, *30*, 350–354. [PubMed]

18. Christensen, E.W.; Spaulding, A.B.; Pomputius, W.F.; Grapentine, S.P. Effects of Hospital Practice Patterns for Antibiotic Administration for Pneumonia on Hospital Lengths of Stay and Costs. *J. Pediatr. Infect. Dis. Soc.* **2019**, *8*, 115–121. [CrossRef]
19. Schmitt, J.P.; Kirfel, A.; Schmitz, M.-T.; Kohlhof, H.; Weisbarth, T.; Wittmann, M. The Impact of Drug Interactions in Patients with Community-Acquired Pneumonia on Hospital Length of Stay. *Geriatrics* **2022**, *7*, 11. [CrossRef]
20. Melgaard, D.; Baandrup, U.; Bøgsted, M.; Bendtsen, M.D.; Kristensen, M.T. Early mobilisation of patients with community-acquired pneumonia reduce length of hospitalisation-a pilot study. *J. Phys. Ther. Sci.* **2018**, *30*, 926–932. [CrossRef]
21. Chen, H.; Hara, Y.; Horita, N.; Saigusa, Y.; Kaneko, T. An Early Screening Tool for Discharge Planning Shortened Length of Hospital Stay for Elderly Patients with Community-Acquired Pneumonia. *Clin. Interv. Aging* **2021**, *16*, 443–450. [CrossRef]
22. Capelastegui, A.; España, P.P.; Quintana, J.M.; Gallarreta, M.; Gorordo, I.; Esteban, C.; Urrutia, I.; Bilbao, A. Declining length of hospital stay for pneumonia and postdischarge outcomes. *Am. J. Med.* **2008**, *121*, 845–852. [CrossRef] [PubMed]
23. Li, X.; Blais, J.E.; Wong, I.C.K.; Tam, A.W.Y.; Cowling, B.J.; Hung, I.F.N.; Chan, E.W.Y. Population-based estimates of the burden of pneumonia hospitalizations in Hong Kong, 2011–2015. *Eur. J. Clin. Microbiol. Infect. Dis.* **2019**, *38*, 553–561. [CrossRef] [PubMed]
24. Fang, Y.-Y.; Ni, J.-C.; Wang, Y.; Yu, J.-H.; Fu, L.-L. Risk factors for hospital readmissions in pneumonia patients: A systematic review and meta-analysis. *World J. Clin. Cases* **2022**, *10*, 3787–3800. [CrossRef]
25. Mucherino, A.; Papajorgji, P.J.; Pardalos, P.M. k-Nearest Neighbor Classification. In *Data Mining in Agriculture*; Mucherino, A., Papajorgji, P.J., Pardalos, P.M., Eds.; Springer: New York, NY, USA, 2009; pp. 83–106. ISBN 978-0-387-88614-5.
26. Beretta, L.; Santaniello, A. Nearest neighbor imputation algorithms: A critical evaluation. *BMC Med. Inform. Decis. Mak.* **2016**, *16* (Suppl. S3), 74. [CrossRef] [PubMed]
27. De-Miguel-Díez, J.; López-de-Andrés, A.; Hernández-Barrera, V.; de-Miguel-Yanes, J.M.; Carabantes-Alarcón, D.; Ji, Z.; Zamorano-Leon, J.J.; Jiménez-García, R. Sex-differences in incidence of hospitalizations and in hospital mortality of community-acquired pneumonia among children in Spain: A population-based study. *Eur. J. Pediatr.* **2022**, *181*, 2705–2713. [CrossRef]
28. Corica, B.; Tartaglia, F.; D'Amico, T.; Romiti, G.F.; Cangemi, R. Sex and gender differences in community-acquired pneumonia. *Intern. Emerg. Med.* **2022**, *17*, 1575–1588. [CrossRef]
29. Arnold, F.W.; Wiemken, T.L.; Peyrani, P.; Mirsaeidi, M.; Ramirez, J.A. Outcomes in females hospitalised with community-acquired pneumonia are worse than in males. *Eur. Respir. J.* **2013**, *41*, 1135–1140. [CrossRef]
30. Seymour, C.W.; Liu, V.X.; Iwashyna, T.J.; Brunkhorst, F.M.; Rea, T.D.; Scherag, A.; Rubenfeld, G.; Kahn, J.M.; Shankar-Hari, M.; Singer, M.; et al. Assessment of Clinical Criteria for Sepsis: For the Third International Consensus Definitions for Sepsis and Septic Shock (Sepsis-3). *JAMA* **2016**, *315*, 762–774. [CrossRef]
31. Breuer, O.; Picard, E.; Benabu, N.; Erlichman, I.; Reiter, J.; Tsabari, R.; Shoseyov, D.; Kerem, E.; Cohen-Cymberknoh, M. Predictors of Prolonged Hospitalizations in Pediatric Complicated Pneumonia. *Chest* **2018**, *153*, 172–180. [CrossRef]
32. Raith, E.P.; Udy, A.A.; Bailey, M.; McGloughlin, S.; MacIsaac, C.; Bellomo, R.; Pilcher, D.V. Prognostic Accuracy of the SOFA Score, SIRS Criteria, and qSOFA Score for In-Hospital Mortality Among Adults With Suspected Infection Admitted to the Intensive Care Unit. *JAMA* **2017**, *317*, 290–300. [CrossRef]
33. Freund, Y.; Lemachatti, N.; Krastinova, E.; van Laer, M.; Claessens, Y.-E.; Avondo, A.; Occelli, C.; Feral-Pierssens, A.-L.; Truchot, J.; Ortega, M.; et al. Prognostic Accuracy of Sepsis-3 Criteria for In-Hospital Mortality Among Patients With Suspected Infection Presenting to the Emergency Department. *JAMA* **2017**, *317*, 301–308. [CrossRef] [PubMed]
34. Grudzinska, F.S.; Aldridge, K.; Hughes, S.; Nightingale, P.; Parekh, D.; Bangash, M.; Dancer, R.; Patel, J.; Sapey, E.; Thickett, D.R.; et al. Early identification of severe community-acquired pneumonia: A retrospective observational study. *BMJ Open Respir. Res.* **2019**, *6*, e000438. [CrossRef] [PubMed]
35. Koch, C.; Edinger, F.; Fischer, T.; Brenck, F.; Hecker, A.; Katzer, C.; Markmann, M.; Sander, M.; Schneck, E. Comparison of qSOFA score, SOFA score, and SIRS criteria for the prediction of infection and mortality among surgical intermediate and intensive care patients. *World J. Emerg. Surg.* **2020**, *15*, 63. [CrossRef] [PubMed]
36. Womack, J.; Kropa, J. Community-Acquired Pneumonia in Adults: Rapid Evidence Review. *Am. Fam. Physician* **2022**, *105*, 625–630.
37. Lanks, C.W.; Musani, A.I.; Hsia, D.W. Community-acquired Pneumonia and Hospital-acquired Pneumonia. *Med. Clin. N. Am.* **2019**, *103*, 487–501. [CrossRef]
38. Ota, K.; Iida, R.; Ota, K.; Sakaue, M.; Taniguchi, K.; Tomioka, M.; Nitta, M.; Takasu, A. An atypical case of atypical pneumonia. *J. Gen. Fam. Med.* **2018**, *19*, 133–135. [CrossRef]
39. Miyashita, N. Atypical pneumonia: Pathophysiology, diagnosis, and treatment. *Respir. Investig.* **2022**, *60*, 56–67. [CrossRef]
40. Amati, F.; Bindo, F.; Stainer, A.; Gramegna, A.; Mantero, M.; Nigro, M.; Bussini, L.; Bartoletti, M.; Blasi, F.; Aliberti, S. Identify Drug-Resistant Pathogens in Patients with Community-Acquired Pneumonia. *Adv. Respir. Med.* **2023**, *91*, 224–238. [CrossRef]
41. Bartlett, J.G. Is activity against "atypical" pathogens necessary in the treatment protocols for community-acquired pneumonia? Issues with combination therapy. *Clin. Infect. Dis.* **2008**, *47* (Suppl. S3), S232–S236. [CrossRef]
42. Garin, N.; Marti, C.; Skali Lami, A.; Prendki, V. Atypical Pathogens in Adult Community-Acquired Pneumonia and Implications for Empiric Antibiotic Treatment: A Narrative Review. *Microorganisms* **2022**, *10*, 2326. [CrossRef]
43. Hedlund, J. Community-acquired pneumonia requiring hospitalisation. Factors of importance for the short-and long term prognosis. *Scand. J. Infect. Dis. Suppl.* **1995**, *97*, 1–60. [PubMed]
44. Bohannon, R.W.; Maljanian, R.D. Hospital readmissions of elderly patients hospitalized with pneumonia. *Conn. Med.* **2003**, *67*, 599–603. [PubMed]

45. Prescott, H.C.; Sjoding, M.W.; Iwashyna, T.J. Diagnoses of early and late readmissions after hospitalization for pneumonia. A systematic review. *Ann. Am. Thorac. Soc.* **2014**, *11*, 1091–1100. [CrossRef] [PubMed]
46. Averin, A.; Shaff, M.; Weycker, D.; Lonshteyn, A.; Sato, R.; Pelton, S.I. Mortality and readmission in the year following hospitalization for pneumonia among US adults. *Respir. Med.* **2021**, *185*, 106476. [CrossRef]
47. Tokioka, F.; Okamoto, H.; Yamazaki, A.; Itou, A.; Ishida, T. The prognostic performance of qSOFA for community-acquired pneumonia. *J. Intensive Care* **2018**, *6*, 46. [CrossRef]
48. Brunetti, V.C.; Ayele, H.T.; Yu, O.H.Y.; Ernst, P.; Filion, K.B. Type 2 diabetes mellitus and risk of community-acquired pneumonia: A systematic review and meta-analysis of observational studies. *CMAJ Open* **2021**, *9*, E62–E70. [CrossRef]
49. Martins, M.; Boavida, J.M.; Raposo, J.F.; Froes, F.; Nunes, B.; Ribeiro, R.T.; Macedo, M.P.; Penha-Gonçalves, C. Diabetes hinders community-acquired pneumonia outcomes in hospitalized patients. *BMJ Open Diabetes Res. Care* **2016**, *4*, e000181. [CrossRef]
50. Chen, S.; Hou, C.; Kang, Y.; Li, D.; Rong, J.; Li, Z. Factors affecting hospital discharge outcomes in patients with community-acquired pneumonia: A retrospective epidemiological study (2014–2021). *Am. J. Med. Sci.* **2023**, *366*, 143–149. [CrossRef]
51. Kim, S.J.; Lee, J.H.; Han, B.; Lam, J.; Bukowy, E.; Rao, A.; Vulcano, J.; Andreeva, A.; Bertelson, H.; Shin, H.P.; et al. Effects of Hospital-Based Physical Therapy on Hospital Discharge Outcomes among Hospitalized Older Adults with Community-Acquired Pneumonia and Declining Physical Function. *Aging Dis.* **2015**, *6*, 174–179. [CrossRef]
52. Chen, H.; Hara, Y.; Horita, N.; Saigusa, Y.; Hirai, Y.; Kaneko, T. Is rehabilitation effective in preventing decreased functional status after community-acquired pneumonia in elderly patients? Results from a multicentre, retrospective observational study. *BMJ Open* **2022**, *12*, e051287. [CrossRef]
53. José, A.; Dal Corso, S. Inpatient rehabilitation improves functional capacity, peripheral muscle strength and quality of life in patients with community-acquired pneumonia: A randomised trial. *J. Physiother.* **2016**, *62*, 96–102. [CrossRef] [PubMed]
54. Sawada, Y.; Sasabuchi, Y.; Nakahara, Y.; Matsui, H.; Fushimi, K.; Haga, N.; Yasunaga, H. Early Rehabilitation and In-Hospital Mortality in Intensive Care Patients With Community-Acquired Pneumonia. *Am. J. Crit. Care* **2018**, *27*, 97–103. [CrossRef] [PubMed]
55. Andreychenko, S.A.; Bychinin, M.V.; Clypa, T.V.; Yeremenko, A.A. Effect of rehabilitation initiation timing in the intensive care unit on outcomes in patients with pneumonia. *Vopr. Kurortol. Fizioter. Lech. Fiz. Kult.* **2021**, *98*, 11–16. [CrossRef] [PubMed]
56. Kolditz, M.; Tesch, F.; Mocke, L.; Höffken, G.; Ewig, S.; Schmitt, J. Burden and risk factors of ambulatory or hospitalized CAP: A population based cohort study. *Respir. Med.* **2016**, *121*, 32–38. [CrossRef] [PubMed]
57. Wadhera, R.K.; Joynt Maddox, K.E.; Wasfy, J.H.; Haneuse, S.; Shen, C.; Yeh, R.W. Association of the Hospital Readmissions Reduction Program With Mortality Among Medicare Beneficiaries Hospitalized for Heart Failure, Acute Myocardial Infarction, and Pneumonia. *JAMA* **2018**, *320*, 2542–2552. [CrossRef]
58. Bruns, A.H.W.; Oosterheert, J.J.; Cucciolillo, M.C.; El Moussaoui, R.; Groenwold, R.H.H.; Prins, J.M.; Hoepelman, A.I.M. Cause-specific long-term mortality rates in patients recovered from community-acquired pneumonia as compared with the general Dutch population. *Clin. Microbiol. Infect.* **2011**, *17*, 763–768. [CrossRef]
59. Holter, J.C.; Ueland, T.; Jenum, P.A.; Müller, F.; Brunborg, C.; Frøland, S.S.; Aukrust, P.; Husebye, E.; Heggelund, L. Risk Factors for Long-Term Mortality after Hospitalization for Community-Acquired Pneumonia: A 5-Year Prospective Follow-Up Study. *PLoS ONE* **2016**, *11*, e0148741. [CrossRef]
60. Glöckner, V.; Pletz, M.W.; Rohde, G.; Rupp, J.; Witzenrath, M.; Barten-Neiner, G.; Kolditz, M. Early post-discharge mortality in CAP: Frequency, risk factors and a prediction tool. *Eur. J. Clin. Microbiol. Infect. Dis.* **2022**, *41*, 621–630. [CrossRef]
61. Uhlmann, M.; Lécureux, E.; Griesser, A.-C.; Duong, H.D.; Lamy, O. Prediction of potentially avoidable readmission risk in a division of general internal medicine. *Swiss Med. Wkly.* **2017**, *147*, w14470. [CrossRef]

Disclaimer/Publisher's Note: The statements, opinions and data contained in all publications are solely those of the individual author(s) and contributor(s) and not of MDPI and/or the editor(s). MDPI and/or the editor(s) disclaim responsibility for any injury to people or property resulting from any ideas, methods, instructions or products referred to in the content.

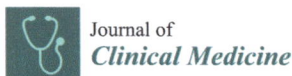
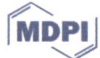

Article

Nebulized Recombinant Tissue Plasminogen Activator (rt-PA) for Acute COVID-19-Induced Respiratory Failure: An Exploratory Proof-of-Concept Trial

Pratima Chowdary [1,2,*], Banwari Agarwal [3], Maria Rita Peralta [1,2], Sanjay Bhagani [4], Simon Lee [4], James Goldring [5], Marc Lipman [5,6], Emal Waqif [1], Mark Phillips [1,2], Helen Philippou [7], Jonathan H. Foley [8], Nicola J. Mutch [9], Robert A. S. Ariëns [7], Kathleen A. Stringer [10,11], Federico Ricciardi [12], Marie Watissée [13], Derralynn Hughes [2], Amit Nathwani [1,2], Anne Riddell [1,14], David Patch [15], Jim Buckley [3], Mark De Neef [3], Rahul Dimber [3], Cecilia Diaz-Garcia [1], Honey Patel [1], Aarti Nandani [16], Upuli Dissanayake [1], Nick Chadwick [1], Ahmed A. A. M. M. Alkhatip [17,18], Peter Watkinson [19], Eamon Raith [20,21], Suveer Singh [22,23,24], Tony Wolff [3], Rajeev Jha [3], Simon E. Brill [6], Ameet Bakhai [3,25], Alison Evans [26], Farhat Gilani [26] and Keith Gomez [1,2]

1. Katharine Dormandy Haemophilia and Thrombosis Centre, Royal Free London NHS Foundation Trust, London NW3 2QG, UK
2. Cancer Institute, University College London, London WC1E 6DD, UK
3. Department of Intensive Care and Anaesthesia, Royal Free London NHS Foundation Trust, London NW3 2QG, UK
4. Department of Infectious Diseases, Royal Free London NHS Foundation Trust, London NW3 2QG, UK
5. Respiratory Medicine, Royal Free London NHS Foundation Trust, London NW1 2BU, UK
6. UCL Respiratory, University College London, London WC1E 6JF, UK; simon.brill@nhs.net
7. Discovery and Translational Science Department, Leeds Institute of Cardiovascular and Metabolic Medicine, University of Leeds, Leeds LS2 9JT, UK
8. Freeline Therapeutics, London SG1 2BP, UK
9. Aberdeen Cardiovascular & Diabetes Centre, School of Medicine, Medical Sciences & Nutrition, Institute of Medical Sciences, University of Aberdeen, Aberdeen AB25 2ZD, UK
10. Department of Clinical Pharmacy, College of Pharmacy University of Michigan, Ann Arbor, MI 48109, USA
11. Division of Pulmonary and Critical Care Medicine, School of Medicine, University of Michigan, Ann Arbor, MI 48109, USA
12. Department of Statistical Science, University College London, London WC1E 6BT, UK
13. WStats Limited, Winchester SO23 8GH, UK
14. Haemophilia & Thrombosis Laboratory (Health Services Laboratories), Royal Free Hospital, London WC1H 9AX, UK
15. Department of Hepatology, Royal Free London NHS Foundation Trust, London NW3 2QG, UK
16. Clinical Trials Pharmacy, Royal Free London NHS Foundation Trust, London NW3 2QG, UK
17. Department of Anaesthesia, Birmingham Children's Hospital, Birmingham B4 6NH, UK
18. Department of Anaesthesia, Faculty of Medicine, Beni-Suef University Hospital, Beni-Suef University, Beni-Suef 2721562, Egypt
19. NIHR Biomedical Research Centre Oxford, Oxford University Hospitals NHS Trust, University of Oxford, Oxford OX3 9DU, UK
20. Bloomsbury Institute for Intensive Care Medicine, Department of Experimental and Translational Medicine, University College London, London WC1E 6JF, UK
21. Discipline of Acute Care Medicine, School of Medicine, The University of Adelaide, Adelaide, SA 5005, Australia
22. Department of Respiratory and Critical Care Medicine, Chelsea & Westminster Hospital, London SW10 9NH, UK
23. Department of Adult Intensive Care, Royal Brompton Hospital, London SW3 6NP, UK
24. Department of Surgery and Cancer, Imperial College London, London SW7 2AZ, UK
25. Department of Cardiology, Royal Free London NHS Foundation Trust, London NW3 2PS, UK
26. University College London (UCL)/University College London Hospitals NHS Trust (UCLH) Joint Research Office, London WC1E 6BT, UK; a.j.evans@ucl.ac.uk (A.E.)
* Correspondence: p.chowdary@ucl.ac.uk; Tel.: +44-207-472-6835

Abstract: Acute lung injury in COVID-19 results in diffuse alveolar damage with disruption of the alveolar-capillary barrier, coagulation activation, alveolar fibrin deposition and pulmonary capillary thrombi. Nebulized recombinant tissue plasminogen activator (rt-PA) has the potential to facilitate localized thrombolysis in the alveolar compartment and improve oxygenation. In this proof-of-concept safety study, adults with COVID-19-induced respiratory failure and a <300 mmHg PaO_2/FiO_2 (P/F) ratio requiring invasive mechanical ventilation (IMV) or non-invasive respiratory support (NIRS) received nebulized rt-PA in two cohorts (C1 and C2), alongside standard of care, between 23 April–30 July 2020 and 21 January–19 February 2021, respectively. Matched historical controls (MHC; n = 18) were used in C1 to explore efficacy. Safety co-primary endpoints were treatment-related bleeds and <1.0–1.5 g/L fibrinogen reduction. A variable dosing strategy with clinical efficacy endpoint and minimal safety concerns was determined in C1 for use in C2; patients were stratified by ventilation type to receive 40–60 mg rt-PA daily for ≤14 days. Nine patients in C1 (IMV, 6/9; NIRS, 3/9) and 26 in C2 (IMV, 12/26; NIRS, 14/26) received nebulized rt-PA for a mean (SD) of 6.7 (4.6) and 9.1(4.6) days, respectively. Four bleeds (one severe, three mild) in three patients were considered treatment related. There were no significant fibrinogen reductions. Greater improvements in mean P/F ratio from baseline to study end were observed in C1 compared with MHC (C1; 154 to 299 vs. MHC; 154 to 212). In C2, there was no difference in the baseline P/F ratio of NIRS and IMV patients. However, a larger improvement in the P/F ratio occurred in NIRS patients (NIRS; 126 to 240 vs. IMV; 120 to 188) and fewer treatment days were required (NIRS; 7.86 vs. IMV; 10.5). Nebulized rt-PA appears to be well-tolerated, with a trend towards improved oxygenation, particularly in the NIRS group. Randomized clinical trials are required to demonstrate the clinical effect significance and magnitude.

Keywords: acute respiratory illness; critical care; recombinant tissue plasminogen activator; nebulization; fibrinolytics; COVID-19 pandemic; inhaled medication; targeted therapy

1. Introduction

SARS-CoV-2 (COVID-19)-induced respiratory failure is the leading cause of COVID-19 mortality [1,2]. The respiratory failure in severe COVID-19 starts as acute lung injury (ALI) progressing to acute respiratory distress syndrome (ARDS), multiorgan failure and death [3]. ALI and ARDS are characterized by extravascular fibrin deposition in the alveolar compartment due to alveolar cell damage and disruption of the alveolar-capillary barrier [4]. This fibrin deposition is essential for maintaining the temporary integrity of the alveolar-capillary barrier and its subsequent repair [5]. SARS-CoV-2 infection is also characterized by cytokine storm or cytokine response syndrome (CRS), with pronounced elevations of pro-inflammatory cytokines [6]. The relative contribution of the viral cytotoxicity and CRS to the diffuse alveolar damage is not well understood. However, the reduction in mortality with immunomodulation, including steroids and JAK-2 inhibitors, confirms the significant contribution of inflammation to mortality [7,8].

The fibrin deposits in ALI in COVID-19 and other conditions with ARDS are associated with cellular debris and infiltration of inflammatory cells [9]. This is facilitated by increased tissue factor expression and coagulation activation, with suppression of fibrinolysis due to a rise in plasminogen activator inhibitor-1 (PAI-1) activity [10,11]. This disruption to the fibrinolytic system and the subsequent enhanced fibrin deposition in the lungs appears to be a major pathophysiological driver of severe lung disease [5].

Fibrinolytic agents including tissue plasminogen activator (tPA), urokinase-type plasminogen activator (uPA), plasminogen and plasmin are being explored to counteract PAI-1-induced dysregulation of the fibrinolytic system [5]. Nebulized recombinant tPA (rt-PA) enhanced the bronchoalveolar fibrinolytic system in rat models of direct and indirect ALI, as reflected by a significant reduction of PAI–1 activity levels in bronchoalveolar lavage fluid, and a consequent increase in plasminogen activator activity (PAA) [12]. A meta-analysis of 22 studies deemed fibrinolytic therapy an effective therapeutic approach for ALI in pre-clinical models due to the observed improvements in lung injury, oxygenation, local neutrophil infiltration, and mortality following treatment [13]. Three cases of off-label use of tPA administered intravenously in patients with COVID-19-related acute respiratory distress syndrome (ARDS) resulted in a temporary improvement in respiratory status, with one durable response [14]. Moreover, intravenous tPA with immediate therapeutic heparin anticoagulation improved oxygenation in a Phase 2 clinical trial among patients with severe COVID-19 respiratory failure [15].

Fibrinolytic agents are usually administered intravenously, resulting in a systemic increase in fibrinolysis [12,16]. Fibrinolytic therapy, therefore, poses a risk of potentially fatal bleeds. In fact, up to 7% of patients exposed to fibrinolytic agents require blood transfusions, and up to 1% die as a consequence of bleeds [17]. Considering that coagulopathy in ALI involves both alveolar and vascular compartments, local administration via nebulization is an attractive option with potentially higher efficacy and reduced bleeding risk [12,16]. In direct and indirect ALI models, nebulization of rt-PA or anti-PAI-1 demonstrated lung-protective effects via promotion of fibrinolysis [12]. Moreover, inhalation of plasminogen improved lung lesion condition and oxygen saturation in patients with clinically moderate to severe COVID-19 [18].

Essentially, COVID-19 is a multi-system disorder with alveolar and pulmonary vascular inflammatory thrombosis that might benefit from combination therapies addressing both inflammation and intravascular thrombosis or alveolar fibrin deposits to improve outcomes [19]. We hypothesized that nebulized rt-PA through local thrombolysis, alongside standard of care, would improve oxygenation without the excess bleeding risk seen with systemic thrombolysis. This proof-of-concept pilot study aimed to test the safety of nebulized rt-PA and investigate its clinical efficacy in patients hospitalized with COVID-19 respiratory failure that required respiratory support.

2. Materials and Methods

2.1. Study Design and Participants

This study (clinicaltrials.gov identifier: NCT04356833) was approved by the National Research Ethics Committee (REC) and Medicines and Healthcare Products Regulatory Agency. Health Research Authority (HRL) approval was granted on 17 April 2020 (REC reference: 20/SC/0187). Procedures followed were in accordance with the ethical standards of the International Council for Harmonisation of Technical Requirements for Registration of Pharmaceuticals for Human Use Good Clinical Practice (ICH GCP) guidelines and with the Declaration of Helsinki of 2013.

Written informed consent was obtained from patients. When a patient could not give written informed consent due to intubation and sedation, the study was discussed with the patient's next of kin, and consent was obtained from an independent professional representative, typically another intensive care consultant not involved in the direct care of the patient or involved in the study. Patients consented at the first opportunity after regaining consciousness and consent could be withdrawn at any time. Supplementary Methods contains the informed consent procedure.

Recruitment for Cohort one (C1) occurred from 23 April to 30 July 2020, during the first COVID-19 surge. Sequential recruitment to the standard of care (SOC) arm originally planned for was not feasible as there were very few COVID-19 admissions to the center after the first COVID-19 surge had subsided by August 2020. Due to low recruitment numbers, the protocol was amended following discussions within the Trial Management Group (TMG) and Independent Data Monitoring Committee (IDMC). This allowed for the recruitment of matched historical controls (MHC) retrospectively for comparison with C1 on 15 October 2020. Recruitment for Cohort two (C2) occurred between 21 January and 19 February 2021 and all patients were assigned to receive rt-PA with SOC to accrue safety data. It is to be noted that SOC itself continued to rapidly evolve through the pandemic with the incorporation of new therapies becoming part of SOC, and our comparison between groups reflects SOC of the time in all study groups (C1, MHC and C2).

Further recruitment details are provided in the Supplementary Methods. After enrolment or the first dose of nebulized rt-PA, patients were followed until the end of the study

(EOS). EOS was day 28 or earlier in the event of death or discharge. Day one for MHC was when patients met the inclusion criteria.

Inclusion criteria in the treatment arm for both cohorts included COVID-19 diagnosis (confirmed by polymerase chain reaction [PCR] or radiologically [C1, n = 0; C2, n/N = 3/26]); ≥16 years of age; and acute COVID-19 respiratory failure determined by a PaO_2/FiO_2 [P/F] ratio of <300 mmHg [20]) that required respiratory support (including invasive mechanical ventilation). A P/F ratio of <300 mmHg was selected to ensure that all severities of respiratory failure from ALI (≤300 mmHg) to ARDs (≤200 mmHg) were included [21]. There was also a recognition that avoiding mechanical ventilation where possible would result in the best possible outcomes. For consistency and anticipating a relatively small recruitment number (given the high number of COVID-related studies at the time) and perceived much poorer outcomes from invasive mechanical ventilation (IMV), the respiratory support was stratified into two broad categories: IMV via an endotracheal tube and non-invasive respiratory support (NIRS) for all other forms of respiratory support. NIRS included non-invasive ventilation (NIV), continuous positive airway pressure (CPAP), high flow nasal oxygen (HFNO) or conventional oxygen therapy (venturi and non-breathing masks). This categorization was to capture a broad range of patients representative of COVID-19 at the time of the study. The type of respiratory support was determined by the clinical team, but the patients had to have a P/F ratio of <300 at study entry.

In IMV patients, the P/F ratio was calculated with the arterial partial pressure of oxygen (PaO_2, P) and fraction of inspired oxygen therapy (FiO_2, F) (Table S1) [22]. In NIRS patients, arterial blood gas analysis was often not performed, and PaO_2 was imputed by non-linear calculation from oxygen saturation on pulse oximetry (SpO_2), with FiO_2 calculated from tables based on oxygen flow and device used (Table S2).

The main exclusion criteria for both cohorts were pregnancy, known allergies to rt-PA or excipients of rt-PA, patients not being actively treated or not considered suitable by the investigator, and fibrinogen levels of ≤2.0 g/L or <1.5 g/L in C1 and C2 at screening, respectively.

There was no restriction on the use of any intervention except participation in another clinical trial of a novel Investigational Medicinal Product. Participation in a recovery study was not an exclusion criterion; nor was concomitant use of anticoagulation or antiplatelet therapy, as the diffusion into alveolar space was considered to be minimal to non-existent. The Supplementary Methods provides additional exclusion criteria for C1.

2.2. Study Drug and Dosing

Alteplase, rt-PA (Actilyse®, Boehringer Ingelheim, Ingelheim am Rhein, Germany) was reconstituted with 5 mL sterile water (2 mg/mL) and administered using an Aerogen® nebulizer. Supplementary Methods provides details of rt-PA administration.

The initial dosing regimen in C1 was 10 mg every 6 h for 72 h. Recruitment was staggered to ensure patient safety and details are provided in the Supplementary Methods. Dosing was amended after observing significant desaturation in patient three, 36 h after the last dose of the initial three-day block of rt-PA was administered. Desaturation was considered significant if the P/F ratio dropped to <300 mmHg. The patient received a second three-day block of rt-PA (Figure 1). This led to a protocol amendment with dosing to take place for a minimum of five days, and a maximum of 14 days. The rationale was underpinned by the fact that several factors impact the sensitivity of the alveolar fibrin deposits to tPA effect, including volume of the clot, duration of the clot, amount of plasminogen available for conversion to plasmin and inhibitors of tPA inhibitors. This resulted in a move from a fixed treatment regimen to an endpoint-driven treatment regimen; treatment was discontinued if blood fibrinogen levels fell to <1.5 g/L (potential toxicity due to systemic absorption) or patients no longer required oxygen (resolution of the interalveolar clot burden). Treatment could be restarted within five days from the last dose of treatment if there was a recurrence of COVID-19-induced respiratory symptoms or a worsening of

P/F ratio considered related to treatment discontinuation. The frequency of dosing was determined by previous protocols used in plastic bronchitis [23]. Previous pre-clinical studies demonstrated around 50% deposition of the drug with an Aerogen® nebulizer [24,25]. Studies in mice suggest that the clearance rate of intratracheal administered rt-PA is around 4 to 6 h [26].

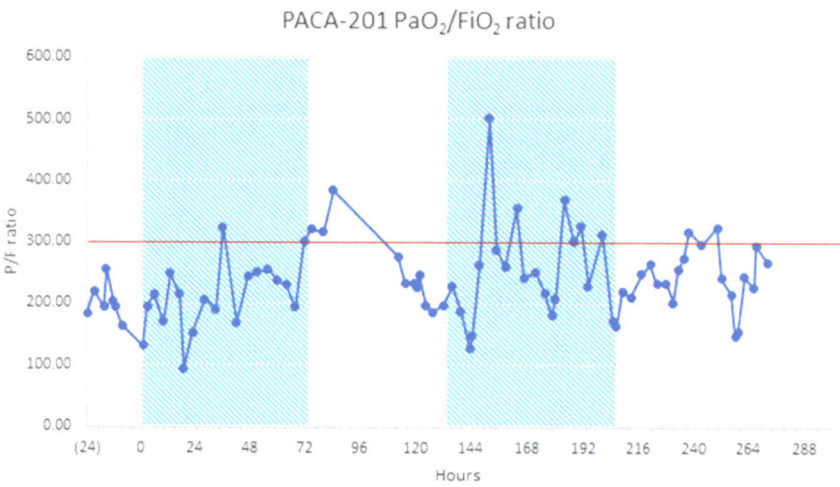

Figure 1. Cohort 1 sample mean PaO$_2$/FiO$_2$ (P/F) ratio over time of relapsed patient on NIRS (HFNO) requiring two blocks of treatment. Red line indicates severe acute COVID-19 respiratory failure determined by a PaO$_2$/FiO$_2$ [P/F] ratio of <300 mmHg [20]). HFNO, high-flow nasal oxygen; NIRS, non-invasive respiratory support; P/F, PaO$_2$/FiO$_2$.

3. Details of the C2 Treatment Regimen

C2 on IMV received 20 mg rt-PA every eight hours (60 mg daily) for a maximum of 14 treatment days. For patients on NIRS, a loading dose of 20 mg every eight hours was administered for the first two days (60 mg daily) followed by 20 mg every 12 h (twice daily; 40 mg total) for a total of 14 days. Patients on IMV were given a higher dose to account for wastage in the circuit. If patients deteriorated and required IMV, they could receive a higher treatment dose. Treatment was discontinued if blood fibrinogen levels fell to <1.0 g/L or if the patient maintained normal SpO$_2$ on room air for 48 h.

3.1. Study Endpoints

Primary endpoints to assess safety were (1) the incidence and severity of major bleeding events directly attributable to the study drug; (2) decrease in fibrinogen levels to <1.0 gm/L (in C1, the threshold was 1.5 gm/L) during treatment period and 48 h after the last dose of treatment; and (3) number and nature of serious adverse events causally related to the treatment. For endpoint (2), a lower threshold was chosen in C2 as there was no evidence of systemic absorption. Patients were reviewed daily for bleeding events, use of anticoagulation, intensity, and antiplatelet drugs. Safety blood tests included a daily coagulation screen with fibrinogen. Treatment was stopped for any major bleed and if the fibrinogen level dropped to <1–1.5 gm/L. All bleeding events were categorized as adverse events (AE) of special interest and evaluated for severity (mild, moderate and severe) and causality; the International Society of Haemostasis and Thrombosis (ISTH) Scientific and Standardisation Committee definition of major bleeding events in patients on anti-hemostatic medications was used to grade severity (Table S3) [27]. A bleeding event was evaluated for relatedness if it occurred within 30 h of the last rt-PA dose. This timeframe was determined based on the estimated 4-to-6-h clearance rate of rt-PA via intratracheal administration, based on pre-clinical data [26]. A conservative 6-h clearance rate estimate was assumed in this study and, therefore, bleeding events were evaluated for relatedness if they occurred within 5 clearance rates (30 h) of rt-PA administration.

The secondary endpoint of efficacy was determined as the change in P/F ratio from baseline (BL), which was assessed daily during treatment, at treatment cessation, and at three- and five-days post-treatment cessation. Other secondary endpoints included changes in clinical status assessed by a 7-point World Health Organization (WHO) ordinal scale until EOS (Table S4), the outcome (discharge, in-patient or death) at EOS, changes in lung compliance (defined as tidal volume/peak inspiratory pressure from BL and absolute values), Sequential Organ Failure Assessment (SOFA) during treatment and through five days after the end of treatment, number of oxygen-, ventilator- and intensive care-free days at EOS, and the number of new oxygen or ventilation requirements before EOS.

3.2. Biomarkers of Fibrinolysis

Blood samples were taken for exploratory assessment of potential biomarkers to investigate systemic absorption of tPA. These included, but were not restricted to, plasminogen, alpha-2 antiplasmin (α2AP), tissue plasminogen activator (t-PA), PAI-1 and a range of inflammatory cytokines and coagulation proteins. All other monitoring was done as per routine SOC.

3.3. Statistical Analysis

Since the study was conducted early in the pandemic, the planned recruitment numbers were based on feasibility and planned recruitment rate rather than statistical considerations. An Independent Data Monitoring Committee was established to provide oversight of the conduct of the study. This was particularly in relation to the causality of bleeding events, dose escalation strategies and to provide recommendations on the continuation of the study.

Descriptive statistics were used for all AEs, including bleeding events of special interest. In C1, the efficacy analysis compared P/F ratios between the rt-PA group and MHC at the EOS, adjusting for the BL P/F ratio, using a linear regression model. A sensitivity analysis was performed, fitting a similar model that controlled for the length of follow-up, as well as the BL P/F ratio. In a further sensitivity analysis, a mixed effects linear regression model was used to compare groups over time and account for the clustering of ratios within patients using a random effect. The model incorporated all P/F ratio measurements over time, with treatment allocation, time, and BL P/F ratio as fixed effects, together with a random slope for time and a random effect at the patient level.

Analyses of C1 and C2 were undertaken separately. C2 analysis was limited to descriptive statistics. Continuous variables were summarized using a number of observations, mean, standard deviation (SD), median, interquartile range (IQR) and minimum and maximum values. Categorical data were summarized using a number of observations and percentages. Further exploratory and post hoc analyses were conducted, and details of all statistical analyses are provided in Supplementary Methods.

4. Results

4.1. Cohort 1

In total, 27 patients enrolled in Cohort 1 (Figure S2a); nine patients received nebulized rt-PA with SOC and 18 patients were recruited as MHC receiving SOC only. In the rt-PA group, six (66.6%) patients received IMV, and three (33.3%) patients received NIRS, none of whom progressed to IMV. Patient characteristics of C1 are shown in Table 1.

Table 1. Details of patient characteristics at baseline in Cohort 1 and Cohort 2.

		Cohort 1		Cohort 2
Patient Characteristics		rt-PA Group (n = 9)	MHC Group (n = 18)	rt-PA Groups (n = 26)
Sex, n (%)	Male	4 (44.4)	9 (50.0)	19 (73.1)
Age, years	Mean	65	67	64
Race, n (%)	Asian	3 (33.3)	4 (22.2)	9 (34.6)
	Black	0	0	1 (3.8)
	White Caucasian	6 (66.7)	10 (55.6)	8 (30.8)
	Other	0	0	5 (19.2)
	Not available/not reported	0	4 (22.2)	3 (11.5)
Ventilation type, n (%)	IMV	6 (66.7)	12 (66.7)	12 (46.2)
	NIRS *	3 (33.3)	6 (33.3)	14 (53.9)
Duration of illness before enrolment	Mean	14.5	8.8	13.1
	Median (min./max.)	8.0 (3/63)	7.0 (0/21)	12.5 (4/27)
Comorbidities of interest, n (%)	Chronic lung disorder	3 (33.3)	0	2 (7.7)
	Chronic heart or circulatory disease	4 (44.4)	9 (50.0)	13 (50)
	Gastrointestinal	2 (22.2)	5 (27.8)	3 (11.5)
	Neurological	1 (11.1)	3 (16.7)	2 (7.7)
	Endocrine	3 (33.3)	4 (22.2)	7 (26.9)
	Chronic haematological	0	1 (5.6)	3 (11.5)
	AIDS/HIV	0	0	0
	Diabetes	3 (33.3)	2 (11.1)	10 (38.5)
	Cancer in the last 12 months	3 (33.3)	1 (5.6)	0
	Rheumatological	2 (22.2)	1 (5.6)	9 (34.6)
	Chronic kidney disease	1 (11.1)	2 (11.1)	0
	Obesity	0	0 [†]	3 (11.5)
	Dementia	0	2 (11.1)	0
	Immunosuppression	2 (22.2)	2 (11.1)	0

* NIRS included non-invasive ventilation (NIV), continuous positive airway pressure (CPAP), high flow nasal oxygen (HFNO) or conventional oxygen therapy (venturi and non-breathing masks); [†] Includes 7 unknown. AIDS, acquired immune deficiency syndrome; ECMO, extracorporeal membrane oxygenation; HIV, human immunodeficiency virus; IMV, invasive mechanical ventilation; MHC, matched historical control; NIRS, non-invasive respiratory support; RRT, renal replacement therapy; WHO, World Health Organization.

Seven bleeding events occurred in four of the nine patients during rt-PA treatment (Tables 2 and S6). These events were reported as AE of special interest and categorized as five mild and two moderate; all resolved completely. All bleeds and AEs were deemed unrelated to rt-PA. The MHC group were not reviewed for bleeding events. In addition, there were no measured decreases in plasma fibrinogen levels (<1.5 g/L) during the treatment period and 48 h after the last dose of rt-PA, nor was there any suggestion of increases in tPA-PAI-1 and plasmin-α2-antiplasmin complexes.

Table 2. Safety data on bleeding events in Cohort 1 and Cohort 2.

Cohort	Type of Bleed	Events (Patients)	AE Categorisation (Events)	Relatedness to rt-PA (Events) *	Outcome (Events)
1	All	7 (4)	–	–	–
	Central venous catheters insertion site	2 (2)	Mild (2)	NR (2)	Resolved (2)
	Gastro-intestinal bleed	1 (1)	Moderate (1)	NR	Resolved
	Blood-stained tracheobronchial secretion	1 (1)	Mild (1)	NR	Resolved
	Tracheostomy site bleed	2 (2)	Mild (1); Moderate (1)	NR (2)	Resolved (2)
	Other	1 (1)	Mild (1)	NR	Resolved
2	All	25 (13)	–	–	–
	Cerebral bleed [†]	1 (1)	Severe	NR	Not assessable
	Chest-drain relate [†]	1 (1)	Severe	R	Not assessable
	GI bleed	2 (2)	Moderate (2)	NR (2)	Resolved (2)
	Blood-stained tracheobronchial secretion	14 (8)	Mild (13); Moderate (1)	R (1)	Resolved (13); Not assessable (1)
	Tracheostomy site bleed	1 (1)	Moderate	NR	Resolved
	Epistaxis	3 (1)	Mild (3)	NR (3)	Resolved (3)
	Other	3 (3)	Mild (2); Moderate (1)	R (2) NR (1)	Resolved (2); Not assessable (1)

* A bleed was evaluated for relatedness if it occurred within 30 h of the last rt-PA dose. Bleeds categorized above minor were managed with stopping of anticoagulation followed by cessation of antiplatelet therapy. Supportive treatment was provided as necessary where there was significant blood loss. Patients were scheduled to receive fibrinogen concentrate if the fibrinogen level dropped to <1.0 g/L. [†] This patient developed a tension pneumothorax that required chest drains. Initially, treatment was continued, but three days after the insertion of chest drains, due to ongoing bleeding, both anticoagulation and rt-PA were stopped. The patient was receiving therapeutic anticoagulation for bilateral deep vein thrombosis along with aspirin and the fibrinogen decreased to 1 gm/L concurrent with the administration of tocilizumab. This was considered a moderate, possibly related event. The patient subsequently went on to develop a brain bleed five days after stopping therapy, which was considered unrelated to rt-PA. AE, adverse event; GI, gastrointestinal; ISTH, International Society of Haemostasis and Thrombosis; NR, not related; NSB, non-significant bleeds; R, related; rt-PA, recombinant tissue plasminogen activator.

The P/F ratio improved during the 28-day study period in the rt-PA and MHC groups (Table 3). One patient that improved to a P/F ratio > 400 on oxygen supplementation by nasal cannula deteriorated 24 to 36 h after the 12th and final dose of rt-PA (Figure 1). This patient was not a candidate for IMV because of previous bronchiectasis; instead, they were treated twice with rt-PA. This observation prompted a change in the dosing schedule for the remaining three patients in C1.

A sensitivity analysis using a linear mixed effects model showed a higher mean P/F ratio in the rt-PA group compared to the MHC group, with an estimated mean difference of 50.6 (95% confidence interval [CI], 6.7–94.4).

Among the rt-PA group, at the EOS, three (33.3%) patients were discharged before Day 28, five (55.6%) remained as in-patients and one patient (11.1%) had died. In the MHC group, six (33.3%) patients had been discharged before Day 28, two (11.1%) were in-patients and ten (55.6%) had died. Patients in the rt-PA group (n = 9) received treatment for a mean (SD) duration of 6.7 (4.6) days (Tables 4 and S5).

Table 3. Summary statistics for the P/F ratio for Cohort 1, stratified by treatment group and the lowest daily P/F ratio for Cohort 2, stratified by ventilation received alongside rt-PA.

	Parameters	Cohort 1 * (N = 27)		Cohort 2 [†] (N = 26)	
		rt-PA Group (n = 9)	MHC Group (n = 18)	IMV Group (n = 12)	NIRS Group (n = 14)
Baseline	n	9	18	12	14
	Mean (SD)	154 (53)	149 (72)	120 (28)	126 (42)
	Median (min./max.)	137 (84/263)	131 (63/268)	121 (71/170)	117 (75/203)
Day 3	n	9	13	12	12
	Mean (SD)	187 (77)	128 (35)	123 (43)	148 (90)
	Median (min./max.)	164 (118/351)	123 (67/202)	112 (43/194)	113 (65/319)
Day 7	n	8	9	10	9
	Mean (SD)	239 (90)	151 (90)	137 (78)	183 (83)
	Median (min./max.)	228 (109/390)	118 (52/305)	150 (30/266)	183 (59/281)
Day 14 [‡]	n	2	4	8 [‡]	5 [‡]
	Mean (SD)	227 (83)	209 (49)	155 (104)	248 (89)
	Median (min./max.)	197 (165/350)	221 (142/262)	149 (43/362)	253 (124/362)
Last On-Treatment Day [§]	n	9	N/A	12	14
	Mean (SD)	218 (73)	N/A	169 (108)	240 (104)
	Median (min./max.)	211 (1114/338)	N/A	149 (53/362)	281 (60/391)
End of Study [¶]	n	9	18	12	14
	Mean (SD)	299 (102)	212 (118)	188 (128)	239 (111)
	Median (min./max.)	319 (136/433)	189 (9/433)	173 (43/391)	288 (40/362)

* All available P/F ratio values were extracted per day and summarized every 4 h (±2 h). Time 0 is the baseline and a single time point on the previous day was chosen to illustrate the changes over time. [†] Up to six P/F ratio values were extracted per day, including the worst P/F ratio over the preceding day; however, the analysis for Cohort 2 includes only the lowest value for the day. [‡] Only thirteen patients (IMV, n = 8; NIRS, n = 5) had an observed measure on Day 14 due to patient discharge or death. [§] The last value available on treatment regardless of the duration of treatment (death or discharge may have occurred within the 14 days). [¶] Last value available regardless of when this measure occurred (discharge or death may have occurred within 28 days). IMV, invasive mechanical ventilation; MHC, matched historical control; N/A, not applicable; NIV, non-invasive respiratory support; P/F, PaO_2/FiO_2; SD, standard deviation; rt-PA, recombinant tissue plasminogen activator.

4.2. Cohort 2

Twenty-six patients were enrolled on the second cohort, and all received rt-PA (Figure S2b). At the time of screening, 12 (46.2%) were on IMV and 14 (53.9%) were on NIRS. Of the latter, four required IMV for variable periods. Additional patient characteristics for C2 are shown in Table 1.

Among the 26 patients, there were 25 bleeding events (Tables 2 and S6); seventeen were in the IMV group, and eight were in the NIRS group. These events were reported as AE of special interest and categorized as 18 mild, five moderate, and two severe. Of these, four bleeding events in three patients were considered possibly related to rt-PA treatment, with one being categorized as a severe AE and the other three as mild (Table 2). No patients experienced fibrinogen levels <1.0 g/L at any time during the study. One patient had a fibrinogen value of 1.0 g/L two and three days after the initiation of rt-PA treatment, which prompted withholding a dose of rt-PA.

Table 4. Secondary endpoints for Cohort 1 and Cohort 2.

Secondary Endpoint		Cohort 1		Cohort 2	
		rt-PA Group (n = 9)	MHC Group (n = 18)	IMV Group (n = 12)	NIRS Group (n = 14)
End of study outcomes (≤28 days), n (%)					
Discharge		3 (33.3)	6 (33.3)	3 (25.0)	9 (64.3)
Inpatient		5 (55.6)	2 (11.1)	4 (33.3)	2 (14.3)
Death		1 (11.1)	10 (55.6)	5 (41.7)	3 (21.4)
End of study clinical outcomes (≤28 days)–exploratory post-hoc analyses					
Number of oxygen-free days (with imputation *)	Mean (SD)	6.1 (9.6)	N/A	4.42 (8.1)	13.43 (11.1)
	Median (min./max.)	0 (0/24)	N/A	0 (0/20)	17.5 (0/26)
Number of ventilator-free days (with imputation *)	Mean (SD)	11.8 (13)	N/A	5.75 (9.9)	21.4 (9.7)
	Median (min./max.)	10 (0/28)	N/A	0 (0/25)	26.5 (0/28)
New oxygen use (relapse)	Patient, n (%)	0	N/A	1 (8.3%)	0
Progression to IMV		NA	NA	NA	4 (24.6)
Duration of treatment					
n		9	18	12	14
Mean (SD)		6.7 (4.6)	N/A	10.5 (4.2)	7.9 (4.6)
Median (min./max.)		5 (3/14)	N/A	12.8 (2.0/13.7)	8.2 (1.7/13.5)
Important concomitant treatments, n (%) †					
Steroids		7 (77.8)	3 (15.8)	12 (100)	14 (100)
Tocilizumab		0	0 (0)	11 (91.7)	12 (85.7)
Remdesivir		4 (44.4)	0 (0)	8 (66.7)	11 (78.6)
1 type of antibiotic		2 (22.2)	7 (36.8)	2 (16.7)	6 (42.9)
2 types of antibiotics		0	2 (10.5)	2 (16.7)	0
≥3 more types of antibiotics		5 (55.6)	2 (10.5)	8 (66.7)	6 (42.9)
Anakinra		1 (22.2)	2 (10.5)	0	0
Anti-platelet		3 (33.3)	5 (26.3)	3 (25)	5 (35.7)
Anticoagulation–highest intensity		9 (100)	17 (89.5)	12 (100)	14 (100)
Therapeutic		6/9	4 (21.1)	7/12	10/14
Intermediate		1/9	2 (10.5)	5/12	2/14
Prophylactic		2/9	11 (57.9)	0	2/14

* Post-hoc calculation where days post-patient discharge are assumed to be days without oxygen or ventilation; † Exploratory post-hoc analyses. HFNO, high flow nasal oxygen; IMV, invasive mechanical ventilation; MHC, matched historical control; NIV, non-invasive respiratory support; rt-PA, recombinant tissue plasminogen activator; SOFA, Sequential Organ Failure Assessment; SD, standard deviation; WHO, World Health Organization.

In the IMV group, the mean (SD) P/F ratio was 120 (28) the day before the first dose of rt-PA, and a small increase was seen for most patients by their last day of treatment, with a mean increase from BL (SD) of 48 (126) (Table 2 and Figure S4). In patients on NIRS, the mean (SD) P/F ratio was 126 (42) the day before the first dose of rt-PA, and an increase was seen for most patients by their last day of treatment, with a mean change (SD) of 114 (92).

The EOS outcomes (28d) for patients on IMV and NIRS, respectively, were as follows: 33.3% and 14.3% remained as inpatients, 25% and 64.3% had been discharged and 41.7% and 21.4% died. The total mean (SD) treatment duration for C1 (n = 26) was 9.1 (4.6) days. Patients on IMV (n = 12) and NIRS (n = 14) received rt-PA for a mean (SD) of 10.5 (4.2) and 7.9 (4.6) days, respectively (Tables 4 and S5).

4.2.1. 7-Point World Health Organization (WHO) Scale

To explore the treatment effect, a post hoc exploration of the data was conducted to describe the time to recovery from COVID-19 for each patient in the study using the WHO's minimal common outcome measure set for COVID-19. Recovery was defined as achieving an absolute WHO ordinal score of 1 or 2, or discharge [28]. Data for patients who did not recover or died were censored on Day 28. The exploration of the data aligns with the published literature [29]. The cumulative incidences of recovery during the 28-day study period are shown in Figure 2. In C1, patients on rt-PA had a more rapid recovery compared with MHC patients. In C2, NIRS patients recovered more rapidly than IMV patients. This is likely due to patients on NIRS having lower initial WHO scores, so less recovery was required to achieve a score of 1 or 2 compared with patients on IMV who had higher initial WHO scores (Table S4; Figure 2).

4.2.2. Assessment of Fibrinolysis Biomarkers

The activity of plasminogen, α2AP, PAI-1 antigen (Ag), t-PA Ag and t-PA/PAI complex during rt-PA treatment is presented in the Supplemental Results (Figure S5). There were no significant changes or obvious patterns induced by rt-PA treatment.

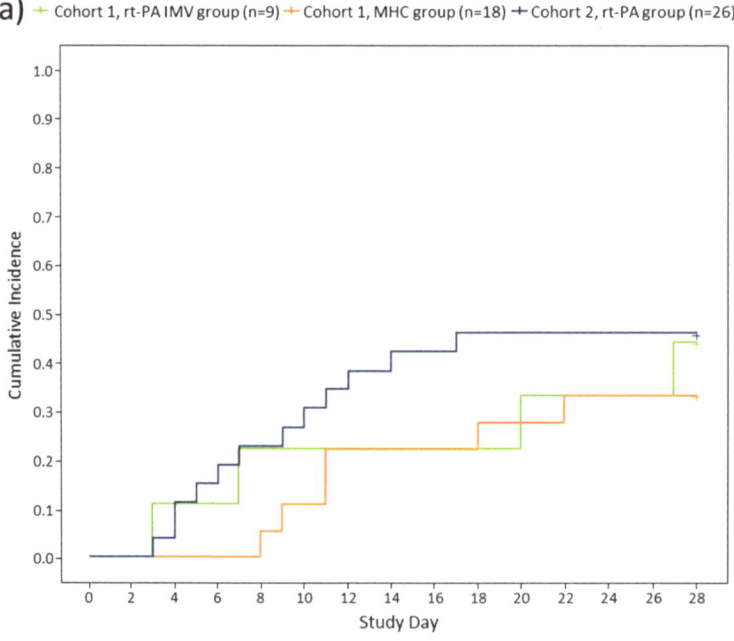

Figure 2. *Cont.*

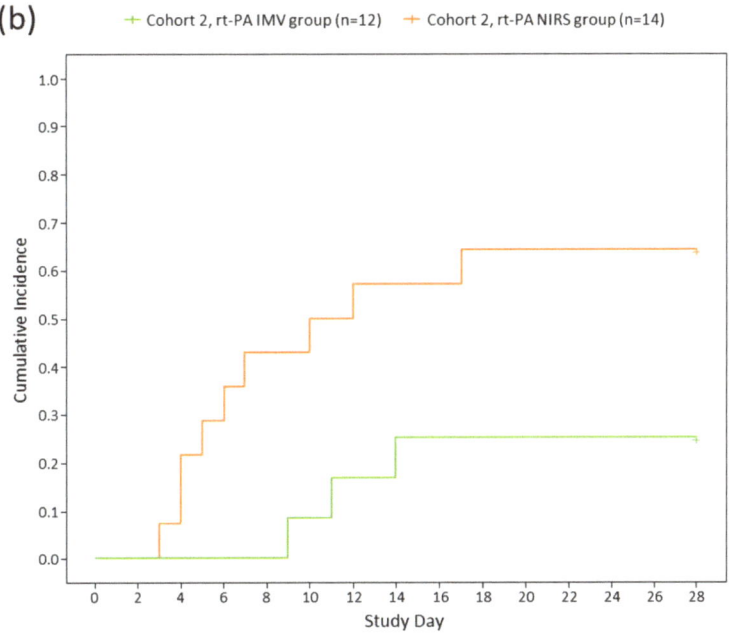

Figure 2. Time to recovery among Cohorts 1 and 2 (**a**); IMV/NIRS subgroups in Cohort 2 (**b**). The graph shows time to recovery, the cumulative incidence of recovery among Cohort 1 and Cohort 2 (**a**) and IMV and NIRS subgroups in Cohort 2 (**b**) (post hoc exploratory results). Time to recovery was defined as the time to achieve a 7-point WHO ordinal score of 1 or 2, or discharge. A breakdown of the WHO ordinal score is provided in Table S4. Data for patients who did not recover and data for patients who died were censored on Day 28. IMV, invasive mechanical ventilation; NIRS, non-invasive respiratory support; rt-PA, recombinant tissue plasminogen activator; MHC, matched historical control.

5. Discussion

This proof-of-concept study is the first clinical trial investigating the use of nebulized rt-PA in patients with COVID-19-induced respiratory failure. Previous reports were limited to intravenous administration of tPA in patients with COVID-19-related respiratory failure [14,15]. Nebulized rt-PA was not associated with any severe excess bleeding and showed an improvement in the P/F ratio among patients with a range of respiratory dysfunction severity. Importantly, the study established a dosing regimen of nebulized rt-PA that was feasible with a tolerable safety profile.

For EOS clinical outcomes, in C1, only one patient (11.0%) receiving rt-PA died during the 28-day study period compared with ten (55.6%) in the MHC group. In C2, five (41.7%) and three (21.4%) patients on IMV and NIRS, respectively, died during the study period. While these findings and an improvement in the P/F ratio were found in the C1 cohort compared with MHC, given the small sample size, they should be viewed as hypothesis-generating and proof-of-concept to support the rationale for a larger, randomized trial.

Alteplase requires plasminogen for its mechanism of action, and therefore, significant bleeding is unlikely due to the low availability of plasminogen. Indeed, the administration of nebulized rt-PA did not appear to induce an increase in systemic markers of fibrinolysis. No patients experienced pulmonary hemorrhage or had clinically significant decreases in systemic fibrinogen. Only a small number of bleeding events and no SAEs of special interest were attributable to rt-PA. In all patients with significant bleeding considered related to rt-PA, concurrent therapeutic anticoagulation with low-molecular-weight heparin (LMWH) was in use, which might have contributed to the bleeding risk. Therapeutic anticoagulation increases the risk of bleeding generally, and this has also been demonstrated in the context of COVID-19 [19,30–32]. Furthermore, the safety of nebulized rt-PA has been demonstrated in patients with plastic bronchitis, with a range of doses and durations that did not result in bleeding complications [33]. The use of clinical response for early termination of treatment and an upper limit for treatment duration improves the safety profile. Moreover, our post hoc, exploratory analyses of key fibrinolysis pathway inhibitors revealed that rt-PA treatment did not result in increased systemic fibrinolysis, suggesting minimal absorption, potentially contributing to the favourable safety profile.

Given that this study was conducted in unprecedented times during the COVID-19 pandemic, there are several limitations to this study that may have been prevented if the study was conducted in less unpredictable circumstances.

- The nature of the study population meant that a change in a patient's condition could result in an alteration in ventilation type post-enrolment. Although all patients had a P/F ratio of <300 at enrolment, the P/F ratio for NIRS and IMV was calculated by different methods: for those on NIRS, the P/F ratio was determined by converting SpO_2 and oxygen flow rate and using imputed values [22,34], whereas the P/F ratio was readily available for those on IMV. Further, the NIRS group was heterogeneous to the device used to improve oxygen concentration;
- The use of MHC for comparison in C1 is a limitation as patients who consented to participate in trials may differ, potentially leading to selection bias; this has been reviewed extensively [35]. The retrospective, non-randomized nature of the control group makes the efficacy comparison between the control and treatment groups exploratory. Additionally, we acknowledge that the use of historical controls in the absence of randomization may introduce confounding bias. However, one of the main study aims was to generate adequate data for a sample size calculation for a future study;
- This study was not blinded due to the practicalities around blinding this type of intervention, especially in the midst of a pandemic. Due to the lack of blinding, there may be potential biases introduced; however, the aim of this study was to investigate safety and not to demonstrate superiority or gold standard comparisons;
- There were differences in the patients enrolled in the C1 and C2 cohorts, with a higher number of bacterial co-infections in C2 patients, most of whom received steroids and interleukin-6 inhibitors. At the time of the study, both cohorts received the SOC, which was rapidly evolving, as demonstrated by the differences in concomitant treatments (Table 4). It is possible that concomitant treatments received by patients may have impacted the study outcomes. These potential cofounding factors should be explored in future randomized studies;
- The duration of illness before enrolment was shorter in C2; this could have impacted the duration of respiratory support. Reactive protocol amendments were required to incorporate learnings associated with the novel administration route;
- Direct administration of drugs into the airways is challenging, particularly in breathless patients despite the perceived advantages. Dosing of inhaled drugs needs to account for the loss in the ventilation circuit, ambient aerosolization and varying disease severity, and conventional drugs tend to have wide therapeutic windows. Protein-based therapeutics typically have narrow therapeutic windows and tend to be expensive. Whilst the delivery of rt-PA with an Aerogen nebulizer has been investigated extensively [23], the following challenges were experienced in NIRS patients, which may impact the feasibility and effectiveness of nebulized rt-PA treatment in real world settings: (1) Difficulty in continuing to support oxygen whilst using the Aerogen nebulizer for drug administration; (2) the loss of the drug through long circuits used for CPAP and HNFO; (3) trapping of the drug in the filters used for CPAP; (4) taste of the drug when a mouthpiece was used for direct inhalation. Administration with

mechanical ventilation was easier due to side ports, but the wastage appeared to be high;
- The assessment of bleeding was complicated by concurrent anticoagulant therapy; whilst this was not a confounder for assessing efficacy, it is an important contributor to the determination of the safety of rt-PA. Indeed, the challenges of the assessment of efficacy and bleeding secondary to anticoagulation in COVID-19 have been extensively reviewed [19,30];
- Lastly, as COVID-19 variants evolve and new therapeutic strategies are developed, the role of salvage therapies like nebulized rt-PA needs careful thought.

Despite these limitations, this study serves as a proof-of-concept that nebulized rt-PA delivery to the airways has a favorable safety profile, even in patients receiving therapeutic anticoagulation with LMWH. The magnitude of clinical impact in relation to the duration of oxygen support, duration of ventilation and need for invasive ventilation needs further assessment. Moreover, the use of nebulized rt-PA for COVID-19-induced respiratory failure, and where this therapy fits into the current COVID-19 disease and treatment landscape will need further exploration.

6. Conclusions

In this proof-of-concept study, nebulized rt-PA demonstrated favorable safety with no excess bleeding in patients hospitalized with COVID-19-induced respiratory failure. This requires further investigation in randomized studies to understand both the magnitude and significance of benefit. In addition, there is also a need to better understand the bronchopulmonary hemostatic disturbances and if alveolar fibrin is an appropriate target. These results should be utilized as a first step towards more extended research in the field and will provide valuable scientific knowledge and direction to optimize the design of future studies.

Supplementary Materials: The following supporting information can be downloaded at: https://www.mdpi.com/article/10.3390/jcm12185848/s1, Table S1. Look up table for imputed PaO_2 for a given SpO_2 based on a non-linear equation. Table S2. Oxygen flow rate calculation (used for calculating FiO_2 in patients receiving NIRS). Table S3. Assessment of adverse events for severity, causality, seriousness, and expectedness. Table S4. 7-point WHO ordinal score. Table S5. Secondary endpoints for Cohort 1 and Cohort 2. Table S6. Full safety data on bleeding events in Cohort 1 and Cohort 2. Figure S1. Schematic diagram of overall trial design. Figure S2. CONSORT diagram for Cohort 1 (a) and Cohort 2 (b) study. Figure S3. Cohort 1–Mean P/F ratio over time (days since baseline) stratified by trial arm. Figure S4. Cohort 2–Lowest daily P/F ratio over time for IMV and NIRS subgroups. Figure S5. Biomarker activity during rt-PA treatment in Cohort 1, Cohort 2 IMV, and Cohort 2 NIRS.

Author Contributions: P.C. takes responsibility for the content of the manuscript, including the data analysis, and manuscript preparation. P.C., B.A., K.G., J.H.F., R.A.S.A., N.J.M. and H.P. (Helen Philippou) conceived this study. P.C., B.A., M.W., K.A.S., M.L., S.B., E.W. and K.G. commented on the paper, oversaw the analysis and edited the final manuscript. P.C., B.A., M.W., E.W. and K.G. led the writing of the paper, with editorial support Meridian HealthComms, in compliance with good publishing practice (GPP3) guidelines. M.W., E.W. and F.R. accessed and verified the underlying data and were responsible for data cleaning and analysis. All authors contributed to drafting the paper and revised the manuscript for important intellectual content. All authors had full access to summary data reported in this study. All authors have read and agreed to the published version of the manuscript.

Funding: Royal Free Charity Trust Fund 35 provided funding for this study. The study drug was provided by Boehringer Ingelheim (BI). BI had no role in the design, analysis, or interpretation of the results. They were given the opportunity to review the manuscript for medical and scientific accuracy since it relates to BI substances and intellectual property considerations.

Institutional Review Board Statement: This study was approved by the National Research Ethics committee and Medicines and Healthcare Products Regulatory Agency and performed in accordance with good clinical practice. Adult consent to participate was obtained. Health Research Authority (HRL) approval was granted on 17 April 2020 (REC reference: 20/SC/0187).

Informed Consent Statement: Not applicable.

Data Availability Statement: All data generated or analysed during this study are included in this published article and its Supplementary Information files. Anonymous, individual participant data that underline the results reported in this article will be made available to others, along with the study protocol, statistical analysis plans and information sheets at publication, with no end date. The data will be made available on application to the corresponding author, with permissions from the Chief Investigator and study sponsor (p.chowdary@ucl.ac.uk; a.j.evans@ucl.ac.uk). Applications for data sharing will need to explain what the data will be used for. If the application is approved by the authors, the data will be shared. Data request proposals should be directed to the CI, p.chowdary@ucl.ac.uk. To gain access, data requestors will need to sign a data-sharing agreement. The following abstract has previously been published: A pilot, open-label, phase II clinical trial of nebulized recombinant tissue-plasminogen activator in patients with COVID-19 acute respiratory distress syndrome: the PACA trial. Presented at the British Society for Haemostasis and Thrombosis conference. Aberdeen, United Kingdom. 2022. Abstract OC-15.

Acknowledgments: We would like to extend our sincerest gratitude to all the colleagues and hospital staff who worked tirelessly throughout the pandemic and without whom this work would not have been possible. Firstly, we would like to thank our colleagues in the intensive care unit (ICU), in particular the matrons, Sean Carroll and Sinead Hanton, and research nurses, Filipe Helder and Amitaa Maharajh for their support, and bedside nurses who bore the responsibility of drug administration. We would also like to extend our thanks to ICU consultants who acted as professional legal consultees on behalf of critical care patients. Equally, we would like to thank colleagues within the respiratory team. Their expertise was instrumental to our role in treating patients on 8N and 8E wards. A special mention to lead Nurse Mary Emerson; we were grateful for her knowledge, support and for facilitating the training for the nebulizer and drug administration on the wards. We would like to thank Aarti Nandani and all the staff in the Royal Free clinical trials pharmacy for their immense support throughout the whole pandemic, especially considering their ever-increasing workload at the time. Thanks also to the HSL coagulation laboratory, the Trust R&D department and all the staff working to cover during a very challenging time. We are also very grateful to the Royal Free charity for funding this study. Finally, we would like to thank all the clinical nurses, physiotherapists, research data managers and healthcare professionals within the Haemophilia department (and wider hospital) for all their many efforts in supporting this study. This trial was overseen by an independent data monitoring committee, chaired by Najib Rahman, Director of the Oxford Respiratory Trials Unit, University of Oxford and comprises the following committee members: Mike Makris, Jonathan Silversides and Henry Watson.

Conflicts of Interest: P.W. declares grants from the NIHR, Wellcome and Sensyne Health (now Arcturis Data). He was previously Chief Medical Officer for Sensyne Health and holds shares in the company. He provides consultancy for Arcturis Data. H.P. is a founder and director of LUNAC Therapeutics, which is currently developing a novel anticoagulant. K.A.S. declares research funding from the US Food and Drug Administration (R01 FD005393) that provides support for a clinical trial of inhaled t-PA in children with acute plastic bronchitis and the US National Institutes of Health (R35 GM136312); she also serves as a paid consultant for FHI Clinical. S.S. has served on an advisory board for Ambu A/S. A.B. is the founder of Amore Health Ltd. and receives an honorarium from Daiichi Sankyo, Pfizer, BMS, Bayer, Novartis, Roche, Napp, Boehringer Ingelheim, Lilly, Astra Zeneca, Novartis and Amgen for lecturing and scientific advice. All other authors declare no conflict of interest.

References

1. Lu, S.; Huang, X.; Liu, R.; Lan, Y.; Lei, Y.; Zeng, F.; Tang, X.; He, H. Comparison of COVID-19 Induced Respiratory Failure and Typical ARDS: Similarities and Differences. *Front. Med.* **2022**, *9*, 829771. [CrossRef] [PubMed]
2. Ruan, Q.; Yang, K.; Wang, W.; Jiang, L.; Song, J. Clinical predictors of mortality due to COVID-19 based on an analysis of data of 150 patients from Wuhan, China. *Intensive Care Med.* **2020**, *46*, 846–848. [CrossRef] [PubMed]

3. Hussain, M.; Syed, S.K.; Fatima, M.; Shaukat, S.; Saadullah, M.; Alqahtani, A.M.; Alqahtani, T.; Bin Emran, T.; Alamri, A.H.; Barkat, M.Q.; et al. Acute Respiratory Distress Syndrome and COVID-19: A Literature Review. *J. Inflamm. Res.* **2021**, *14*, 7225–7242. [CrossRef] [PubMed]
4. Matthay, M.A.; Zemans, R.L.; Zimmerman, G.A.; Arabi, Y.M.; Beitler, J.R.; Mercat, A. Acute respiratory distress syndrome. *Nat. Rev. Dis. Primers* **2019**, *5*, 18. [CrossRef] [PubMed]
5. Idell, S. Coagulation, fibrinolysis, and fibrin deposition in acute lung injury. *Crit. Care Med.* **2003**, *31* (Suppl. S4), S213–S220. [CrossRef]
6. Montazersaheb, S.; Khatibi, S.M.H.; Hejazi, M.S.; Tarhriz, V.; Farjami, A.; Sorbeni, F.G.; Farahzadi, R.; Ghasemnejad, T. COVID-19 infection: An overview on cytokine storm and related interventions. *Virol. J.* **2022**, *19*, 92. [CrossRef] [PubMed]
7. Recovery Collaborative Group; Horby, P.; Lim, W.S.; Emberson, J.R.; Mafham, M.; Bell, J.L.; Linsell, L.; Staplin, N.; Brightling, C.; Ustianowski, A.; et al. Dexamethasone in Hospitalized Patients with COVID-19. *N. Engl. J. Med.* **2021**, *384*, 693–704.
8. Kalil, A.C.; Patterson, T.F.; Mehta, A.K.; Tomashek, K.M.; Wolfe, C.R.; Ghazaryan, V.; Marconi, V.C.; Ruiz-Palacios, G.M.; Hsieh, L.; Kline, J.; et al. Baricitinib plus Remdesivir for Hospitalized Adults with COVID-19. *N. Engl. J. Med.* **2021**, *384*, 795–807. [CrossRef]
9. Bellingan, G.J. The pulmonary physician in critical care * 6: The pathogenesis of ALI/ARDS. *Thorax* **2002**, *57*, 540–546. [CrossRef]
10. Idell, S.; James, K.K.; Coalson, J.J. Fibrinolytic activity in bronchoalveolar lavage of baboons with diffuse alveolar damage: Trends in two forms of lung injury. *Crit. Care Med.* **1992**, *20*, 1431–1440. [CrossRef]
11. Whyte, C.S.; Morrow, G.B.; Mitchell, J.L.; Chowdary, P.; Mutch, N.J. Fibrinolytic abnormalities in acute respiratory distress syndrome (ARDS) and versatility of thrombolytic drugs to treat COVID-19. *J. Thromb. Haemost.* **2020**, *18*, 1548–1555. [CrossRef] [PubMed]
12. Hofstra, J.J.; Cornet, A.D.; Declerck, P.J.; Dixon, B.; Aslami, H.; Vlaar, A.P.J.; Roelofs, J.J.; van der Poll, T.; Levi, M.; Schultz, M.J. Nebulized fibrinolytic agents improve pulmonary fibrinolysis but not inflammation in rat models of direct and indirect acute lung injury. *PLoS ONE* **2013**, *8*, e55262. [CrossRef] [PubMed]
13. Liu, C.; Ma, Y.; Su, Z.; Zhao, R.; Zhao, X.; Nie, H.-G.; Xu, P.; Zhu, L.; Zhang, M.; Li, X.; et al. Meta-Analysis of Preclinical Studies of Fibrinolytic Therapy for Acute Lung Injury. *Front. Immunol.* **2018**, *9*, 1898. [CrossRef] [PubMed]
14. Wang, J.; Hajizadeh, N.; Moore, E.E.; McIntyre, R.C.; Moore, P.K.; Veress, L.A.; Yaffe, M.B.; Moore, H.B.; Barrett, C.D. Tissue plasminogen activator (tPA) treatment for COVID-19 associated acute respiratory distress syndrome (ARDS): A case series. *J. Thromb. Haemost.* **2020**, *18*, 1752–1755. [CrossRef] [PubMed]
15. Barrett, C.D.; Moore, H.B.; Moore, E.E.; Wang, J.; Hajizadeh, N.; Biffl, W.L.; Lottenberg, L.; Paterl, P.R.; Truitt, M.S.; Mclntyre, R.C.; et al. Study of Alteplase for Respiratory Failure in SARS-CoV-2 COVID-19: A Vanguard Multicenter, Rapidly Adaptive, Pragmatic, Randomized Controlled Trial. *Chest* **2022**, *161*, 710–727. [CrossRef]
16. Camprubí-Rimblas, M.; Tantinyà, N.; Bringué, J.; Guillamat-Prats, R.; Artigas, A. Anticoagulant therapy in acute respiratory distress syndrome. *Ann. Transl. Med.* **2018**, *6*, 36. [CrossRef]
17. Global Use of Strategies to Open Occluded Coronary Arteries (GUSTO III) Investigators. A comparison of reteplase with alteplase for acute myocardial infarction. *N. Engl. J. Med.* **1997**, *337*, 1118–1123. [CrossRef]
18. Wu, Y.; Wang, T.; Guo, C.; Zhang, D.; Ge, X.; Huang, Z.; Zhou, X.; Li, Y.; Peng, Q.; Li, J. Plasminogen improves lung lesions and hypoxemia in patients with COVID-19. *QJM* **2020**, *113*, 539–545. [CrossRef]
19. Chowdary, P. COVID-19 coagulopathy—What should we treat? *Exp. Physiol.* **2022**, *107*, 749–758. [CrossRef]
20. Ranieri VI, T.O.; Rubenfeld, G.D.; Thompson, B.T.; Ferguson, N.D.; Caldwell, E.; Fan, E.; Camporota, L. Acute respiratory distress syndrome: The Berlin Definition. *JAMA* **2012**, *307*, 2526–2533.
21. Bilan, N.; Dastranji, A.; Ghalehgolab Behbahani, A. Comparison of the spo$_2$/fio$_2$ ratio and the pao$_2$/fio$_2$ ratio in patients with acute lung injury or acute respiratory distress syndrome. *J. Cardiovasc. Thorac. Res.* **2015**, *7*, 28–31. [CrossRef] [PubMed]
22. Brown, S.M.; Duggal, A.; Hou, P.C.; Tidswell, M.; Khan, A.; Exline, M.; Park, P.K.; Schoenfeld, D.; Liu, M.; Grissom, C.K.; et al. Nonlinear Imputation of PaO$_2$/FIO$_2$ from SpO$_2$/FIO$_2$ among Mechanically Ventilated Patients in the ICU: A Prospective, Observational Study. *Crit. Care Med.* **2017**, *45*, 1317–1324. [CrossRef] [PubMed]
23. Dunn, J.S.; Nayar, R.; Campos, J.; Hybertson, B.M.; Zhou, Y.; Manning, M.C.; Repine, J.E.; Stringer, K.A. Feasibility of tissue plasminogen activator formulated for pulmonary delivery. *Pharm. Res.* **2005**, *22*, 1700–1707. [CrossRef] [PubMed]
24. Labiris, N.R.; Dolovich, M.B. Pulmonary drug delivery. Part II: The role of inhalant delivery devices and drug formulations in therapeutic effectiveness of aerosolized medications. *Br. J. Clin. Pharmacol.* **2003**, *56*, 600–612. [CrossRef] [PubMed]
25. O'Callaghan, C.; Barry, P.W. The science of nebulised drug delivery. *Thorax* **1997**, *52* (Suppl. S2), S31–S44. [CrossRef]
26. Lackowski, N.P.; Pitzer, J.E.; Tobias, M.; Van Rheen, Z.; Nayar, R.; Mosharaff, M.; Stringer, K.A. Safety of prolonged, repeated administration of a pulmonary formulation of tissue plasminogen activator in mice. *Pulm. Pharmacol. Ther.* **2010**, *23*, 107–114. [CrossRef]
27. Schulman, S.; Kearon, C.; The Subcommittee on Control of Anticoagulation of the Scientific and Standardization Committee of the International Society on Thrombosis and Haemostasis. Definition of major bleeding in clinical investigations of antihemostatic medicinal products in non-surgical patients. *J. Thromb. Haemost.* **2005**, *3*, 692–694. [CrossRef]
28. Marshall, J.C.; Murthy, S.; Diaz, J.; Adhikari, N.K.; Angus, D.C.; Arabi, Y.M.; Baillie, K.; Buer, M.; Berry, S.; Blackwood, B.; et al. A minimal common outcome measure set for COVID-19 clinical research. *Lancet Infect. Dis.* **2020**, *20*, e192–e197. [CrossRef]

29. Beigel, J.H.; Tomashek, K.M.; Dodd, L.E.; Mehta, A.K.; Zingman, B.S.; Kalil, A.C.; Elizabeth Hohmann, M.P.H.; Chu, H.Y.; Annie Luetkemeter, M.P.H.; Kline, S.; et al. Remdesivir for the Treatment of Covid-19—Final Report. *N. Engl. J. Med.* **2020**, *383*, 1813–1826. [CrossRef]
30. Connors, J.M.; Moll, M.; Levy, J.H. Interpreting recent clinical studies for COVID-19: A continual process with more new data. *Anaesth. Crit. Care Pain. Med.* **2021**, *41*, 101016. [CrossRef]
31. Musoke, N.; Lo, K.B.; Albano, J.; Peterson, E.; Bhargav, R.; Gul, F.; DeJoy, R.; Salacup, G.; Pelayo, J.; Tipparaju, P.; et al. Anticoagulation and bleeding risk in patients with COVID-19. *Thromb. Res.* **2020**, *196*, 227–230. [CrossRef] [PubMed]
32. Klok, F.A.; Huisman, M.V. How I assess and manage the risk of bleeding in patients treated for venous thromboembolism. *Blood* **2020**, *135*, 724–734. [CrossRef] [PubMed]
33. Colaneri, M.; Quarti, A.; Pozzi, M.; Gasparini, S.; Carloni, I.; de Benedictis, F.M. Management of plastic bronchitis with nebulized tissue plasminogen activator: Another brick in the wall. *Ital. J. Pediatr.* **2014**, *40*, 18. [CrossRef]
34. Brown, S.M.; Grissom, C.K.; Moss, M.; Rice, T.W.; Schoenfeld, D.; Hou, P.C.; Thompson, B.T.; Brower, R.G.; NIH/NHLBI PETAL Network Collaborators. Nonlinear Imputation of PaO_2/FIO_2 From SpO_2/FIO_2 Among Patients with Acute Respiratory Distress Syndrome. *Chest* **2016**, *150*, 307–313. [CrossRef] [PubMed]
35. Arabi, Y.M.; Cook, D.J.; Zhou, Q.; Smith, O.; Hand, L.; Turgeon, A.F.; Matte, A.; Mehta, S.; Graham, R.; Brierley, K.; et al. Characteristics and Outcomes of Eligible Nonenrolled Patients in a Mechanical Ventilation Trial of Acute Respiratory Distress Syndrome. *Am. J. Respir. Crit. Care Med.* **2015**, *192*, 1306–1313. [CrossRef]

Disclaimer/Publisher's Note: The statements, opinions and data contained in all publications are solely those of the individual author(s) and contributor(s) and not of MDPI and/or the editor(s). MDPI and/or the editor(s) disclaim responsibility for any injury to people or property resulting from any ideas, methods, instructions or products referred to in the content.

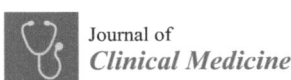 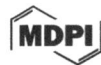

Case Report

Severe Bacterial Superinfection of Influenza Pneumonia in Immunocompetent Young Patients: Case Reports

Szymon Białka [1], Michał Zieliński [2], Magdalena Latos [2,*], Marlena Skurzyńska [3], Michał Żak [4], Piotr Palaczyński [1] and Szymon Skoczyński [2]

- [1] Department of Anaesthesiology and Intensive Care, Faculty of Medical Sciences in Zabrze, Medical University of Silesia in Katowice, 41-803 Zabrze, Poland; szymon.bialka@gmail.com (S.B.); piotr.palaczynski@gmail.com (P.P.)
- [2] Department of Lung Diseases and Tuberculosis, Faculty of Medical Sciences in Zabrze, Medical University of Silesia in Katowice, 41-803 Zabrze, Poland; michal.zielinski1@interia.pl (M.Z.); sz.skoczynski@sum.edu.pl (S.S.)
- [3] Clinical Department of Anaesthesiology and Intensive Care, Independent Public Clinical Hospital No. 1., 41-800 Zabrze, Poland; marlena.skurzynska1998@gmail.com
- [4] Student Scientific Society at the Department of Anaesthesiology and Intensive Care, Faculty of Medical Sciences in Zabrze, Medical University of Silesia in Katowice, 41-800 Zabrze, Poland; michal181297@gmail.com
- * Correspondence: latos.magdalena93@gmail.com

Abstract: Influenza can lead to or coexist with severe bacterial pneumonia, with the potential to permanently damage lung tissue, refractory to conservative treatment in the post-COVID-19 period. It can lead to serious complications; therefore, annual vaccinations are recommended. This case series with a literature review pertains to two young female patients with an insignificant past medical history, who required emergency lobectomy due to bacterial complications after influenza infection. Urgent lobectomy proves to be a feasible therapeutic option for selected patients with pleural complications.

Keywords: respiratory infections; lobectomy; influenza; intensive care; bacterial coinfection; unvaccinated; young patients; infectious diseases; viral infection

1. Introduction

Respiratory viruses have played a significant role in causing community-acquired pneumonia. It was reported that before the COVID-19 pandemic, such agents were detected in 10–30% of patients with the aforementioned condition [1]. Viral epidemiology in this aspect has changed with the occurrence of severe acute respiratory syndrome coronavirus 2 (SARS-CoV-2) [2]. A global pandemic was declared by World Health Organization (WHO) on 11 March 2020, and it remained an international public health emergency until May 2023 [3]. During the pandemic, various interventions were undertaken in order to mitigate the effects of the disease. Pre-emptive measures such as avoiding physical contact with infected individuals, wearing face masks, and aerosol elimination by proper air treatment proved effective, not only for limiting the spread of coronavirus but also by affecting the prevalence of remaining microbial agents [4]. For some viruses, the prevalence increased in the second half of pandemic when restrictions eased [2]. An increase in influenza infections among children along with a concomitant decrease in COVID-19 cases was observed in March 2022 and reported by a Romanian pediatric hospital [5]. This may serve as a warning that while restrictions are relaxed, we should keep being vigilant.

Rhinovirus/enterovirus were the predominant respiratory viruses (excluding SARS-CoV-2) during COVID-19 pandemic, with a pooled prevalence of 5.05%. Influenza virus followed in these statistics as the second most prevalent with 3.27%, with a significantly higher prevalence of influenza A than influenza B species observed [2].

Influenza virus has always been described as one of the most common causes of severe viral pneumonia. Moreover, due to its high mortality and rapid transmission, it has been associated with a significant healthcare burden [6,7]. It was estimated that influenza virus accounted for approximately 500,000 deaths each year before the COVID-19 pandemic, with the majority of the deceased being either less than 5 years old or more than 75 years old [8,9]. Significant antigenic drift due to a segmented genome allows the virus to cause seasonal outbreaks every year [9,10]. Furthermore, strain dominance differs depending on the region of the world, and it is closely monitored and reported by the World Health Organization [6].

2. Case Series

This case series pertains to two young, female patients with an insignificant past medical history, who required emergency lobectomy due to bacterial complications after influenza infection. Detailed timelines of their clinical courses are presented in Figure 1. Both patients were treated at the same Polish facility in the spring of 2024. During the patients' stay, a total of 25 patients were hospitalized in the ICU, including 17 with respiratory failure. Among them, 7 showed an exacerbation of chronic respiratory failure and 10 had acute respiratory failure. In our center, for the first time, we encountered cases presenting a need for surgical treatment due to complications of pneumonia in people so young. The doses of catecholamines were continuously adjusted depending on the current indications of hemodynamic monitoring. The Cardiac Index (CI), Stroke Volume Index (SVI), Preload—Global End-Diastolic Volume Index (GEDI), and Afterload—Systemic Vascular Resistance Index (SVRI) were continuously monitored using a hemodynamic monitoring device (HemoSphere, Edwards Lifesciences, Irvine, CA, USA). The Cardiac Function Index (CFI), Stroke Volume Variation (SVV), Pulse Pressure Variation (PPV), Extravascular lung Water Index (ELWI), and Pulmonary Vascular Permeability Index (PVPI) were also employed. Continuous veno-venous renal replacement therapy was performed with the Baxter PrisMax system using citrate regional anticoagulation. The parameters of acid–base balance, electrolytes (K^+, Na^+ Ca^{2+}, total Ca, P^{2+}), and kidney function were regularly monitored, and water balance was calculated twice a day. Based on the data obtained, the therapy settings were modified by regulating the flow: blood flow rate, flow before the blood pump, dialysate flow, replacement fluid flow, and CRRT dose.

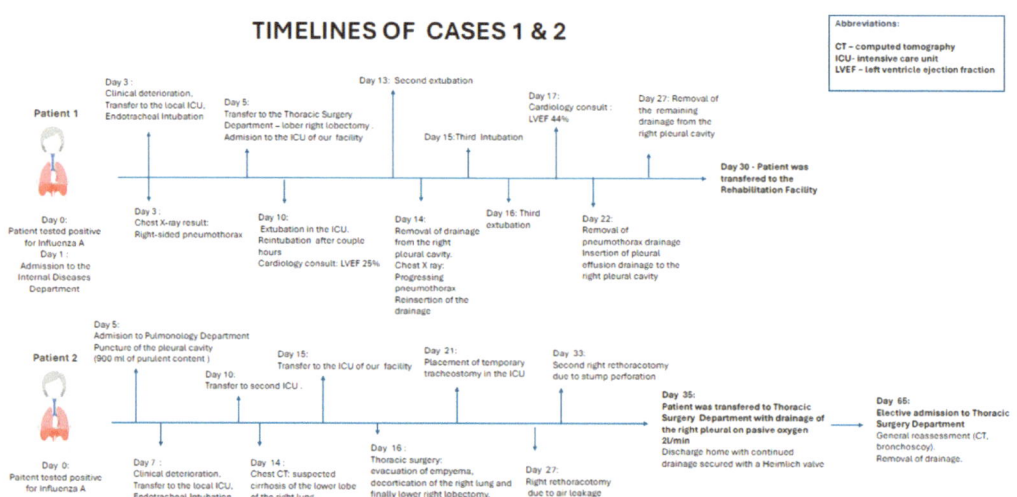

Figure 1. Timelines of the clinical courses of both patients.

Mechanical ventilation (ventilation with two-phase positive airway pressure) was used in accordance with the principles of lung protective ventilation so that the tidal volume was 4–6 mL/kg of the ideal body weight and the driving pressure (ΔP) < 14 cm H20.

2.1. Case 1

The first patient was a 36-year-old female who was initially hospitalized in the Department of Internal Diseases in the district hospital in a nearby city from day 1 to day 3 due to influenza infection. Her past medical history consisted of asthma and irritable bowel syndrome. She was admitted due to the worsening of respiratory symptoms despite antiviral treatment (oseltamiwir). On day 3, hemoptysis occurred, and decreased oxygen saturation was detected. Her clinical deterioration required admission to the ICU, where she was intubated and mechanically ventilated. Chest X-ray revealed right-sided pneumothorax, which was treated twice with pleural drainage—without the effect of lung expansion. She was then transferred for surgical treatment to the Thoracic Surgery Department in Zabrze due to suspected pleural empyema, lung abscesses, and pneumothorax with air leak. The chest X-ray performed at admission is presented in Figure 2.

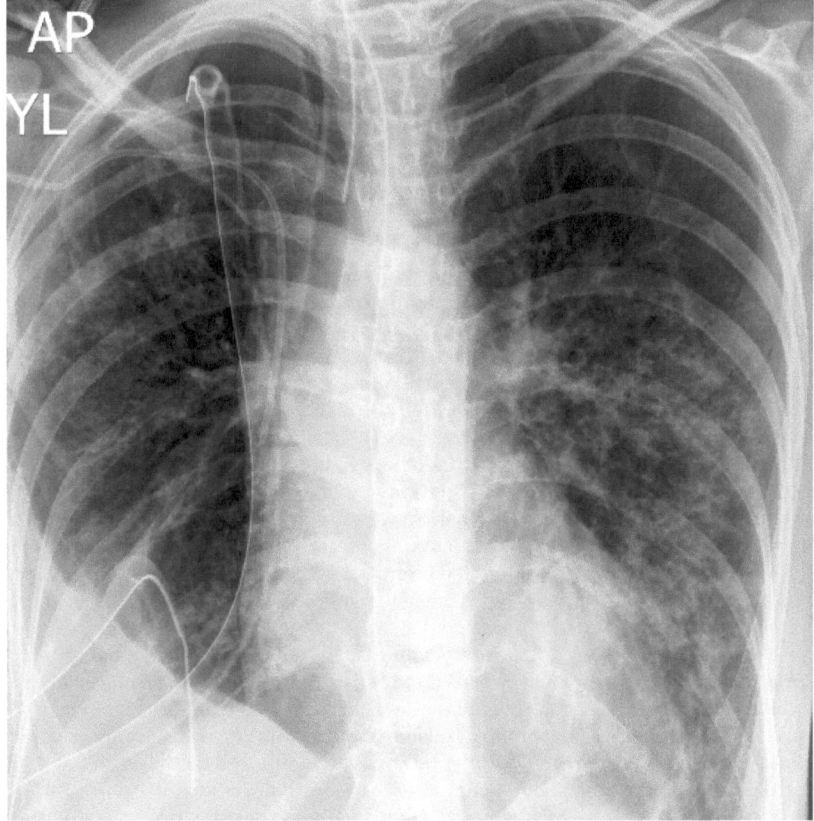

Figure 2. Chest X-ray of patient 1 at admission to the intensive care unit.

After admission, bronchofiberoscopy was performed—sticky, mucopurulent secretion was aspirated and the BAL sample was collected for culture. After connecting to an active drainage system, the leakage of the breathing mixture was 4500 mL/min. It was changed to passive underwater drainage. Due to severe coagulation disorders, Octaplex was administered. The patient underwent emergency surgery due to ventilation problems and a severe septic condition. During the procedure, a right lower lobectomy was performed. After the procedure, she was transferred to the ICU in the same hospital in Zabrze for further treatment.

At post-operative admission to the ICU, the patient was in acute cardiorespiratory failure. Hemodynamic and vital signs' monitoring was implemented. Mechanical ventilation, intensive anti-shock treatment, and targeted antibiotic therapy were continued, which were modified according to the results of microbiological tests. An assessment of the fungal pathogens was performed. A negative result was obtained for both patients. The detailed microbiological findings and antibiotic therapy are presented in Table 1. Based on the recruitment maneuvers performed, and determination of the optimal PEEP values and acid–base balance parameters, the mechanical ventilation settings were modified. Due to the increasing features of septic shock that did not respond to fluid therapy and norepinephrine infusion, argipressin infusion was added to the therapy. The treatment included antifungal drugs, analgesics, sedatives, mucolytics, antacids, steroids, inhaled bronchodilators, neuro- and hepatoprotective drugs, antiarrhythmics, diuretics, antithrombotic prophylaxis, vitamins, probiotics, enteral nutrition under the control of indirect calorimetry, and balanced water–electrolyte and acid–base therapies. Blood morphological deficiencies were supplemented. Anti-decubitus prophylaxis was used. Due to atelectasis, bronchofiberoscopy of the respiratory tract was performed several times. Due to arrhythmias and an increase in myocardial necrosis parameters as well as high NTproBNP values, the patient was consulted by a cardiologist. Cardiac ultrasound was performed—the valves showed no organic changes and vegetation, the left ventricle ejection fraction was 25%, and there was a normoechoic, round structure (suspected thrombus/vegetation) in the middle part of the right ventricle. Diagnosis of inflammatory cardiomyopathy with generalized hypokinesis was made. An infusion of dobutamine was added, which resulted in an improvement in hemodynamic parameters. In the following days, clinical improvement was noted. The infusion of vasoconstricting amines was gradually reduced. During hospitalization, the patient underwent cardiological consultation three more times (on the fifth, seventh, and twelfth postoperative day), which revealed an improvement in left ventricular function (LVEF approximately 44%) and the absence of vegetation previously visible in the right ventricular lumen. Respiratory improvement allowed for a reduction in mechanical ventilation support. On the fifth day of postoperative hospitalization, the patient was extubated with subsequent passive oxygen therapy.

After extubation, despite intensive kinesiotherapy, the patient presented an ineffective cough, leading to the accumulation of secretions in the respiratory tract and increasing respiratory effort with desaturation. The patient was intubated and mechanical ventilation was started. After intubation, a significant amount of serous content was aspirated from the airway. Bronchofiberoscopic cleaning of the bronchial tree performed on subsequent days revealed a patent bronchus intermedius and residual mucous content, which was aspirated. On the eighth day, the patient was extubated again, followed by passive oxygen therapy via a face mask. Due to repeated respiratory areflexia, secretion retention in the respiratory tract, and increased respiratory effort and desaturation, the patient was reintubated after approximately 38 h and mechanical ventilation was started. In the double drainage of the right pleural cavity, a decreasing value of leakage of the respiratory mixture was observed, and as a result the drain from the right pleural cavity was removed on the ninth day. Due to the progression of the right-sided pneumothorax visible in the follow-up chest X-ray, the patient was consulted by a thoracic surgeon again and drainage of the right pleural cavity was performed to observe the leakage of the respiratory mixture. The aforementioned chest X-ray is presented in Figure 3.

Table 1. Microbiological assessment, antibiotic treatment, and histopathological findings of both patients.

Culture Origin	Patient 1	Patient 2
Anal swab	Enterococcus faecalis HLAR, VRE Staphylococcus haemolyticus Pseudomonas aeruginosa	Escherichia coli OXA-48 Escherichia coli ESBL Klebsiella pneumoniae KPC Pseudomonas aeruginosa Candida spp.
Nasal swab	no data	Klebsiella pneumoniae
Pleural fluid culture	Candida dubliniensis	Candida glabrata Klebsiella pneumoniae KPC
Urine culture	Pseudomonas aeruginosa	no data
Blood culture	Staphylococcus epidermidis	Klebsiella pneumoniae KPC
PCR respiratory panel	Staphylococcus spp. Staphylococcus epidermidis	Acinetobacter calcoaceticus-baumannii Klebsiella pneumoniae Streptococcus pyogen
Antibiotic treatment during intensive care stay	Colistin 3 × 3 million iv (for 10 days), colistin 3 × 2 million inhalations (for 10 days), meropenem 3 × 1 g iv (for 8 days), tigecycline 2 × 50 mg iv (for 11 days), ampicillin + sulbactam 1 g + 0.5 g × 4 (for 10 days), avibactam + ceftazidime 2 g + 0.5 g × 3 iv (for 10 days), amikacin 1.2 g × 1 iv (for 7 days).	Clindamycin 900 mg × 3 iv (for 9 days), vancomycin 2 times a day iv according to blood levels, meropenem 3 × 1 g iv (for 5 days), penicillin 24 mL iv in continuous infusion (for 8 days).
Histopathological findings from the resected lobes	Purulent bronchopneumonia with foci of parenchymal necrosis and formation of abscesses, fibroblastic foci in the lumen of the alveoli, and purulent pleuritis.	Purulent lobar pneumonia with foci of necrosis, purulent pleurisy, and purulent inflammation around the vessels.

Legends: ESBL—extended-spectrum beta-lactamases, HLAR—high-level aminoglycoside resistance, KPC—*Klebsiella pneumoniae* carbapenemase, OXA-48—oxacillinase 48, VRE—vancomycin-resistant enterococcus.

On the eleventh day of stay, after a thorough cleaning of the bronchial tree and meeting the necessary criteria, the patient was extubated again with subsequent passive oxygen therapy. In a follow-up ultrasound examination, the presence of free fluid in the right pleural cavity was observed. On the seventeenth day of ICU stay, and as a result of a thoracic surgical consultation, the drainage from the apex of the right lung was removed due to the lack of leakage of the respiratory mixture, and a Seldinger drain was placed to decompress the free fluid (in ultrasound >50 mm). On the twenty-third day, the drain from the right pleural cavity was removed. During the subsequent thoracic surgery consultation, a follow-up chest X-ray confirmed that the lungs had expanded and the patient did not require any surgical intervention. Histopathological findings from the resected lobe are presented in Table 1. Due to the symptoms of significant muscle weakness, mainly manifested by swallowing and breathing disorders, the patient was consulted by a neurologist—generalized muscle adynamia was diagnosed and blood was taken to determine the level of antibodies against Ach receptors (the result was negative). Pyridostigmine was added to the pharmacotherapy, with a marked improvement in the patient's condition.

At this point, the patient was conscious, in full logical contact. She complied with quadriplegic commands with dominant muscle weakness in the lower limbs and could perform spontaneous breathing through natural channels with periodically applied passive oxygen therapy through a nasal cannula 1–2 L/min. The patient then returned to the Pulmonology Department of the District Hospital in a nearby city for treatment continuation.

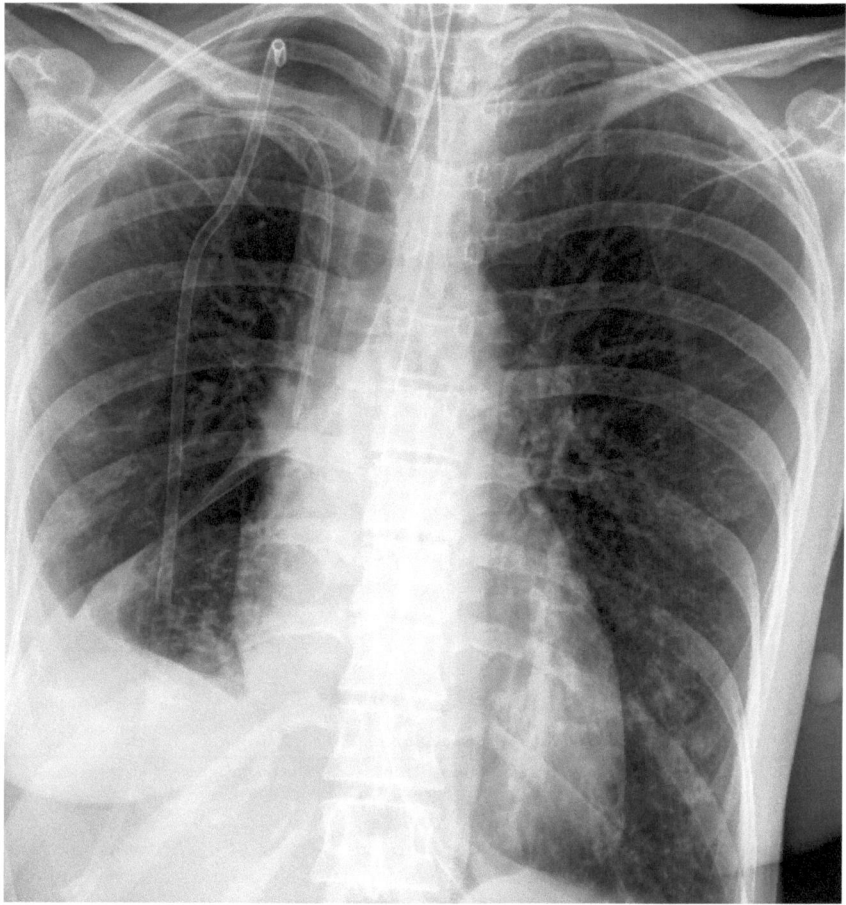

Figure 3. Chest X ray of patient 1 during treatment—progression of right-sided pneumothorax, which resulted in drainage of right pleural cavity.

2.2. Case 2

Another case pertains to a 35-year-old female patient who was transferred to our facility from the ICU of the Medical University Hospital in Katowice due to suspected cirrhosis of the right lower lobe. In the referral department, the patient was hospitalized due to acute cardiorespiratory failure due to pneumonia of mixed etiology (influenza A virus with secondary *S. pyogenes* infection) complicated by pleural empyema.

On day 0, the patient had a positive swab test for influenza virus. She began taking oseltamiwir instantly. However, her condition deteriorated to the point of that she admitted to the pulmonology department in a nearby city on day 5, where she underwent puncture of the pleural cavity (900 mL of purulent content was obtained). During her stay, she started developing symptoms of septic shock. On day 7, she was admitted to the ICU of the local hospital. At the beginning, she required high-flow nasal oxygen therapy, but her condition worsened. She was intubated with subsequent mechanical ventilation in place. She was then transferred to the Medical University Hospital in Katowice and admitted in critical condition to the ICU, with profound respiratory failure, hypoxemia, and hypercapnia despite invasive ventilation with FiO2 1.0. Intensive, multidirectional treatment was used (mechanical ventilation, circulatory support with catecholamine infusion, empirical and then targeted antibiotic therapy, RRT-CVVHDF with CytoSorb, right pleural drainage), achieving an initial stabilization of the patient's general condition, improvement in ventilation conditions, reduction in the number and dose of catecholamines, and a temporary decrease in inflammatory parameters. On the 14th day, there was another increase in inflammatory parameters, and a follow-up CT scan of the chest revealed an increase in fluid in both pleural cavities. The consulting thoracic surgeon suspected cirrhosis of the lower lobe of the right lung, and a preliminary positive qualification for right lower lobectomy was made.

The patient was then transferred to the ICU in our facility. Cultures obtained from her nasal swab as well as her anal swab were positive for Klebsiella pneumoniae. The remaining microbiological findings as well as her antibiotic therapy are presented in Table 1. She had also been surgically evaluated and underwent evacuation of empyema, decortication of the right lung, and finally lower right lobectomy, on the 16th day of hospitalization. She was transferred back to the ICU with drainage of the right pleural cavity. A CT scan image is presented in Figure 4.

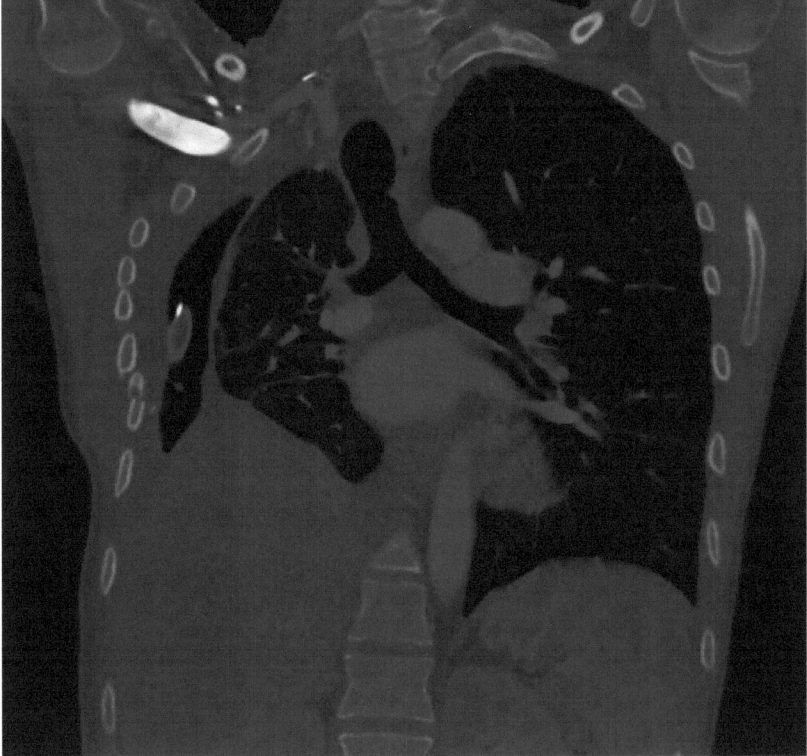

Figure 4. CT scan of the patient 2 at admission to the ICU.

Her pleural fluid and blood cultures were positive for *Klebsiella pneumoniae*. Her condition improved slightly, but extubating was still not feasible. On day 21, temporary tracheostomy was performed. Further microbiological assessments were positive for *K. pneumoniae*, but also for *Acinetobacter calcoaceticus*–baumannii and *Streptococcus pyogenes*. The patient needed a rethoracotomy twice. The first one was performed on day 27 as air leakage was found from the upper lobe parenchyma at the back, near the upper lobe bronchus. The second one pertained to suturing of the bronchial stump due to perforation and took place on the 33rd day. Purulent tissues of the right pulmonary hilum were observed and managed. During the ICU stay, she underwent cardiac assessment. Cardiac ultrasound did not reveal any significant abnormalities. She was then transferred to the thoracic surgery department for further treatment. On transfer day, the patient was conscious, mobilized, and upright, and respiratory rehabilitation was continued. With passive oxygen therapy of 2 L/min, there was a reduced vesicular sound over the lung fields at the base of the left lung and over the entire right lung field. Drainage of the right pleural cavity with air leak was maintained. After observation, she was discharged home with continued drainage secured with a Heimlich valve. She was again electively admitted for follow-up diagnostics, including CT scan, bronchoscopy, and general reassessment after a month. Significant improvements in lung aeration and low inflammation parameters were observed. The drain was removed. She was discharged home in quite good general condition. Histopathological findings from the resected lobe are presented in Table 1.

3. Discussion

Recent WHO report pertaining to influenza virus in the European region shows a continuous predominance of influenza A. However, its proportion increased to 96% in the studied period of 2023–2024, compared with 72% in 2022–2023. Currently, influenza B is sporadically detected in Europe (4%) [6]. The relative frequencies of influenza A subtypes have also shifted, with A/H1N1 viruses increasing (74% A/H1N1 vs. 26% A/H3N2) compared to the previous season (61% A/H1N1 vs. 39% A/H3N2) [6]. The majority of countries have reported detections of co-circulation of A/H1N1 and A/H3N2, with predominance of the latter, as well as sporadic detections of influenza B/Victoria. What is more interesting, it was reported that B/Yamagata-lineage viruses may have become extinct after the COVID-19 pandemic, as their circulation has not been verified since March of 2020 [11]. This further emphasizes the changes in the microbiome in the post-pandemic world.

Influenza virus can lead to severe pneumonia, but its mortality is usually attributed to its complications, especially among patients with pre-existing pulmonary or cardiovascular conditions [8,9,12,13]. Patients with asthma, chronic obstructive pulmonary disease (COPD), and cystic fibrosis (CF) are more prone not to only to bacterial or fungal infection but also to developing acute respiratory distress syndrome (ARDS) [7]. Moreover, bacterial infection is a common cause of hospitalization among otherwise healthy individuals with influenza [9,12,14]. Bacterial co-infection during the 2009 H1N1 pandemic was associated with high mortality rates despite proper antibiotic therapy [12,15,16].

It has been documented that severe influenza syndrome may lead to a release of cytokines, which results in the dysregulation of the immune system regardless of secondary infection [15,17]. The mechanisms underlying post-viral bacterial infections include interactions between viruses, bacteria, and a patient's immune system. Antiviral immune response triggered by the influenza virus can be associated with changes in the microbiome of the respiratory tract. It may change immune function to the point of actually enhancing the proliferation of pathogenic bacteria [15].

Among healthy people, microbial communities in the upper respiratory tract are more diverse in comparison to the its lower part. The microbiome of the lungs consists mostly of Bacteroidetes and Firmicutes (mainly *Prevotella*, *Veillonella*, and *Streptococcus*) [15,18]. Proper maintenance of the microbiome of the entire respiratory tract is crucial as bacterial colonization of the upper part is often considered to be the first step in the development of invasive bacterial infections, as well as bacterial infections, which follows respiratory viral infection [15,19]. It is reported that the upper respiratory tract microbiome may be enriched with Proteobacteria (i.a *A. baumanii*, *Pseuomonas* spp.); Firmicutes (i.a. *S. aureus*, *S. pneumoniae*); and *H. influenzae*, *M. catarrhalis*, and *K. pneumoniae* after confirmed influenza infection [20–22].

Despite the aforementioned microbiome changes, influenza virus can moderate a host's immune response. It was reported that A/H1N1 has the ability to cause a cytokine storm that may be associated with ARDS and severe multi-organ failure [23]. Additionally, various types of white blood cells have also been shown to have a reduced phagocytic capacity during influenza infection [9].

What is more, immune system dysfunction can progress further during bacterial coinfection/secondary bacterial infections, as a synergic disruptive effect was reported, particularly with *S. aureus* and *S. pneumoniae* [24]. Mice models that were assessed following pneumonia in the lungs and mediastinal lymph nodes showed increased virus titers and bacterial cell counts, a decreased level of virus-specific immunoglobulins, and certain types of white blood cells. In the mediastinal lymph nodes of mice, a significantly decreased amount of germinal center B cells, T follicular helper cells, and plasma cells were detected in lethal cases of coinfection [24]. An unfortunate fatal coinfection of influenza and *S. aureus* was also reported in previously healthy 17-year-old, which confirmed the significant immunosuppressive abilities of both the A/H1N1 strain and bacterial agents [14].

The described characteristics may sometimes lead to a severe clinical course of the disease among patients with comorbidities, but they can also happen among young and relatively healthy people. Patients with respiratory infection due to influenza virus with bacterial coinfection/secondary infection may progress to a clinical state that merits admission to an intensive care unit (ICU). The majority of admitted patients demonstrate pulmonary involvement requiring mechanical ventilation. Moreover, SAPS II score at admission, need for vasoconstricting drugs, and endotracheal intubation within the first 48 h were assessed as significantly increasing the chance of death. Despite proper treatment, ICU mortality is mostly impacted by age (<65 years), history of cancer disease, severity of ARDS, and the presence of bacterial coinfection [25].

Influenza and bacterial coinfection or bacterial pneumonia secondary to influenza can result in significant pulmonary complications, which have mostly been assessed and studied during A/H1N1 outbreaks. Back then, 46.6% of patients had a documented bacterial co-infection, which among all critically-ill patients was 20–32% [7]. Data from 23 French ICUs indicate that they were mostly caused by Streptococcus pneumoniae (54%) or Staphylococcus aureus (31%) [26]. Instances of *K. pneumoniae, S. oralis, H. influenzae, M. catarrhalis,* and *L. pneumophila* were also reported in a Korean study [27]. Coinfection with *S. aureus* or pneumococcus pneumoniae strains during ICU stay was not correlated with mortality. Therefore, it is advised to diagnose the presence of bacterial coinfections at admission to a hospital as well as in the ICU to properly and timely implement effective antibiotic therapy [25].

The majority of data pertaining to influenza viruses focuses on the more prevalent type A. However, it is important to acknowledge a series of case reports of Streptococci and Staphylococcal pneumonia with concomitant influenza B infection, which have since demonstrated potential morbidity and mortality in adults [7]. In the northern hemisphere during the 2017–2018 season, influenza B virus predominantly caused infections [28].

Pulmonary complications over the course of infectious disease may result in focal bronchiectasis or cavitary infectious lung disease, which may require surgical resection. The majority of patients benefiting from such treatment (mostly lobectomy) with the aforementioned lesions were operated on due to active or recurrent mycobacteriosis [29]. Furthermore, pneumonia may progress to necrotizing lung infection or lung abscess, or it may present as permanent atelectasis with pneumothorax [30]. The most common pathogens cultured from lung tissue in a study pertaining to acute necrotizing lung infections requiring thoracic intervention were *Streptococcus pneumoniae* (15/35 cases) and *Staphylococcus aureus* (11/35 cases), with some cases of *Pseudomonas aeruginosa, Klebsiella,* and *Haemophilus* species [30]. In other words, these are the bacterial agents mostly associated with post-viral bacterial infections/viral and bacterial coinfections in course of influenza. It seems that patients with an unfavorable course of influenza may develop pulmonary complications so severe that they require thoracic surgery.

During the COVID-19 pandemic, post-viral bacterial infections/viral and bacterial coinfections over the course of SARS-CoV-2 delivered multiple parallel examples of serious pulmonary complications that require surgical management [31].

Influenza virus poses a global threat each year by causing infections associated with high morbidity and mortality. Public health preventative measures, such as seasonal influenza vaccines, have been routinely used for many decades [32–34]. Vaccine strain selection must be conducted months before vaccine distribution; therefore, it can be challenging [33,34]. A study by Gross et al. confirmed that influenza vaccination is effective in the reduction of pneumonia, hospitalization rate, and death if the vaccine strain and epidemic strain are similar, especially among the older patients [35]. It was associated with less outpatient visits for pneumonia. It also decreased the frequency of hospitalization [7]. Vaccination against other prevalent pathogens may affect the type of bacterial coinfection, as the rate of S. pneumonia seems to be decreasing, likely due to vaccination, and that of H. influenza and P. aeruginosa are on the rise according to observations [7,36]. Both patients have never received their influenza vaccinations by choice. In adults (>18 years old), influenza vaccine effectiveness was 38% (95% CI 30–45%) in those with high-risk conditions versus 44% (95% CI 38–50%) among generally healthy individuals [32].

Patient number 1 had a prior respiratory condition (asthma), which can be exacerbated by influenza. Her clinical course was so severe that she was admitted to the ICU. Verdier et al. performed an analysis of mortality factors among patients hospitalized in the ICU due to influenza. They fortunately demonstrated that asthma does not increase the risk of death among their studied group [25]. It has not been established whether influenza vaccination has the ability to prevent asthma exacerbations [37]. However, using a systematic review and meta-analysis, Vasileiou et al. assessed that vaccination was associated with a 59–78% reduction in asthma episodes, leading to emergency visits or hospitalizations [38]. Patient number 1 also suffered from cardiovascular complications of influenza, with her LVEF decreasing to 25%. It is worth noting the significant association between influenza vaccine and a reduced risk of cardiovascular events, including myocardial infarction [7].

Both female patients were in their 30s and were relatively healthy. They both acquired influenza in the spring of 2024. This means that they became sick after the COVID-19 pandemic. The available literature provides only one similar case of a young, relatively healthy woman with severe pneumonia of H1N1 origin with bacterial superinfection with Staphylococcus aureus. Her clinical course was characterized by a high level of interleukine-6 and a rapid and lethal course [14].

Some studies suggest that susceptibility to influenza virus infection can depend on the host. Susceptible people may have impaired intracellular controls of viral replication, defective interferon responses, or defects in cell-mediated immunity, with an increased systemic inflammation baseline [39]. Other studies indicate that individuals under stress have weakened immunity, making them more prone to more severe courses of viral infection, as reported by a study of stress-induced susceptibility to influenza with the use of corticone among mice [40]. It was also noted that childhood seems to be a crucial time to develop immunity to influenza, as our first exposure to the influenza antigen determines the quality of lifelong antiviral immunity [41]. This is supported by the fact that older patients experienced lower rates of A/H1N1 infection during the 2009 pandemic, as they underwent exposure to A/H1N1 antigens in 1918–1919 during the Spanish flu pandemic [42].

It is difficult to assess which of the aforementioned factors pertains to our patients, as both their cases are described retrospectively. Although individual assessments of influenza susceptibility sound promising, they are currently not a standard of care, especially pre-emptively. It is worth noting that both patients experienced severe bacterial complications, particularly in their lung tissue. The decision to perform lobectomy among patients that young proved to be appropriate in the clinical context. However, the available literature is lacking in this aspect. The majority of publications pertaining to lung resection (pneumectomy or lobectomy) as a treatment measure for infection pertains to tuberculosis and mycobacterium other than tuberculosis [29,43,44].

Mitchel et al. reported that the most common non-mycobacterial agent associated with surgical treatment among 171 patients with bronchiectasis or cavity lung disease was

P. aeruginosa [29]. Contrary to the emergency cases presented here, all patients underwent elective targeted anatomic resection to remove damaged lung parenchyma. The paper proves that lobectomy can be a feasible treatment for the selected group of patients. They reported 0% operative mortality, with 5.6% of patients experiencing prolonged air leak (the most common noted complication) [29]. Patient number 2 also had complicated prolonged air leak, managed with drainage, which was ultimately treated with good outcome. Pneumectomy was also reported as a therapeutic option for infectious lung disease by Blyth, with tuberculosis being the main indication (72% of cases) [44]. This author also describes an emergency pneumectomy performed on a 57-year-old male with tuberculosis due to hemoptysis with unfavorable outcome.

4. Conclusions

Influenza can lead to or coexist with severe bacterial pneumonia, with the potential to permanently damage the lung tissue, refractory to conservative treatment. Urgent lobectomy proves to be a feasible therapeutic option for selected patients with the aforementioned complications.

Author Contributions: All authors participated in the literature review. S.B. and S.S. established the main points of interest and they provided supervision for the entire manuscript, M.Z. prepared figures, co-wrote, and edited the manuscript. M.L. co-wrote and edited manuscript, prepared tables, and serves as a corresponding author. M.S. and M.Ż. were responsible for gathering patients' data and preparing the clinical courses of both patients. All authors have read and agreed to the published version of the manuscript.

Funding: Medical University of Silesia Grants no. PCN-1-25/N/2/K as well as PCN-1-090/N/2/K.

Institutional Review Board Statement: Not applicable.

Informed Consent Statement: Informed consent was obtained from all subjects involved in the study. Written informed consent has been obtained from the patients to publish this paper.

Data Availability Statement: Data is unavailable due to privacy of the patients.

Conflicts of Interest: All authors declare that they have no conflicts of interest regarding this paper.

References

1. Jung, H.S.; Kang, B.J.; Ra, S.W.; Seo, K.W.; Jegal, Y.; Jun, J.B.; Jung, J.; Jeong, J.; Jeon, H.J.; Ahn, J.S.; et al. Elucidation of Bacterial Pneumonia-Causing Pathogens in Patients with Respiratory Viral Infection. *Tuberc. Respir. Dis.* **2017**, *80*, 358–367. [CrossRef] [PubMed]
2. Schüz, M.L.; Dallmeyer, L.; Fragkou, P.C.; Omony, J.; Krumbein, H.; Hünerbein, B.L.; Skevaki, C. Global Prevalence of Respiratory Virus Infections in Adults and Adolescents during the COVID-19 Pandemic: A Systematic Review and Meta-Analysis. *Int. J. Infect. Dis.* **2023**, *137*, 16–24. [CrossRef] [PubMed]
3. COVID-19. Available online: https://www.ecdc.europa.eu/en/covid-19 (accessed on 18 May 2024).
4. Aho Glele, L.S.; de Rougemont, A. Non-Pharmacological Strategies and Interventions for Effective COVID-19 Control: A Narrative Review. *J. Clin. Med.* **2023**, *12*, 6465. [CrossRef] [PubMed]
5. Miron, V.D.; Bar, G.; Filimon, C.; Craiu, M. From COVID-19 to Influenza—Real-Life Clinical Practice in a Pediatric Hospital. *Diagnostics* **2022**, *12*, 1208. [CrossRef] [PubMed]
6. WHO Regional Office for Europe and Stockholm: European Centre for Disease Prevention and Control. *Influenza Virus Characterization: Summary Report, Europe, March 2024*; WHO Regional Office for Europe and Stockholm: Copenhagen, Denmark, 2024. Available online: http://apps.who.int/bookorders (accessed on 2 July 2024).
7. Daoud, A.; Laktineh, A.; Macrander, C.; Mushtaq, A.; Soubani, A.O. Pulmonary Complications of Influenza Infection: A Targeted Narrative Review. *Postgrad. Med.* **2019**, *131*, 299–308. [CrossRef]
8. Iuliano, A.D.; Roguski, K.M.; Chang, H.H.; Muscatello, D.J.; Palekar, R.; Tempia, S.; Cohen, C.; Gran, J.M.; Schanzer, D.; Cowling, B.J.; et al. Estimates of Global Seasonal Influenza-Associated Respiratory Mortality: A Modelling Study. *Lancet* **2018**, *391*, 1285–1300. [CrossRef]
9. Sluijs, K.; Poll, T.; Lutter, R.; Juffermans, N.P.; Schultz, M.J. Bench-to-Bedside Review: Bacterial Pneumonia with Influenza—Pathogenesis and Clinical Implications. *Crit. Care* **2010**, *14*, 219. [CrossRef]
10. Scholtissek, C. Molecular Evolution of Influenza Viruses. *Virus Genes* **1995**, *11*, 209–215. [CrossRef]
11. Paget, J.; Caini, S.; Del Riccio, M.; van Waarden, W.; Meijer, A. Has Influenza B/Yamagata Become Extinct and What Implications Might This Have for Quadrivalent Influenza Vaccines? *Eurosurveillance* **2022**, *27*, 2200753. [CrossRef]

12. Morens, D.M.; Taubenberger, J.K.; Fauci, A.S. Predominant Role of Bacterial Pneumonia as a Cause of Death in Pandemic Influenza: Implications for Pandemic Influenza Preparedness. *J. Infect. Dis.* **2008**, *198*, 962–970. [CrossRef]
13. Mamas, M.A.; Fraser, D.; Neyses, L. Cardiovascular Manifestations Associated with Influenza Virus Infection. *Int. J. Cardiol.* **2008**, *130*, 304–309. [CrossRef] [PubMed]
14. Tomassini, L.; Ferretti, F.; Uvelli, A.; Fedeli, D.; Gualtieri, G. Fatal Viral and Bacterial Septicemia in a Seventeen-Year-Old Woman with Immunodepressive Influenza A H1N1: An Autopsy Case. *Clin. Ter.* **2024**, *175*, 95–100. [CrossRef] [PubMed]
15. Hanada, S.; Pirzadeh, M.; Carver, K.Y.; Deng, J.C. Respiratory Viral Infection-Induced Microbiome Alterations and Secondary Bacterial Pneumonia. *Front. Immunol.* **2018**, *9*, 2640. [CrossRef] [PubMed]
16. Cillóniz, C.; Ewig, S.; Menéndez, R.; Ferrer, M.; Polverino, E.; Reyes, S.; Gabarrús, A.; Marcos, M.A.; Cordoba, J.; Mensa, J.; et al. Bacterial Co-Infection with H1N1 Infection in Patients Admitted with Community Acquired Pneumonia. *J. Infect.* **2012**, *65*, 223–230. [CrossRef] [PubMed]
17. Muscedere, J.; Ofner, M.; Kumar, A.; Long, J.; Lamontagne, F.; Cook, D.; McGeer, A.; Chant, C.; Marshall, J.; Jouvet, P.; et al. The Occurrence and Impact of Bacterial Organisms Complicating Critical Care Illness Associated with 2009 Influenza A(H1N1) Infection. *Chest* **2013**, *144*, 39–47. [CrossRef]
18. Morris, A.; Beck, J.M.; Schloss, P.D.; Campbell, T.B.; Crothers, K.; Curtis, J.L.; Flores, S.C.; Fontenot, A.P.; Ghedin, E.; Huang, L.; et al. Comparison of the Respiratory Microbiome in Healthy Nonsmokers and Smokers. *Am. J. Respir. Crit. Care Med.* **2013**, *187*, 1067–1075. [CrossRef]
19. Wolter, N.; Tempia, S.; Cohen, C.; Madhi, S.A.; Venter, M.; Moyes, J.; Walaza, S.; Malope-Kgokong, B.; Groome, M.; du Plessis, M.; et al. High Nasopharyngeal Pneumococcal Density, Increased by Viral Coinfection, Is Associated with Invasive Pneumococcal Pneumonia. *J. Infect. Dis.* **2014**, *210*, 1649–1657. [CrossRef]
20. Edouard, S.; Million, M.; Bachar, D.; Dubourg, G.; Michelle, C.; Ninove, L.; Charrel, R.; Raoult, D. The Nasopharyngeal Microbiota in Patients with Viral Respiratory Tract Infections Is Enriched in Bacterial Pathogens. *Eur. J. Clin. Microbiol. Infect. Dis.* **2018**, *37*, 1725–1733. [CrossRef]
21. Leung, R.K.-K.; Zhou, J.-W.; Guan, W.; Li, S.-K.; Yang, Z.-F.; Tsui, S.K.-W. Modulation of Potential Respiratory Pathogens by PH1N1 Viral Infection. *Clin. Microbiol. Infect.* **2013**, *19*, 930–935. [CrossRef]
22. Greninger, A.L.; Chen, E.C.; Sittler, T.; Scheinerman, A.; Roubinian, N.; Yu, G.; Kim, E.; Pillai, D.R.; Guyard, C.; Mazzulli, T.; et al. A Metagenomic Analysis of Pandemic Influenza A (2009 H1N1) Infection in Patients from North America. *PLoS ONE* **2010**, *5*, e13381. [CrossRef]
23. Morris, G.; Bortolasci, C.C.; Puri, B.K.; Marx, W.; O'Neil, A.; Athan, E.; Walder, K.; Berk, M.; Olive, L.; Carvalho, A.F.; et al. The Cytokine Storms of COVID-19, H1N1 Influenza, CRS and MAS Compared. Can One Sized Treatment Fit All? *Cytokine* **2021**, *144*, 155593. [CrossRef] [PubMed]
24. Wu, Y.; Tu, W.; Lam, K.-T.; Chow, K.-H.; Ho, P.-L.; Guan, Y.; Peiris, J.S.M.; Lau, Y.-L. Lethal Coinfection of Influenza Virus and Streptococcus Pneumoniae Lowers Antibody Response to Influenza Virus in Lung and Reduces Numbers of Germinal Center B Cells, T Follicular Helper Cells, and Plasma Cells in Mediastinal Lymph Node. *J. Virol.* **2015**, *89*, 2013–2023. [CrossRef] [PubMed]
25. Verdier, V.; Lilienthal, F.; Desvergez, A.; Gazaille, V.; Winer, A.; Paganin, F. Severe Forms of Influenza Infections Admitted in Intensive Care Units: Analysis of Mortality Factors. *Influenza Other Respir. Viruses* **2023**, *17*, e13168. [CrossRef]
26. Cuquemelle, E.; Soulis, F.; Villers, D.; Roche-Campo, F.; Ara Somohano, C.; Fartoukh, M.; Kouatchet, A.; Mourvillier, B.; Dellamonica, J.; Picard, W.; et al. Can Procalcitonin Help Identify Associated Bacterial Infection in Patients with Severe Influenza Pneumonia? A Multicentre Study. *Intensive Care Med.* **2011**, *37*, 796–800. [CrossRef] [PubMed]
27. Song, J.Y.; Cheong, H.J.; Heo, J.Y.; Noh, J.Y.; Yong, H.S.; Kim, Y.K.; Kang, E.Y.; Choi, W.S.; Jo, Y.M.; Kim, W.J. Clinical, Laboratory and Radiologic Characteristics of 2009 Pandemic Influenza A/H1N1 Pneumonia: Primary Influenza Pneumonia versus Concomitant/Secondary Bacterial Pneumonia. *Influenza Other Respir. Viruses* **2011**, *5*, e535–e543. [CrossRef] [PubMed]
28. Geerdes-Fenge, H.F.; Klein, S.; Schuldt, H.M.; Löbermann, M.; Köller, K.; Däbritz, J.; Reisinger, E.C. Complications of Influenza in 272 Adult and Pediatric Patients in a German University Hospital during the Seasonal Epidemic 2017–2018. *Wien. Med. Wochenschr.* **2021**, *172*, 280–286. [CrossRef]
29. Mitchell, J.D.; Yu, J.A.; Bishop, A.; Weyant, M.J.; Pomerantz, M. Thoracoscopic Lobectomy and Segmentectomy for Infectious Lung Disease. *Ann. Thorac. Surg.* **2012**, *93*, 1033–1040. [CrossRef]
30. Ann Reimel, B.; Krishnadasen, B.; Cuschieri, J.; Klein, M.B.; Gross, J.; Karmy-Jones, R.; Reimel, B.; Krishnadasen, B.; Cuschieri, J.; Klein, M.; et al. Surgical Management of Acute Necrotizing Lung Infections. *Can. Respir. J.* **2006**, *13*, 369–373. [CrossRef]
31. Peeters, K.; Mesotten, D.; Willaert, X.; Deraedt, K.; Nauwelaers, S.; Lauwers, G. Salvage Lobectomy to Treat Necrotizing SARS-CoV-2 Pneumonia Complicated by a Bronchopleural Fistula. *Ann. Thorac. Surg.* **2021**, *111*, e241–e243. [CrossRef]
32. Buchy, P.; Badur, S. Who and When to Vaccinate against Influenza. *Int. J. Infect. Dis.* **2020**, *93*, 375–387. [CrossRef]
33. Sekiya, T.; Ohno, M.; Nomura, N.; Handabile, C.; Shingai, M.; Jackson, D.C.; Brown, L.E.; Kida, H. Selecting and Using the Appropriate Influenza Vaccine for Each Individual. *Viruses* **2021**, *13*, 971. [CrossRef] [PubMed]
34. McLean, H.Q.; Belongia, E.A. Influenza Vaccine Effectiveness: New Insights and Challenges. *Cold Spring Harb. Perspect. Med.* **2021**, *11*, a038315. [CrossRef] [PubMed]
35. Gross, P.A. The Efficacy of Influenza Vaccine in Elderly Persons. *Ann. Intern. Med.* **1995**, *123*, 518. [CrossRef] [PubMed]
36. Martin-Loeches, I.; van Someren Gréve, F.; Schultz, M.J. Bacterial Pneumonia as an Influenza Complication. *Curr. Opin. Infect. Dis.* **2017**, *30*, 201–207. [CrossRef]

37. Cates, C.J.; Rowe, B.H. Vaccines for Preventing Influenza in People with Asthma. *Cochrane Database Syst. Rev.* **2013**, *2013*, CD000364. [CrossRef]
38. Vasileiou, E.; Sheikh, A.; Butler, C.; El Ferkh, K.; von Wissmann, B.; McMenamin, J.; Ritchie, L.; Schwarze, J.; Papadopoulos, N.G.; Johnston, S.L.; et al. Effectiveness of Influenza Vaccines in Asthma: A Systematic Review and Meta-Analysis. *Clin. Infect. Dis.* **2017**, *65*, 1388–1395. [CrossRef]
39. Clohisey, S.; Baillie, J.K. Host Susceptibility to Severe Influenza A Virus Infection. *Crit. Care* **2019**, *23*, 303. [CrossRef]
40. Luo, Z.; Liu, L.F.; Jiang, Y.N.; Tang, L.P.; Li, W.; Ouyang, S.H.; Tu, L.F.; Wu, Y.P.; Gong, H.B.; Yan, C.Y.; et al. Novel Insights into Stress-Induced Susceptibility to Influenza: Corticosterone Impacts Interferon-β Responses by Mfn2-Mediated Ubiquitin Degradation of MAVS. *Signal Transduct. Target. Ther.* **2020**, *5*, 202. [CrossRef]
41. Mettelman, R.C.; Thomas, P.G. Human Susceptibility to Influenza Infection and Severe Disease. *Cold Spring Harb. Perspect. Med.* **2021**, *11*, a038711. [CrossRef]
42. Krause, J.C.; Tumpey, T.M.; Huffman, C.J.; McGraw, P.A.; Pearce, M.B.; Tsibane, T.; Hai, R.; Basler, C.F.; Crowe, J.E. Naturally Occurring Human Monoclonal Antibodies Neutralize Both 1918 and 2009 Pandemic Influenza A (H1N1) Viruses. *J. Virol.* **2010**, *84*, 3127–3130. [CrossRef]
43. Nie, G.; Liu, G.J.; Deslauriers, J.; Fan, Z.M. Pneumonectomy for Chronic Inflammatory Lung Disease: Indications and Complications. *Chin. Med. J.* **2010**, *123*, 1216–1219. [CrossRef] [PubMed]
44. Blyth, D.F. Pneumonectomy for Inflammatory Lung Disease☆. *Eur. J. Cardio-Thorac. Surg.* **2000**, *18*, 429–434. [CrossRef] [PubMed]

Disclaimer/Publisher's Note: The statements, opinions and data contained in all publications are solely those of the individual author(s) and contributor(s) and not of MDPI and/or the editor(s). MDPI and/or the editor(s) disclaim responsibility for any injury to people or property resulting from any ideas, methods, instructions or products referred to in the content.

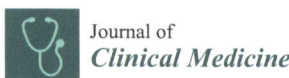
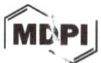

Review

Bronchoscopic Diagnosis of Severe Respiratory Infections

Maire Röder [1], Anthony Yong Kheng Cordero Ng [2] and Andrew Conway Morris [2,3,4,*]

1. School of Clinical Medicine, Addenbrooke's Hospital, University of Cambridge, Hills Road, Cambridge CB2 0QQ, UK; meb85@cam.ac.uk
2. Department of Medicine, Addenbrooke's Hospital, University of Cambridge, Hills Road, Cambridge CB2 0QQ, UK; aykn2@cam.ac.uk
3. Division of Immunology, Department of Pathology, University of Cambridge, Tennis Court Road, Cambridge CB2 0QQ, UK
4. JVF Intensive Care Unit, Addenbrooke's Hospital, Hills Road, Cambridge CB2 0QQ, UK
* Correspondence: ac926@cam.ac.uk

Abstract: The diagnosis of severe respiratory infections in intensive care remains an area of uncertainty and involves a complex balancing of risks and benefits. Due to the frequent colonisation of the lower respiratory tract in mechanically ventilated patients, there is an ever-present possibility of microbiological samples being contaminated by bystander organisms. This, coupled with the frequency of alveolar infiltrates arising from sterile insults, risks over-treatment and antimicrobial-associated harm. The use of bronchoscopic sampling to obtain protected lower respiratory samples has long been advocated to overcome this problem. The use of bronchoscopy further enables accurate cytological assessment of the alveolar space and direct inspection of the proximal airways for signs of fungal infection or alternative pathologies. With a growing range of molecular techniques, including those based on nucleic acid amplification and even alveolar visualisation and direct bacterial detection, the potential for bronchoscopy is increasing concomitantly. Despite this, there remain concerns regarding the safety of the technique and its benefits versus less invasive sampling techniques. These discussions are reflected in the lack of consensus among international guidelines on the topic. This review will consider the benefits and challenges of diagnostic bronchoscopy in the context of severe respiratory infection.

Keywords: bronchoscopy; intensive care; respiratory infections; pneumonia

1. Introduction

Respiratory failure is the most common reason for admission to the intensive care unit (ICU), and identifying its cause is critical for effective management. It is important to differentiate between sterile and infective causes of lung inflammation, and in infective causes, identification of the causative organism helps inform rational antimicrobial therapy. Common differentials for acute respiratory failure are infectious pneumonia, sterile direct lung injury, and acute respiratory distress syndrome (ARDS) arising from extrapulmonary insults.

Globally, the most common cause of respiratory failure requiring ICU admission is pneumonia. Despite its importance, there remains a paucity of evidence-based management of this condition [1]. Pneumonia is also the most common cause of ICU-acquired secondary infection [2]. The distinct categories of pneumonia encountered in the ICU include community-acquired (CAP), hospital-acquired (HAP), and ventilator-associated (VAP) pneumonia. These types of pneumonia differ in their microbial precipitants, and to some extent, the host responses directed against them.

Due to its ubiquity, patients with acute respiratory failure are commonly assumed to have pneumonia and frequently receive empiric antimicrobial therapy. When this therapy is either inappropriate (i.e., does not target the organisms present) or unnecessary (i.e., attempts to treat sterile lung injury), patients may come to harm [3,4]. This also has a negative impact on antimicrobial stewardship and efforts to limit antimicrobial resistance [5].

Invasive respiratory sampling for the diagnosis of severe pneumonia remains an area of active discussion and disagreement in critical care practice. Whether its risks are outweighed by its benefits has not yet been sufficiently systematically examined for a clear consensus to be reached. Furthermore, the impact of the growing suite of optical and molecular diagnostic techniques that can be used alongside bronchoscopy remains to be evaluated. Currently, there is significant heterogeneity in the diagnostic approaches employed by clinicians globally [6], and clinical guidelines are vague or divergent [7,8].

Although international guidelines discuss diagnostic management, their implementation is inconsistent [6] and the evidence underlying these recommendations is relatively sparse. A major decision in the diagnostic process in cases of suspected pneumonia is the method by which lower respiratory tract samples are obtained. Here, we describe the current practice of bronchoscopy and non-invasive respiratory sampling in the ICU; review the existing evidence concerning the utility of bronchoscopy in severe respiratory infections; then reflect on this in the context of current guidelines, highlight areas of uncertainty, and propose directions for future study.

1.1. Definition, Epidemiology, and Importance of Pneumonia

Pneumonia is defined as an inflammatory alveolar infiltrate and is normally triggered by an infectious agent, most commonly of bacterial origin. The global incidence of pneumonia is around 360 million cases per year [9], with a case fatality rate of 0.66%, which rises by at least an order of magnitude in severe cases [10]. It is therefore a leading global cause of death due to infection; in 2016, it was the primary cause of over 2 million deaths worldwide, around 650,000 of which were in children under five years of age. Nearly 5% of all deaths worldwide are due to pneumonia, and the majority of these are bacterial or viral in aetiology, with modest contributions from fungal and parasitic pathogens.

Respiratory viruses and *Streptococcus pneumoniae* are common causes of CAP, whilst nosocomial infections such as HAP and VAP are more commonly caused by Gram-negative bacteria and *Staphylococcus aureus*. A significant challenge in the diagnosis of pneumonia is that microbial cultures are frequently negative and a causal pathogen is only identified in approximately one-third of patients [2]. Additionally, many bacteria that cause pneumonia are also commonly found in the upper respiratory tract as commensal organisms [11].

In ventilated patients, the proximal lower respiratory tract (e.g., the trachea) is similarly rapidly colonised by these commensal organisms [12]. The clinician seeking a microbial diagnosis is therefore faced with the dual dilemmas of missing causal organisms and detection of commensals. This, coupled with the wide range of sterile causes of pulmonary inflammation, illustrates the challenge of diagnosing acute inflammatory respiratory failure.

Consensus criteria to grade the severity of community-acquired and nosocomial respiratory infections remain elusive, partly due to the breadth of causal pathogens, pathophysiologic endotypes of pulmonary infection [5], and international heterogeneity in management. The consensus guidelines for severe CAP [13] and HAP/VAP [14] agreed between the European Respiratory Society, European Society of Intensive Care Medicine, and the European Society of Clinical Microbiology and Infectious Diseases and Latin American Thoracic Association (ERS/ESICM/ESCMID/ALAT) define severe pneumonia pragmatically as cases requiring ICU admission. Separately, the American Thoracic Society (ATS) has defined ten criteria for severe CAP, listed in Table 1 [15]. These criteria were all associated with mortality in a multivariate analysis, except hypoxia. The ATS originally defined pneumonia with one major criterion, which was sensitive (98%) but not specific (32%) for predicting mortality, and no combination of criteria could be found that accurately predicted the outcome. Hence, a unifying definition in the literature remains lacking.

Table 1. ATS severity criteria for community-acquired pneumonia. The ATS define ten criteria that can be used to identify severe community-acquired pneumonia. These are divided into six minor and four major criteria. Three criteria are respiratory (respiratory rate, hypoxia, and mechanical ventilation); three are radiologic (bilateral or multilobar involvement, or radiologic progression); and the remaining four pertain to extrapulmonary organ failure (blood pressure, vasopressor requirement, and renal failure). Adapted from Ewig et al. [15].

Minor Criteria	
Respiratory	Respiratory rate >30 breaths per minute
	Hypoxia (Pa_{O_2}/Fi_{O_2} ratio <250 mm Hg)
Radiologic	Bilateral pneumonia
	Multilobar involvement
Extrapulmonary	Systolic blood pressure <90 mm Hg
	Diastolic blood pressure <60 mm Hg
Major Criteria	
Respiratory	Mechanical ventilation
Radiologic	Increase in infiltrate size by >50% despite treatment
Extrapulmonary	Vasopressor requirement
	New onset renal failure

1.2. Methodology and Literature Review

In order to ensure the breadth of the literature was captured for this review, we employed the Cochrane Handbook for Systematic Reviews search filters, following the 'Highly Sensitive Search Strategy for identifying randomised trials in MEDLINE' [16]. We searched the MEDLINE database for any references containing the keywords 'ICU', 'mechanical ventilation', or 'critical care'. Publications from this search were then filtered for those containing the keyword 'bronchoscopy' and either 'infection' or 'pneumonia'. We considered these terms sufficiently broad to capture the majority of the existing comparative clinical literature, facilitating rigorous scrutiny of contemporary evidence. Despite this relatively non-selective search, only 115 results were identified, which were then manually curated. This further highlights the paucity of systematic evidence guiding the use of this important intervention.

The most widely used guidelines relevant to international practice were selected for discussion. These were often published as collaborative documents involving multiple large multinational societies, for example, the ERS/ESICM/ESCMID/ALAT guidelines described above. Other major guidelines from societies such as the ATS and British Thoracic Society (BTS) were also considered. Regrettably, we could not identify guidelines from many low and middle-income countries, and publications identified in this review were largely from centres in the developed world. This remains a crucial area of unmet clinical need and underscores the importance of supporting clinical research in low-resource settings where the aetiologies of pneumonia may differ significantly.

1.3. Development of Bronchoscopy in Intensive Care

Bronchoscopy has provided a valuable window into the respiratory system since its conception over 150 years ago. It has a wide range of diagnostic and therapeutic indications and its scope has increased alongside technological advances during this time. The first bronchoscopes were rigid; fibreoptic bronchoscopy (FOB) was developed in 1968 and revolutionised the field with its comparative versatility, portability, and reduced risk of cross-infection. The ability conferred by FOB to access the distal airways and lung parenchyma with only local anaesthesia and/or mild sedation makes it an attractive bedside choice. With advances in optics and their miniaturisation, rigid bronchoscopy is nowadays generally limited to highly specialised therapeutic applications. FOB has been useful in the ICU for over 50 years [17].

Single-use disposable bronchoscopes are becoming increasingly available, accelerated by the COVID-19 pandemic, making bronchoscopy an ever more accessible diagnostic and therapeutic tool. Indications for FOB in the ICU include localisation and management of haemorrhage, assisting definitive airway placement, clearance of respiratory secretions, and perhaps most commonly, targeted distal airway sampling for infection. Here, we summarise the relevant anatomy and practice of fibreoptic bronchoscopy in the ICU, followed by a discussion of the current evidence for its use as a diagnostic tool in primary and secondary pulmonary infections, including in specific clinical contexts. Finally, we make recommendations for clinical practice and highlight areas requiring further study.

2. Relevant Anatomy

The respiratory system exhibits a complex branching architecture adapted for optimal air flow and gas exchange. The lower respiratory tract divides sequentially to form a tracheobronchial tree, mirrored by blood and lymphatic vessels, around which the lung parenchyma is centred. This branching commences with the bifurcation of the trachea to give the right and left main bronchi, and continues until 23 generations have been established.

Airways diverge spatially through the lung parenchyma, their numbers roughly doubling at each generation. The conducting systems (generations 0–16) comprise named macroanatomical structures such as the trachea, bronchi, and bronchioles, and do not have any capacity for gas exchange. They deliver inspired gas to the generations 17–23, comprising the respiratory bronchioles, alveolar ducts, and terminal alveoli, where gas exchange occurs. The airways are lined by pseudostratified ciliated columnar or cuboidal epithelium until the respiratory bronchioles, at which point the epithelium becomes squamous to facilitate gas exchange [18].

The typical lobar and bronchial anatomy of the human lung is shown in Figure 1. The right lung is divided into upper, middle, and lower lobes; the left into upper and lower principal lobes, with a small lingula lobe which arises from the left upper lobe bronchus. Each lobe is itself divided into wedge-shaped bronchopulmonary segments, each with its own bronchus, arterial supply, and venous and lymphatic drainage. The nerve supply of the lungs arises from the pulmonary plexi posterior to the hila, themselves derived from vagal fibres and 2nd–4th sympathetic trunk ganglia. Most fibreoptic bronchoscopes are of a calibre which allows airway visualisation to the level of the segmental and subsegmental bronchi, whereupon airway diameter limits further scope progression [7,19]. The visual anatomy of the main and principal segmental carinae is shown in Figure 2.

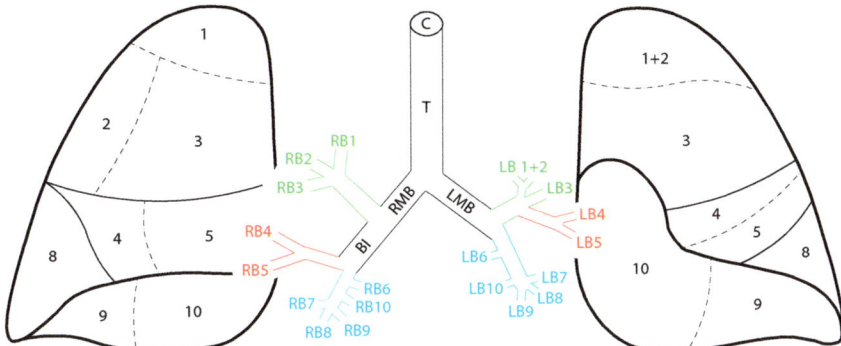

Figure 1. Anatomy of the human lung. The surface anatomy of the human lung divided into bronchopulmonary segments is shown here, viewed from the front. Numbered segments correspond to the airway shown in the bronchial tree (i.e., the right upper lobe apical segment 1 corresponds to its segmental bronchus, RB1). The right upper lobe bronchus is divided into three segmental bronchi (RB1–3), the right middle lobe bronchus into two segmental bronchi (RB4–5), and the right lower lobe

bronchus into five segmental bronchi (RB6–10). The left upper lobe bronchus gives rise to a fused apicoposterior segment (LB1+2) and an anterior segment (LB3). The lingula bronchus is divided into two segmental bronchi (LB4–5), and the left lower lobe bronchus into five segmental bronchi (LB6–10). In the surface anatomy diagram, the apical (6) and medial (7) segments of the lower lobes are not seen as they are posterior. Solid lines indicate major fissures, while dotted lines indicate non-fissural borders between segments. Green segments show the upper lobes, red segments show the middle/lingula lobes and blue segments show the lower lobes. C, cricoid cartilage; T, trachea; RMB, right main bronchus; LMB, left main bronchus; BI, bronchus intermedius.

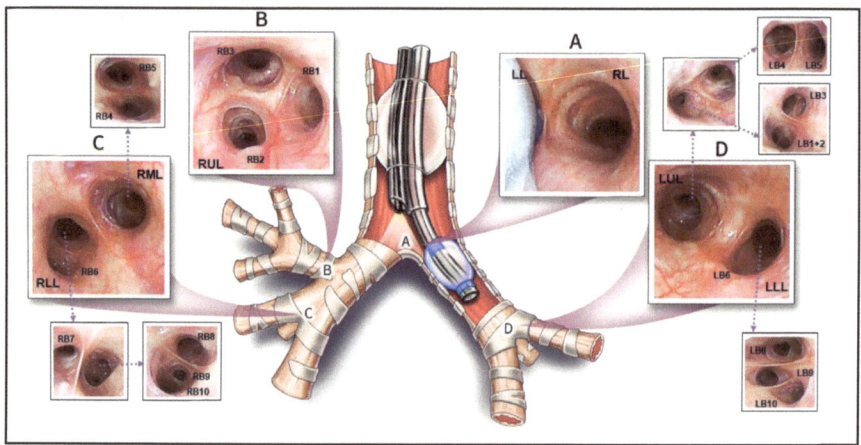

Figure 2. Major carinae of the human bronchial tree. Representative pictures of carinae from the human bronchial tree as seen during selective endobronchial intubation. (**A**) The main carina with the right (RL) and left (LL) main bronchi seen during left main stem intubation. (**B**) Canonical right upper lobe anatomy, with segments RB1-3 shown. (**C**) View from the right bronchus intermedius showing the common right lower lobe (RLL) and right middle lobe (RML) bronchi. Arrows show segmental carinae for segments RB4-10. (**D**) View from the left main bronchus, showing the left upper lobe (LUL) and left lower lobe (LLL) bronchi. Above is the view from the LUL bronchus, leading to the upper lobe proper (LB1+2 and LB3) and lingula (LB4–5). Below this are the LLL basal segments (LB8–10). LB6 is seen at the left main carina, and LB7 is not shown. This figure was adapted from Liang et al. [20] under a creative commons CC BY-NC-ND 4.0 licence (https://creativecommons.org/licenses/by-nc-nd/4.0/).

3. Alveolar and Bronchial Cell Types in Health and Disease

The anatomical complexity of the respiratory system is reflected in its cellular composition. The respiratory epithelium is specified from the ventral foregut endoderm and lines the developing respiratory tract continuously as it undergoes branching morphogenesis. The mature airways consist of a pseudostratified epithelium supported by a basal lamina of smooth muscle, cartilage, and fibroblasts derived from mesoderm cells; the overall pattern of cell types and their numbers within this framework varies over the proximal-distal axis [21]. Over 40 cell types have been identified in the lungs; the Human Cell Atlas Consortium further characterises these with high spatial resolution across a range of biological contexts, aided by high-throughput single-cell genomic and transcriptomic analyses [22]. The major cell type categories are epithelial, endothelial, stromal, and immune cells [23]. Single-cell RNA-seq and differential cell analyses of samples from the upper airways, lower airways, and parenchyma demonstrate that healthy upper airways contain relatively few immune cells. Conversely, the lower airways are more densely populated by immune cells, which are mostly alveolar macrophages [24].

In the context of bronchoscopic sampling, the cellular composition of bronchoalveolar lavage (BAL) fluid (BALF) is clinically useful. The most abundant cells in BALF are immune cells from the alveolar space and analysing their relative abundances aids the diagnosis of various diseases [25]. Over 80% of the cells isolated from BALF from healthy individuals are alveolar macrophages; around 5–15% are lymphocytes; and neutrophils, eosinophils, and mast cells are present in small numbers [26]. Neutrophils predominate in acute inflammation, and whilst sensitive to infectious causes of pneumonia, they are non-specific and cannot reliably differentiate from non-sterile causes of inflammation and ARDS [27]. In conditions with a known cellular aetiology such as eosinophilic pneumonia, lavage cells may be highly specific. Similarly, a preponderance of lymphocytes progressive interstitial diseases may point to specific diagnoses; however, the findings in many disease states overlap with others and are non-specific [7,28]. Thus, although BALF cell composition may be suggestive of the nature of pulmonary inflammation, it is unable to differentiate between specific aetiologies.

4. Bronchoscopic Sampling Techniques

4.1. Bronchoalveolar Lavage and Washings

Bronchoalveolar lavage is a technique for sampling the distal alveolar space that is otherwise not accessible using conventional fibreoptic bronchoscopes. Lavage is performed by first wedging the bronchoscope in the appropriate sub-segmental bronchus, then instilling fluid (usually warmed 0.9% saline) via the working channel to form a continuous column from the bronchoscope to the alveolar space. The fluid is then aspirated, with the initial (bronchial) aliquot discarded and cellular (alveolar) fluid collected. Although practice varies, the consensus is that at least 100 mL is required to reliably reach the alveolar space, and a volume of 100–150 mL is commonly recommended, with consensus statements available to guide optimal bronchoalveolar lavage technique in severe acute respiratory failure [19,29]. This allows for sampling of at least 1×10^6 alveoli [30].

Bronchial washing involves the instillation of small volumes (20–40 mL) of saline via a bronchoscope without wedging. This technique samples the proximal bronchioles and is more subject to contamination by respiratory flora, which may not reflect the causal pathogen in pneumonia. While this technique does not allow true sampling of the alveolar space, it is a relatively rapid procedure which requires minimal operator expertise in comparison to a true directed BAL which requires careful manipulation of the bronchoscope to an anatomically defined location and often hand-driven aspiration to optimise alveolar fluid returns.

4.2. Protected Specimen Brush

Protected specimen brushes (PSB) are sterile brushes that are advanced down the working channel of the bronchoscope and allow sampling of the airways distal to the scope, minimising contamination from the trachea and proximal airways. The brush does not extend much beyond the end of the scope and therefore samples the respiratory surface of the proximal bronchioles. Whilst this shows similar microbiological features to more distal samples from lavage [31], the cellular components are different and reflect the more proximal nature of the sample. Thus, BAL may have greater diagnostic utility in cases of uncertainty as to the aetiology of alveolar infiltrates.

4.3. Blind Bronchial Sampling Techniques

Non-directed mini bronchoalveolar lavage (mini-BAL) was first described in 1987 by Mann and colleagues [32]. It is a blind technique which involves endotracheal advancement of a lavage catheter, instillation of small volumes of saline, and subsequent aspiration to obtain the sample. This may be performed using a bespoke double-lumen lavage catheter as originally described, or by using widely available flexible suction catheters after blind endotracheal instillation of saline flushes [33]. Mini-BAL is a safe, rapid, reproducible, and cost-effective technique which requires minimal operator experience and relies on widely available materials and is effective in diagnosing VAP [34]. However, as it does not sample the true alveolar space, it may be ineffective in the diagnosis of anatomically localised VAP and is susceptible to contamination by commensal airway organisms.

4.4. Direct Bronchial Examination and Novel Optical Techniques for Alveolar Visualisation

Given the drawbacks of current practice in diagnosing VAP, there is a clinical need for tests to more accurately and quickly identify or exclude the presence of a causative organism [35]. One of the advantages inherent to bronchoscopy is the ability it gives clinicians to perform a visual inspection of mucosal surfaces. For example, *Aspergillus* tracheitis has a characteristic macroscopic appearance; the presence of pus within a segment or subsegment of a lung has a high positive predictive value for bacterial pneumonia. Similarly, in cases of bronchial obstruction and lung collapse, endobronchial infection mimics such as obstructing lung tumours can be rapidly identified, biopsied, and confirmed by histopathological examination. However, the resolution of information that can be derived from crude visualisation alone is limited. In recent years, novel optical bronchoscopic technologies for visualising the alveoli have proven promising in addressing these issues. In 2018, Dhaliwal and colleagues developed an imaging method for the detection of Gram-negative bacteria in the distal lung in real time. A fluorophore-conjugated polymyxin probe binds to lipid A on Gram-negative bacterial membranes which are subsequently visualised with optical endomicroscopy [36].

The Translational Healthcare Technologies group has recently developed an optical molecular alveoscopy (OMA) platform that facilitates bedside diagnosis in the ICU. In this method, fluorescent molecular imaging probes directed against important elements of pneumonia (e.g., bacteria, activated neutrophils) are delivered into the distal lung via the working channel of a bronchoscope [35]. Another platform, termed fibered confocal fluorescence microscopy (FCFM), can detect matrix metalloprotease (MMP) activity using a bronchoscope-compatible delivery device. MMP activity is implicated in numerous inflammatory respiratory diseases [37]. Detection of host enzyme activity in the lungs may facilitate better differentiation between sterile and infective causes of respiratory failure and a more personalised impression of a patient's disease process. These technologies are currently undergoing clinical evaluation before being made more widely available in the future.

5. Molecular Microbiology

This growing arsenal of optical tools is complemented by advances in molecular diagnostics. In the conventional diagnostic pipeline, BALF culture and sensitivities incur an obligate delay of up to 72 h. However, an expanding array of rapid polymerase chain reaction (PCR) based molecular diagnostics is increasingly mitigating this critical drawback of conventional practice. Many ICUs globally have access to molecular diagnostics and their availability is likely to increase further [6]. This shifts the risk–benefit balance of bronchoscopy and should prompt a reassessment of its merits in this new context.

In recent years, rapid syndromic tests for bacterial pneumonia have become commercially available [38] and demonstrated great promise. In the INHALE trial, 652 respiratory samples were analysed using conventional microbiology and two multiplex PCR platforms. Both platforms were considerably more sensitive than routine microbiology [39]. The development of a 52-respiratory-pathogen TAQman array card (TAC) allows the rapid and highly sensitive detection of multiple pathogens and alters prescribing. The TAC is also customisable and amenable to rapid modifications so can be adapted to emerging threats [40]. Its utility extends to critically ill children and may facilitate early rationalisation of antimicrobials in the paediatric ICU [41].

The inclusion of viral panels in diagnostic tests further aids differentiation between causes of ARF and reduces antibiotic overuse [42]. Further enhancing their clinical value, several syndromic tests now include assays for key antimicrobial resistance (AMR) genes, including MecA, which induces methicillin resistance, and NDM-1 and blaKPC, which encode key carbapenemases [42]. There is mounting evidence that metagenomics may take on an increasing role in diagnostics in critical care. A recently developed 6 h nanopore sequencing respiratory metagenomics workflow demonstrated great potential in ventilated patients with coronavirus disease (COVID-19). This workflow influenced prescribing decisions in 80% of cases and prompted early immunomodulation for suspected inflammatory lung conditions where infection was excluded [43].

False negative results from molecular tests can have adverse consequences, and a decision to withhold antibiotics in the absence of detected organism needs to be considered in the context of the range of organisms on the test and the pre-test probability of bacterial pneumonia based on the patient presentation [42]. However, this must be balanced with the risk of mistaking detectable colonisation for infection. A combination of highly sensitive molecular diagnostics and protected lower respiratory tract samples that are less likely to detect colonising organisms may represent the optimal balance between sensitivity and specificity. However, the impact on patient outcomes is currently uncertain and the merits of proximal vs. distal sampling in the context of molecular diagnostics remain to be elucidated.

6. Safety of Bronchoscopy

Although semi-invasive in nature, bronchoscopy is widely regarded as safe. Its mortality rate is reported as 0.01–0.04% and its complication rate below 0.3% [19], although this is higher in intensive care settings, where complication rates of up to 10% are reported [44]. The effects on the physiology of the respiratory system—increased airway resistance; reduced lung compliance; hypoxaemia and hypercapnia; and cardiovascular effects—explain the risks of the procedure [19]. Common complications are illustrated in Figure 3.

Hypoxaemia, haemorrhage, and pneumothorax constitute the major risks of bronchoscopy. Hypoxaemia is caused by increased airway resistance, in turn caused by occlusion of a fraction of the trachea by the bronchoscope and potentially endotracheal tube, and alveolar flooding [19]. Appropriate bronchoscope selection can help mitigate this, with a recommendation that the external diameter for the scope should be at least 2 mm smaller than the internal diameter of the endotracheal tube [45]. Additional strategies to avoid hypoxaemia include pre-oxygenation, positioning the patient head-up, and the use of neuromuscular blockade. Airway pressures rise during the procedure, posing the risk of pneumothorax, which can be mitigated by careful monitoring of ventilator settings and efficient technique [7].

Reduced lung compliance is likely caused by distal airway collapse secondary to the effects of suction and saline lavage and resulting changes in surfactant. Hypercapnia is underpinned by hypoventilation due to airway obstruction. Effects on heart rate and blood pressure stem from sympathetic stimulation and the effects of sedatives. Hypotension requiring vasopressors occurs in around 22% of patients in the ICU and can be exacerbated during bronchoscopy. However, high standards of clinician training, careful patient selection, knowledge of the risks, and appropriate mitigation measures allow the procedure to be conducted safely in ventilated, critically ill patients [46]. Concerningly, confidence in bronchoscopy and reported formal training amongst intensivists is highly variable [6,47]. Reported practice in lavage volumes is also highly variable and seldom conforms with consensus standards for bronchoscopy [6]. We suggest this requires urgent attention from training and regulatory bodies worldwide.

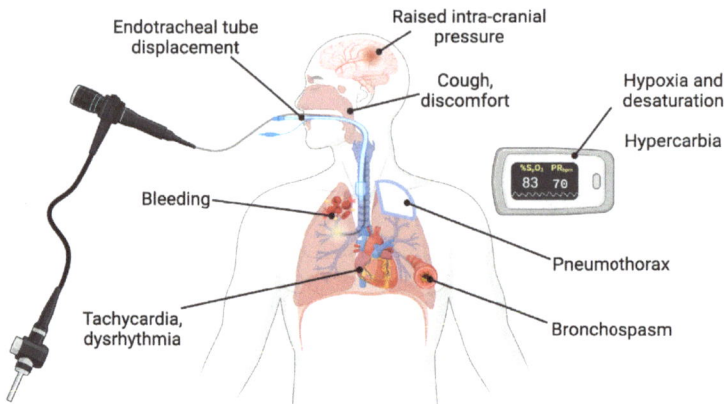

Figure 3. Common complications of ICU bronchoscopy. Categories of complications of bronchoscopy include cardiovascular (bleeding, bradycardia, hypotension); respiratory (hypercapnia, hypoxia, bronchospasm, pneumothorax); and symptomatic (pain, breathlessness, cough). These can be mitigated by measures frequently used in the ICU, such as sedation. Importantly for ICU bronchoscopy, meticulous attention must be given to endotracheal tube security to prevent displacement.

7. Evidence for Bronchoscopic Sampling in Severe Respiratory Infections

7.1. Timing of Bronchoscopy

Ideally, sampling for causative agents in the context of bacterial infections should occur prior to the administration of antibiotics. However, an association between antibiotic timing and mortality constitutes an important caveat; sampling should not delay timely medication [48,49]. For less invasive, technically simpler procedures such as blood cultures, balancing early pre-antibiotic sampling and timely medication is a realistic goal. However, for a specialist technique such as bronchoscopy, appropriately trained clinicians may not be present when infection is identified [6]. Thus, empirical therapy is frequently given prior to bronchoscopy, which may limit the sensitivity of conventional culture techniques.

In a study involving 63 cases of VAP, recent antibiotic administration reduced the sensitivity of BAL from 78% to 38%, highlighting the effects of even short antibiotic courses [50]. Additionally, in a separate study, three days of de novo antibiotic therapy was capable of complete eradication of susceptible organisms in 94% of samples from patients with VAP [51]. These data suggest that earlier timing of bronchoscopy may improve culture yield and organism identification in patients with bacterial aetiologies. This advantage must be balanced with the importance of early antibiotic administration and the availability of trained personnel. The use of molecular diagnostics, discussed below, may help reduce this dilemma.

7.2. Ventilator-Associated Pneumonia

VAP has an incidence of up to 35% among critically ill patients mechanically ventilated for 48 h and carries a mortality rate of up to 27% [19]. Diagnostic practices for VAP vary significantly globally [6,52]. The bulk of the available literature regarding bronchoscopy for diagnosing respiratory infections is in the context of VAP. Invasive sampling may seem intuitive; as BAL captures cells and organisms from the alveolar compartment, it is singular in its ability to confirm or refute the presence of infection at this anatomical level. A single-centre prospective study of BAL for the diagnosis of VAP in a post-surgical population demonstrated an overall sensitivity of 80% and specificity of 66% when compared to the gold standard of histopathologic examination [53]. Subsequent work from this team demonstrated similar diagnostic performance in another cohort [54]. Additionally, an alveolar neutrophil percentage of <50% in BALF combined with a negative Gram stain can exclude bacterial pneumonia with a negative predictive value of close to 100% [7]. However, invasive techniques are likely only beneficial if they alter practices such as antibiotic prescribing; otherwise, they are unlikely to alter outcomes such as ICU length of stay or mortality.

In 2000, Fagon et al. found in a randomised controlled trial that invasive sampling was associated with lower 14-day mortality when antibiotics were held following a negative result on bronchoscopy [55]. However, several subsequent studies demonstrated that negative respiratory cultures alone were insufficient to drive clinicians to discontinue antibiotics, making it less likely that tangible clinical outcomes be affected by bronchoscopy [7,56–58]. A 2006 multi-centre randomised trial comparing ETA and BAL for VAP diagnosis did not reveal any significant differences between the groups in 28-day mortality, ICU length of stay, or organ dysfunction [59]. More patients in the BAL than the ETA group (59.7% vs. 51.9%) had a positive culture. However, patients were treated empirically with broad-spectrum antibiotics, and therapy was continued in some cases of low pre-test probability of VAP and negative culture [59]. Observational studies suggest that discontinuation of antibiotics in VAP can be carried out safely and results in fewer multi-drug resistant superinfections [60].

Fernando et al. concluded in a 2020 systematic review and meta-analysis of 25 studies and 1639 patients that classic clinical indicators including fever, purulent secretions, leukocytosis, chest radiography, ETA, and bronchoscopic samples all have low specificity for diagnosing VAP. However, of these, bronchoscopy has the highest specificity at 79.6%. The authors note that pooled estimates are of low certainty owing to poor study quality, and frequent lack of histopathological gold standard [31]. Importantly, studies often do not disclose whether antibiotics were administered prior to bronchoscopy; this will affect the reported sensitivity. Targeted antibiotic therapy (discontinued or adjusted antibiotics) based on the results of bronchoscopy has been shown to be safe and associated with improved clinical outcomes [61]. A recent large retrospective study found that bronchoscopy was associated with significantly reduced ICU and in-hospital mortality [62]. However, the antibiotic treatment of these patients before and after bronchoscopy was not evaluated. Another study showed that ETA and BAL culture results were concordant in only 53% of patients with VAP diagnosed bronchoscopically [63]. A switch from an endotracheal aspirate to a bronchoscopic diagnostic approach in suspected VAP was associated with a reduction in the microbiological diagnosis of VAP, antibiotic use and mortality [64].

Bronchoscopy and BAL may also be useful in diagnosing early pneumonia in critically ill trauma patients, allowing delineation between traumatic lung injury and VAP and preventing spurious diagnosis of the latter [65]. Combinatorial diagnostic algorithms incorporating early BALF parameters and clinical and radiological data may outperform the sensitivity and specificity of any variable alone [66].

Overall, the evidence for bronchoscopy in the diagnosis of VAP is not strongly compelling. However, this is likely largely attributable to antibiotic prescribing practices and low-quality studies. A recurring caveat to otherwise high-quality studies is that negative results on bronchoscopy often fail to translate to modified antibiotic therapy. A recent randomised controlled trial (VAPrapid2) across 24 UK ICUs reconfirmed this pattern: despite BALF biomarker-informed recommendations to discontinue antibiotics, antibiotic use was not changed and no significant changes in clinical outcome were observed [67].

Where antibiotics are targeted following bronchoscopy, bronchoscopy is associated with improved clinical outcomes [55,62]. In light of this, a review article published in 2022 concluded that, all things considered, invasive sampling is favourable [7]. High-quality randomised trials would clarify the extent of the clinical utility of bronchoscopy in VAP diagnosis. Additionally, standardised clinical guidelines regarding antibiotic usage following bronchoscopy would allow this knowledge to translate to improved outcomes.

7.3. Immunocompromised Patients in the ICU

Immunocompromised patients are especially at risk of developing severe respiratory infections, which are associated with high mortality in this group. This population of patients includes those with prolonged neutropaenia, allogenic haematopoietic stem cell or solid organ transplant recipients, those with inherited or acquired immunodeficiencies, and those who have been treated with high-dose or prolonged corticosteroids [68]. A multi-centre study of 1611 immunocompromised patients admitted to the ICU for acute respiratory failure found that fungal infections were responsible for 14% of these [69,70]. Due to the scale of the clinical problem presented by invasive fungal respiratory infections, along with their increasing incidence in immunocompetent patients [71], they will be discussed in a separate section.

In a general non-HIV immunocompromised critically ill population, a 2018 prospective observational study concluded that flexible bronchoscopy is safe and its yield is improved when performed prior to empirical antibiotic administration [72]. The impact of bronchoscopy on management was most notable in patients receiving corticosteroids and those who had recently received chemotherapy, and lowest in patients receiving non-corticosteroid immunosuppressive therapy. Focal, rather than interstitial or diffuse, radiological findings are predictive of higher diagnostic yield. Authors suggest that bronchoscopy be performed within 24 h of ICU admission due to improved diagnostic yield in this window [72].

Among high-risk immunocompromised patients with haematological malignancies, pulmonary complications are a significant source of morbidity and mortality. Around 85% of patients undergoing antileukaemic chemotherapy develop infections and/or fever [73]. However, pulmonary infiltrates may also be caused by haemorrhage, neoplasia, or treatment-related toxicity. In acute respiratory failure (ARF), early identification of pulmonary infiltrate aetiology is associated with better outcomes [74], and is crucial in the face of emerging aetiologies of sterile infiltration in this population, notably from checkpoint inhibition [75].

Bronchoscopy is safe and valuable in the diagnosis of respiratory infections in this group; its diagnostic yield was 47.9% and its utilisation led to antimicrobial modification in 38.2% of cases [73]. An earlier study reported an overall diagnostic yield of 49% and a higher yield in those with chemotherapy-induced neutropaenia [76]. Within the umbrella of patients with haematological malignancies admitted to the ICU for ARF, bronchoscopy has a lower diagnostic yield in acute myeloid leukaemia (AML) than lymphoid malignancies including non-Hodgkin's lymphoma, Hodgkin's lymphoma, chronic lymphocytic leukaemia, and multiple myeloma [74]. In a retrospective study of febrile neutropaenic patients with lung infiltrates, 85.6% of whom had haematological malignancies and the remaining had solid organ malignancies, bronchoscopy was safe and useful. It exhibited sufficient diagnostic yield to alter management in the majority [77].

Similarly, bronchoscopic sampling led to altered antibiotic prescription in 35% of critically unwell lung transplant recipients [78]. Furthermore, bronchoscopy was the best investigation for diagnosing non-ventilator ICU-acquired pneumonia following cardiothoracic surgery and preventing excessive antibiotic treatment [79].

High-quality randomised controlled trials examining the merits of bronchoscopy among immunocompromised patients in the ICU are lacking. However, the available evidence suggests that bronchoscopy is a safe means of aiding the diagnosis of respiratory infections and affects antimicrobial prescribing across a wide range of aetiologies of immune dysfunction. As in VAP, empirical antibiotics likely affect the diagnostic yield.

7.4. Invasive Fungal Infections

Among immunocompromised patients, fungal infections constitute a significant threat. However, invasive fungal diseases can also present in previously immunocompetent patients without the associated classical host factors. The immune dysfunction that occurs paradoxically in concert with hyperinflammation in sepsis is implicated in the higher risk of contracting opportunistic infections that critically ill patients face [80]. Furthermore, the medications and clinical procedures patients are exposed to in the ICU may affect their susceptibility to fungal infections [71,81,82].

Invasive fungal infections of the respiratory system carry very high mortality of >80% if not met with sufficiently aggressive treatment [19], partially attributable to non-specific signs and symptoms and their resulting under-diagnosis in the ICU [69]. As such, re-evaluating the merits of invasive respiratory sampling in this context is worthwhile. Infections with *Aspergillus* species constitute the most commonly encountered invasive respiratory fungal infections in the critical care setting and are therefore the focus of this section. Mucormycosis is rare but growing in prevalence. *Candida* species are commonly isolated from the lungs of critically ill patients but are seldom thought to cause pneumonia. They may, however, represent heavy candidal colonisation, a known risk factor for candidaemia.

The lungs are the most common site of *Aspergillus* infection, and *Aspergillus fumigatus* is the most frequent causative species [69]. The incidence of invasive aspergillosis (IA) in the ICU is up to 5.8%, although this varies globally. BAL cultures have a sensitivity of around 50%, with histopathological examination remaining the gold standard for diagnosis, despite its invasive nature and the resulting high threshold for carrying it out in this vulnerable population [69].

Differentiating IA from colonisation can be a challenge, so clinical reasoning should encompass clinical signs and patient risk factors. The polysaccharide galactomannan (GM) is a a fungal cell wall component that may be quantified by enzyme-linked immunosorbent assay (ELISA) on serum or BALF. The latter has a reported sensitivity of up to 86%, specificity of up to 91%, and positive and negative predictive values of 80% and 95%, respectively. However, among other factors, beta-lactam antibiotic medications may result in false positives [69]. Lateral flow test devices that sample serum or BALF have become available, enabling results within 1 h.

A recent meta-analysis found no difference between the accuracy of lateral flow assay (LFA) alone and a combination of GM and LFA in diagnosing IA; LFA is advisable if timely results are of the essence [83]. A prospective study of critically ill non-neutropaenic patients found that bronchoscopy is a reliable procedure with high sensitivity and specificity for the diagnosis of tracheobronchial aspergillosis (TBA), a form of IA limited to the tracheobronchial tree, in this cohort. However, this applies to macroscopic assessment on bronchoscopy in addition to BALF analysis [84].

The COVID-19 pandemic accelerated investigations into the merits of bronchoscopy in diagnosing fungal infections because IA emerged as a common complication among critically ill COVID-19 patients. COVID-19-associated pulmonary aspergillosis (CAPA) is discussed in detail in the following section, and the insights these studies yielded are applicable to non-COVID-19-associated IA.

7.5. COVID-19

International recommendations regarding the use of bronchoscopy were issued from expert panels and scientific societies in 2020; however, technical guidance was vague and clinical practice was heterogeneous [85–88]. Bronchoscopy appears safe and of both therapeutic and diagnostic value in patients with SARS-CoV-2 pneumonia [89,90]. In patients with clinical and radiological signs but negative nasopharyngeal swab results, it aids differentiation between COVID-19 and its mimics [88], and is also useful in detecting bacterial superinfections. Targeted antibiotic therapy can then be initiated to prevent over-treatment with broad-spectrum antibiotics. However, concerns regarding aerosol generation and risk of transmission limited the use of bronchoscopy during the pandemic [91], despite published strategies for mitigating these risks [92].

As the COVID-19 pandemic evolved, it became apparent that CAPA is a common complication of COVID-19 among critically ill patients and confers very high mortality [93]. Respiratory viruses damage the respiratory epithelium, permitting fungal invasion [91]. The incidence of CAPA among critically unwell COVID-19 patients was roughly 2% in one large prospective observational study [91]. As such, timely diagnosis of CAPA is important. BALF GM testing had a high sensitivity (84.9%) and BALF metagenomic next-generation sequencing facilitated earlier diagnosis, leading to authors recommending timely bronchoscopy in patients with suspected CAPA [94]. ETA was shown to be inferior to BAL, albeit with a high negative predictive value, so is recommended where bronchoscopy is not possible [95].

Testing BALF with an *Aspergillus* lateral flow device (AspLFD) is reasonably sensitive and highly specific for CAPA, also enabling rapid diagnosis [93]. Metagenomic and meta-transcriptomic analyses of the lower respiratory microbiome and host immune profiling were conducted on BALF from critically ill mechanically ventilated COVID-19 patients. SARS-CoV-2 abundance was identified as a predictor of mortality, along with certain host transcriptomic signatures and immune cell abundances. Authors were able to discern that poor specific antibody responses and SARS-CoV-2 replication, rather than secondary infections, drove increased mortality [96].

The role of the lung microbiota in severe COVID-19 infections was further clarified in 2022; increased bacterial and fungal burden on BAL correlated with lower probability of extubation and higher mortality [97]. Bronchoscopy is also useful in diagnosing viral superinfections, revealing high rates of HSV and CMV reactivation in the lung; however, these were not associated with altered outcomes [98]. One study found that mini-BAL is a useful tool for screening for CAPA, despite not being as effective as BAL for diagnosis [99].

7.6. Bronchoscopy in Critically Ill Paediatric Patients

The literature concerning bronchoscopy in paediatric populations is more sparse compared to that for adults. However, one 2008 UK study concluded that flexible bronchoscopy "should be seen as a routine diagnostic and therapeutic tool in paediatric intensive care" [46]. This is reiterated in later studies. One 2023 paper studying bronchoscopy in 229 children in a Chinese paediatric ICU found that early BAL reduced the duration of ICU stay but not mortality; the authors plan to conduct a larger multi-centre trial to further investigate the role of bronchoscopy in this population [100]. Among neonates, bronchoscopy has diagnostic and therapeutic value and affects antimicrobial prescription [101]. In a resource-limited setting, authors concluded from a small prospective study that non-bronchoscopic blind BAL in children in the paediatric ICU is most appropriate for diagnosing VAP [102].

8. Bronchoscopic Sampling in Differentiating Infective from Sterile Inflammatory Disease

Identifying and treating the underlying cause of critical illness is vital. However, diagnosis in the ICU is often imprecise despite complex pathophysiology and marked individual variation in the way patients react to critical illness of both infectious and sterile aetiologies. In the context of the respiratory system, ARDS is often used as a diagnosis but is comprised of a collection of diseases which necessitate specific treatment. Although infective and sterile causes of ARDS warrant distinct treatment paradigms, the clinical and immunological responses they elicit from the host exhibit significant overlap due to converging molecular pathways centred on pattern recognition receptors (PRRs). Profiling the host immune response to inflammation promises to aid differentiation between sterile and infective inflammation and disentangle the latter from colonisation [5]. A variety of means of transcriptional, proteomic, and functional profiling are available [5]. These methods may help bring a precision medicine revolution to the ICU.

Exemplifying the importance of delineating sterile inflammatory lung injury from infection is that non-infective exacerbations of interstitial lung disease (ILD) mimic ARDS, where disease modification by immunosuppressive therapies is necessary. Differential cell counts may show lymphocyte-rich BALF, which in conjunction with high-resolution CT scanning may support a diagnosis of ILD subtypes such as sarcoidosis or hypersensitivity pneumonitis [103]. However, similar BALF findings are common in viral pneumonia, so this is an imperfect method for identifying sterile inflammation. Similarly, interstitial eosinophilia is highly suggestive of primary pulmonary eosinophilic disease, but may also occur in parasitic lung infections. Thus, BALF cellularity must be carefully interpreted when used to rule out severe respiratory infection.

9. Current Clinical Guidelines

The most recent British Thoracic Society (BTS) guidelines concerning diagnostic flexible bronchoscopy in adults were published in 2013. They state that directed non-invasive diagnostic strategies should be used first line in the diagnosis of VAP, but that when such non-invasive diagnostic techniques fail to identify a responsible organism, bronchoscopy should be considered for the diagnosis of VAP [104]. This advice overlooks that ETA is likely to identify an organism, but it is difficult to distinguish tracheal colonisation from infection. Contraindications to bronchoscopy include active myocardial ischaemia and continuous ECG monitoring is recommended where there is a high clinical risk of arrhythmia [104]. Current guidelines suggest that bronchoscopy with lavage can be performed with platelet counts of over 20,000 per μL. However, platelet transfusion prior to diagnostic bronchoscopy does not reduce bleeding risk in thrombocytopaenic patients, and overall bleeding complications are low even for patients with platelet counts under 20,000 per μL [105]. This suggests this target may be unduly conservative and warrants further systematic study.

The Infectious Diseases Society of America (IDSA) and ATS published guidelines on the management of adults with HAP and VAP in 2016. These guidelines suggest non-invasive sampling (ETA) with semi-quantitative cultures but designate this as a weak recommendation based on low-quality evidence. However, the guidelines also emphasise antibiotic de-escalation to minimise patient harm, exposure to unnecessary antibiotics, and the development of antibiotic resistance. They suggest that antibiotics be held if invasive quantitative cultures are below the diagnostic threshold for VAP. Again, this is designated a weak recommendation and the included remarks highlight the importance of clinical judgement [106]. Overall, the guidelines note that the literature does not reveal a significant difference between outcomes after invasive and non-invasive sampling but fails to question whether this is due to prescribing practices.

The 2017 ERS/ESICM/ESCMID/ALAT guidelines for the management of HAP and VAP [13,14] are the most recently published. They suggest obtaining distal quantitative samples prior to antibiotic treatment to reduce antibiotic exposure in stable patients with suspected VAP. The authors highlight differences between these European/Latin American guidelines and the US guidelines and give reasoning as to why this divergence exists. Firstly, it is acknowledged that definitions of HAP and VAP differ somewhat. Additionally, authors point out that while ventilator-associated complications are widely used as a surrogate measure of VAP in the USA, a lack of sensitivity and specificity has precluded this in Europe [14].

Overall, there is a dearth of evidence-based guidelines regarding bronchoscopic sampling in respiratory infections in the ICU. The guidelines are also at least 7 years old. This is significant as the COVID-19 pandemic saw an increased output of studies evaluating the use of diagnostic bronchoscopy and recognition of CAPA in the ICU. The past decade has also seen significant developments in optical bronchoscopic techniques and molecular diagnostics. Furthermore, despite sharing a common body of literature, the recommendations in the three different guidelines diverge notably. Future directions for the field should include the generation of high-quality studies along with up-to-date guidelines.

10. Conclusions, Future Directions, and Recommendations for Clinical Practice

In conclusion, although not universally implemented, diagnostic bronchoscopy is well established in the ICU. It offers clinicians the ability to perform directed, protected sampling for infection, cellular makeup, and haemorrhage at the bedside. It is clear that at the heart of the debate surrounding its application to respiratory infections in the ICU is a risk–benefit calculation based on a trade-off between sensitivity and specificity. Non-invasive sampling is likely to identify organisms, but these may be colonising, and patients may then be exposed to unnecessary broad-spectrum antibiotics. In the case of bronchoscopy, the procedure itself is semi-invasive and confers a further degree of risk to already vulnerable patients. However, high standards of clinical practice allow mitigation of the risk this procedure confers and its appropriate use has the potential to identify the precise aetiology of ARF.

The combination of bronchoscopic sampling and rapid molecular diagnostics may allow simultaneously high specificity and sensitivity. Importantly, this might circumvent the clinical harm of irrational antibiotic use. High-quality studies and up-to-date guidelines are warranted and their generation should be a priority for the field. It is also important that standards for training and practice be agreed upon to maximise the safety of this technique. Currently, evidence suggests that bronchoscopy is of particular benefit in VAP, where there is a high risk of sample contamination, among immunocompromised patients, and in invasive aspergillosis. In all cases, informed by these complexities and their patient's unique situation, clinicians must use their judgement to weigh up which diagnostic process has the most favourable risk–benefit profile.

Author Contributions: Conceptualisation, writing of the original draft, and review and editing were performed by M.R., A.Y.K.C.N. and A.C.M. Supervision was provided by A.C.M. All authors have read and agreed to the published version of the manuscript.

Funding: A.Y.K.C.N. was supported by a Wellcome Trust PhD Fellowship Grant (222919/Z/21/Z). A.C.M. was supported by an MRC Clinician Scientist Fellowship (MR/V006118/1).

Conflicts of Interest: A.C.M. has received speaking fees from Boston Scientific, Biomerieux and ThermoFisher. All other authors declare no conflicts of interest.

References

1. Salluh, J.I.F.; Póvoa, P.; Beane, A.; Kalil, A.; Sendagire, C.; Sweeney, D.A.; Pilcher, D.; Polverino, E.; Tacconelli, E.; Estenssoro, E.; et al. Challenges for a broad international implementation of the current severe community-acquired pneumonia guidelines. *Intensive Care Med.* **2024**, *50*, 526–538. [CrossRef] [PubMed]
2. Conway Morris, A.; Gadsby, N.; McKenna, J.P.; Hellyer, T.P.; Dark, P.; Singh, S.; Walsh, T.S.; McAuley, D.F.; Templeton, K.; Simpson, A.J.; et al. 16S pan-bacterial PCR can accurately identify patients with ventilator-associated pneumonia. *Thorax* **2017**, *72*, 1046–1048. [CrossRef] [PubMed]
3. Iregui, M.; Ward, S.; Sherman, G.; Fraser, V.J.; Kollef, M.H. Clinical importance of delays in the initiation of appropriate antibiotic treatment for ventilator-associated pneumonia. *Chest* **2002**, *122*, 262–268. [CrossRef] [PubMed]
4. Arulkumaran, N.; Routledge, M.; Schlebusch, S.; Lipman, J.; Conway Morris, A. Antimicrobial-associated harm in critical care: A narrative review. *Intensive Care Med.* **2020**, *46*, 225–235. [CrossRef]
5. Jeffrey, M.; Denny, K.J.; Lipman, J.; Conway Morris, A. Differentiating infection, colonisation, and sterile inflammation in critical illness: The emerging role of host-response profiling. *Intensive Care Med.* **2023**, *49*, 760–771. [CrossRef]
6. Reyes, L.F.; Mayorga, C.; Zhang, Z.; Tsuji, I.; De Pascale, G.; Prieto, V.; Mer, M.; Sheehan, E.; Nasa, P.; Zangana, G.A.S.; et al. D-PRISM, a Global Study of Diagnostic Approaches in Severe Pneumonia. *Res. Sq.* **2024**, preprint. [CrossRef]
7. Martin-Loeches, I.; Chastre, J.; Wunderink, R.G. Bronchoscopy for diagnosis of ventilator-associated pneumonia. *Intensive Care Med.* **2023**, *49*, 79–82. [CrossRef]
8. Morris, A.C. Management of pneumonia in intensive care. *J. Emerg. Crit. Care Med.* **2018**, *2*, 101. [CrossRef]
9. GBD 2016 Lower Respiratory Infections Collaborators. Estimates of the global, regional, and national morbidity, mortality, and aetiologies of lower respiratory infections in 195 countries, 1990–2016: A systematic analysis for the Global Burden of Disease Study 2016. *Lancet Infect. Dis.* **2018**, *18*, 1191–1210. [CrossRef]
10. Garcia-Vidal, C.; Fernández-Sabé, N.; Carratalà, J.; Díaz, V.; Verdaguer, R.; Dorca, J.; Manresa, F.; Gudiol, F. Early mortality in patients with community-acquired pneumonia: Causes and risk factors. *Eur. Respir. J.* **2008**, *32*, 733–739. [CrossRef]
11. Bogaert, D.; De Groot, R.; Hermans, P.W.M. Streptococcus pneumoniae colonisation: The key to pneumococcal disease. *Lancet Infect. Dis.* **2004**, *4*, 144–154. [CrossRef] [PubMed]
12. Ewig, S.; Torres, A.; El-Ebiary, M.; Fábregas, N.; Hernández, C.; González, J.; Nicolás, J.M.; Soto, L. Bacterial colonization patterns in mechanically ventilated patients with traumatic and medical head injury. Incidence, risk factors, and association with ventilator-associated pneumonia. *Am. J. Respir. Crit. Care Med.* **1999**, *159*, 188–198. [CrossRef] [PubMed]
13. Martin-Loeches, I.; Torres, A.; Nagavci, B.; Aliberti, S.; Antonelli, M.; Bassetti, M.; Bos, L.; Chalmers, J.D.; Derde, L.; de Waele, J.; et al. ERS/ESICM/ESCMID/ALAT guidelines for the management of severe community-acquired pneumonia. *Eur. Respir. J.* **2023**, *61*, 2200735. [CrossRef] [PubMed]

14. Torres, A.; Niederman, M.S.; Chastre, J.; Ewig, S.; Fernandez-Vandellos, P.; Hanberger, H.; Kollef, M.; Li Bassi, G.; Luna, C.M.; Martin-Loeches, I.; et al. International ERS/ESICM/ESCMID/ALAT guidelines for the management of hospital-acquired pneumonia and ventilator-associated pneumonia: Guidelines for the management of hospital-acquired pneumonia (HAP)/ventilator-associated pneumonia (VAP) of the European Respiratory Society (ERS), European Society of Intensive Care Medicine (ESICM), European Society of Clinical Microbiology and Infectious Diseases (ESCMID) and Asociación Latinoamericana del Tórax (ALAT). *Eur. Respir. J.* **2017**, *50*, 1700582. [PubMed]
15. Ewig, S.; Ruiz, M.; Mensa, J.; Marcos, M.A.; Martinez, J.A.; Arancibia, F.; Niederman, M.S.; Torres, A. Severe community-acquired pneumonia. Assessment of severity criteria. *Am. J. Respir. Crit. Care Med.* **1998**, *158*, 1102–1108. [CrossRef]
16. Higgins, J.P.T.; Thomas, J.; Chandler, J.; Cumpston, M.; Li, T.; Page, M.; Welch, V.A. *Cochrane Handbook for Systematic Reviews of Interventions Version 6.5 (Updated August 2024)*; Cochrane: London, UK, 2024.
17. Amikam, B.; Landa, J.; West, J.; Sackner, M. Bronchofiberscopic observations of the tracheobronchial tree during intubation. *Am. Rev. Respir. Dis.* **1972**, *105*, 747–755.
18. Luks, A. *West's Respiratory Physiology: The Essentials*; LWW: Saint Paul, MN, USA, 2020.
19. Singh, S. Bronchoscopy in critical care. In *Oxford Textbook of Respiratory Critical Care*; Oxford University Press: Oxford, UK, 2023; pp. 183–194.
20. Liang, C.; Jiang, L.; Liu, Y.; Yao, M.; Cang, J.; Miao, C. The anatomical landmarks for positioning of double lumen endotracheal tube using flexible bronchoscopy: A prospective observational study. *Heliyon* **2022**, *8*, e11779. [CrossRef]
21. Hogan, B.L.M.; Barkauskas, C.E.; Chapman, H.A.; Epstein, J.A.; Jain, R.; Hsia, C.C.W.; Niklason, L.; Calle, E.; Le, A.; Randell, S.H.; et al. Repair and regeneration of the respiratory system: Complexity, plasticity, and mechanisms of lung stem cell function. *Cell Stem Cell* **2014**, *15*, 123–138. [CrossRef]
22. Schiller, H.B.; Montoro, D.T.; Simon, L.M.; Rawlins, E.L.; Meyer, K.B.; Strunz, M.; Vieira Braga, F.A.; Timens, W.; Koppelman, G.H.; Budinger, G.R.S.; et al. The Human Lung Cell Atlas: A high-resolution reference map of the human lung in health and disease. *Am. J. Respir. Cell Mol. Biol.* **2019**, *61*, 31–41. [CrossRef]
23. Madissoon, E.; Oliver, A.J.; Kleshchevnikov, V.; Wilbrey-Clark, A.; Polanski, K.; Richoz, N.; Ribeiro Orsi, A.; Mamanova, L.; Bolt, L.; Elmentaite, R.; et al. A spatially resolved atlas of the human lung characterizes a gland-associated immune niche. *Nat. Genet.* **2023**, *55*, 66–77. [CrossRef]
24. Vieira Braga, F.A.; Kar, G.; Berg, M.; Carpaij, O.A.; Polanski, K.; Simon, L.M.; Brouwer, S.; Gomes, T.; Hesse, L.; Jiang, J.; et al. A cellular census of human lungs identifies novel cell states in health and in asthma. *Nat. Med.* **2019**, *25*, 1153–1163. [CrossRef] [PubMed]
25. Meyer, C. Bronchoalveolar lavage as a diagnostic tool. *Semin. Respir. Crit. Care Med.* **2007**, *28*, 546–560. [CrossRef] [PubMed]
26. Pouwels, S.; Burgess, J.; Verschuuren, E.; Slebos, D. The cellular composition of the lung lining fluid gradually changes from bronchus to alveolus. *Respir. Res.* **2021**, *22*, 285. [CrossRef] [PubMed]
27. Walter, J.; Ren, Z.; Yacoub, T.; Reyfman, P.; Shah, R.; Abdala-Valencia, H.; Nam, K.; Morgan, V.; Anekalla, K.; Joshi, N.; et al. Multidimensional Assessment of the Host Response in Mechanically Ventilated Patients with Suspected Pneumonia. *Am. J. Respir. Crit. Care Med.* **2019**, *199*, 1225–1237. [CrossRef]
28. Davidson, K.R.; Ha, D.M.; Schwarz, M.I.; Chan, E.D. Bronchoalveolar lavage as a diagnostic procedure: A review of known cellular and molecular findings in various lung diseases. *J. Thorac. Dis.* **2020**, *12*, 4991–5019. [CrossRef]
29. Mikacenic, C.; Fussner, L.A.; Bell, J.; Burnham, E.L.; Chlan, L.L.; Cook, S.K.; Dickson, R.P.; Almonor, F.; Luo, F.; Madan, K.; et al. Research bronchoscopies in critically ill research participants: An official American thoracic society workshop report. *Ann. Am. Thorac. Soc.* **2023**, *20*, 621–631. [CrossRef]
30. Patel, P.; Antoine, M.; Sankari, A.; Ullah, S. Bronchoalveolar Lavage. In *Bronchoalveolar Lavage*; StatPearls Publishing: Treasure Island, FL, USA, 2024.
31. Fernando, S.; Tran, A.; Cheng, W.; Klompas, M.; Kyeremanteng, K.; Mehta, S.; English, S.; Muscedere, J.; Cook, D.; Torres, A.; et al. Diagnosis of ventilator-associated pneumonia in critically ill adult patients-a systematic review and meta-analysis. *Intensive Care Med.* **2020**, *46*, 1170–1179. [CrossRef]
32. Mann, J.M.; Altus, C.S.; Webber, C.A.; Smith, P.R.; Muto, R.; Heurich, A.E. Nonbronchoscopic lung lavage for diagnosis of opportunistic infection in AIDS. *Chest* **1987**, *91*, 319–322. [CrossRef]
33. Bonvento, B.V.; Rooney, J.A.; Columb, M.O.; McGrath, B.A.; Bentley, A.M.; Felton, T.W. Non-directed bronchial lavage is a safe method for sampling the respiratory tract in critically ill patient. *J. Intensive Care Soc.* **2019**, *20*, 237–241. [CrossRef]
34. Papazian, L.; Thomas, P.; Garbe, L.; Guignon, I.; Thirion, X.; Charrel, J.; Bollet, C.; Fuentes, P.; Gouin, F. Bronchoscopic or blind sampling techniques for the diagnosis of ventilator-associated pneumonia. *Am. J. Respir. Crit. Care Med.* **1995**, *152*, 1982–1991. [CrossRef]
35. Jones, W.; Suklan, J.; Winter, A.; Green, K.; Craven, T.; Bruce, A.; Mair, J.; Dhaliwal, K.; Walsh, T.; Simpson, A.; et al. Diagnosing ventilator-associated pneumonia (VAP) in UK NHS ICUs: The perceived value and role of a novel optical technology. *Diagn. Progn. Res.* **2022**, *6*, 5. [CrossRef] [PubMed]

36. Akram, A.R.; Chankeshwara, S.V.; Scholefield, E.; Aslam, T.; McDonald, N.; Megia-Fernandez, A.; Marshall, A.; Mills, B.; Avlonitis, N.; Craven, T.H.; et al. In situ identification of Gram-negative bacteria in human lungs using a topical fluorescent peptide targeting lipid A. *Sci. Transl. Med.* **2018**, *10*, eaal0033. [CrossRef] [PubMed]
37. Megia-Fernandez, A.; Marshall, A.; Akram, A.R.; Mills, B.; Chankeshwara, S.V.; Scholefield, E.; Miele, A.; McGorum, B.C.; Michaels, C.; Knighton, N.; et al. Optical Detection of Distal Lung Enzyme Activity in Human Inflammatory Lung Disease. *BME Front.* **2021**, *2021*, 9834163. [CrossRef] [PubMed]
38. Poole, S.; Clark, T.W. Rapid syndromic molecular testing in pneumonia: The current landscape and future potential. *J. Infect.* **2020**, *80*, 1–7. [CrossRef]
39. Enne, V.; Aydin, A.; Baldan, R.; Owen, D.; Richardson, H.; Ricciardi, F.; Russell, C.; Nomamiukor-Ikeji, B.; Swart, A.; High, J.; et al. Multicentre evaluation of two multiplex PCR platforms for the rapid microbiological investigation of nosocomial pneumonia in UK ICUs: The INHALE WP1 study. *Thorax* **2022**, *77*, 1220–1228. [CrossRef]
40. Navapurkar, V.; Bartholdson, S.; Maes, M.; Hellyer, T.; Higginson, E.; Forrest, S.; Pereira-Dias, J.; Parmar, S.; Heasman-Hunt, E.; Polgarova, P.; et al. Development and implementation of a customised rapid syndromic diagnostic test for severe pneumonia. *Wellcome Open Res.* **2022**, *12*, 256. [CrossRef]
41. Clark, J.A.; Conway Morris, A.; Curran, M.D.; White, D.; Daubney, E.; Kean, I.R.L.; Navapurkar, V.; Bartholdson Scott, J.; Maes, M.; Bousfield, R.; et al. The rapid detection of respiratory pathogens in critically ill children. *Crit. Care* **2023**, *27*, 11. [CrossRef]
42. Conway Morris, A.; Bos, L.; Nseir, S. Molecular diagnostics in severe pneumonia: A new dawn or false promise? *Intensive Care Med.* **2022**, *48*, 740–742. [CrossRef]
43. Charalampous, T.; Alcolea-Medina, A.; Snell, L.; Alder, C.; Tan, M.; Williams, T.; Al-Yaakoubi, N.; Humayun, G.; Meadows, C.; Wyncoll, D.; et al. Routine Metagenomics Service for ICU Patients with Respiratory Infection. *Am. J. Respir. Crit. Care Med.* **2024**, *209*, 164–174. [CrossRef]
44. Schnabel, R.M.; van der Velden, K.; Osinski, A.; Rohde, G.; Roekaerts, P.M.H.J.; Bergmans, D.C.J.J. Clinical course and complications following diagnostic bronchoalveolar lavage in critically ill mechanically ventilated patients. *BMC Pulm. Med.* **2015**, *15*, 107. [CrossRef]
45. Estella, A. Bronchoscopy in Mechanically Ventilated Patients. In *Global Perspectives on Bronchoscopy*; Haranath, S.P., Razvi, S., Eds.; IntechOpen: Rijeka, Croatia, 2012; Chapter 5.
46. Davidson, M.G.; Coutts, J.; Bell, G. Flexible bronchoscopy in pediatric intensive care. *Pediatr. Pulmonol.* **2008**, *43*, 1188–1192. [CrossRef] [PubMed]
47. Browne, E.; Hellyer, T.P.; Baudouin, S.V.; Conway Morris, A.; Linnett, V.; McAuley, D.F.; Perkins, G.D.; Simpson, A.J. A national survey of the diagnosis and management of suspected ventilator-associated pneumonia. *BMJ Open Respir. Res.* **2014**, *1*, e000066. [CrossRef] [PubMed]
48. Seymour, C.W.; Gesten, F.; Prescott, H.C.; Friedrich, M.E.; Iwashyna, T.J.; Phillips, G.S.; Lemeshow, S.; Osborn, T.; Terry, K.M.; Levy, M.M. Time to treatment and mortality during mandated emergency care for sepsis. *New Engl. J. Med.* **2017**, *376*, 2235–2244. [CrossRef] [PubMed]
49. Evans, L.; Rhodes, A.; Alhazzani, W.; Antonelli, M.; Coopersmith, C.M.; French, C.; Machado, F.R.; Mcintyre, L.; Ostermann, M.; Prescott, H.C.; et al. Surviving sepsis campaign: International guidelines for management of sepsis and septic shock 2021. *Crit. Care Med.* **2021**, *49*, e1063–e1143. [CrossRef] [PubMed]
50. Souweine, B.; Veber, B.; Bedos, J.P.; Gachot, B.; Dombret, M.C.; Regnier, B.; Wolff, M. Diagnostic accuracy of protected specimen brush and bronchoalveolar lavage in nosocomial pneumonia: Impact of previous antimicrobial treatments. *Crit. Care Med.* **1998**, *26*, 236–244. [CrossRef]
51. Montravers, P.; Fagon, J.Y.; Chastre, J.; Lecso, M.; Dombret, M.C.; Trouillet, J.L.; Gibert, C. Follow-up protected specimen brushes to assess treatment in nosocomial pneumonia. *Am. Rev. Respir. Dis.* **1993**, *147*, 38–44. [CrossRef]
52. Koulenti, D.; Lisboa, T.; Brun-Buisson, C.; Krueger, W.; Macor, A.; Sole-Violan, J.; Diaz, E.; Topeli, A.; DeWaele, J.; Carneiro, A.; et al. Spectrum of practice in the diagnosis of nosocomial pneumonia in patients requiring mechanical ventilation in European intensive care units. *Crit. Care Med.* **2009**, *37*, 2360–2368. [CrossRef]
53. Rouby, J.J.; Rossignon, M.D.; Nicolas, M.H.; Martin de Lassale, E.; Cristin, S.; Grosset, J.; Viars, P. A prospective study of protected bronchoalveolar lavage in the diagnosis of nosocomial pneumonia. *Anesthesiology* **1989**, *71*, 679–685. [CrossRef]
54. Rouby, J.J.; de Lassales, E.M.; Poete, P.; Nicolas, M.H.; Bodin, L.; Jarlier, V.; Le Charpentier, Y.; Grosset, J.; Viars, P. Nosocomial bronchopneumonia in the critically ill. Histologic and bacteriologic aspects. *Am. Rev. Respir. Dis.* **1992**, *146*, 1059–1066. [CrossRef]
55. Fagon, J.Y.; Chastre, J.; Wolff, M.; Gervais, C.; Parer-Aubas, S.; Stéphan, F.; Similowski, T.; Mercat, A.; Diehl, J.L.; Sollet, J.P.; et al. Invasive and noninvasive strategies for management of suspected ventilator-associated pneumonia. *Ann. Intern. Med.* **2000**, *132*, 621. [CrossRef]
56. Sanchez-Nieto, J.M.; Torres, A.; Garcia-Cordoba, F.; El-Ebiary, M.; Carrillo, A.; Ruiz, J.; Nuñez, M.L.; Niederman, M. Impact of invasive and noninvasive quantitative culture sampling on outcome of ventilator-associated pneumonia: A pilot study. *Am. J. Respir. Crit. Care Med.* **1998**, *157*, 371–376. [CrossRef] [PubMed]

57. Ruiz, M.; Torres, A.; Ewig, S.; Marcos, M.; Alcón, A.; Lledó, R.; Asenjo, M.; Maldonaldo, A. Noninvasive versus invasive microbial investigation in ventilator-associated pneumonia: Evaluation of outcome. *Am. J. Respir. Crit. Care Med.* **2000**, *162*, 119–125. [CrossRef] [PubMed]
58. Solé Violán, J.; Fernández, J.; Benítez, A.; Cardeñosa Cendrero, J.; Rodríguez de Castro, F. Impact of quantitative invasive diagnostic techniques in the management and outcome of mechanically ventilated patients with suspected pneumonia. *Crit. Care Med.* **2000**, *28*, 2737–2741. [CrossRef] [PubMed]
59. Canadian Critical Care Trials Group. A randomized trial of diagnostic techniques for ventilator-associated pneumonia. *New Engl. J. Med.* **2006**, *355*, 2619–2630. [CrossRef]
60. Raman, K.; Nailor, M.D.; Nicolau, D.F.; Aslanzadeh, J.; Nadeau, M.; Kuti, J.L. Early Antibiotic Discontinuation in Patients with Clinically Suspected Ventilator-Associated Pneumonia and Negative Quantitative Bronchoscopy Cultures. *Crit. Care Med.* **2013**, *47*, 1656–1663. [CrossRef]
61. Joffe, A.R.; Muscedere, J.; Marshall, J.C.; Su, Y.; Heyland, D.K.; Canadian Critical Care Trials Group. The safety of targeted antibiotic therapy for ventilator-associated pneumonia: A multicenter observational study. *J. Crit. Care* **2008**, *23*, 82–90. [CrossRef]
62. Zhang, L.; Li, S.; Yuan, S.; Lu, X.; Li, J.; Liu, Y.; Huang, T.; Lyu, J.; Yin, H. The association between bronchoscopy and the prognoses of patients with ventilator-associated pneumonia in Intensive Care units: A retrospective study based on the MIMIC-IV database. *Front. Pharmacol.* **2022**, *13*, 868920. [CrossRef]
63. Tezcan, A.H.; Yagmurdur, H.; Karakurt, O.; Leblebici, F. The efficiency of routine endotracheal aspirate cultures compared to bronchoalveolar lavage cultures in ventilator-associated pneumonia diagnosis. *Niger. J. Clin. Pract.* **2016**, *19*, 46. [CrossRef]
64. Morris, A.C.; Kefala, K.; Simpson, A.J.; Wilkinson, T.S.; Everingham, K.; Kerslake, D.; Raby, S.; Laurenson, I.F.; Swann, D.G.; Walsh, T.S. Evaluation of the effect of diagnostic methodology on the reported incidence of ventilator-associated pneumonia. *Thorax* **2009**, *64*, 516–522. [CrossRef]
65. Harrell, K.N.; Lee, W.B.; Rooks, H.J.; Briscoe, W.E.; Capote, W.; Dart, B.W., 4th; Hunt, D.J.; Maxwell, R.A. Early pneumonia diagnosis decreases ventilator-associated pneumonia rates in trauma population. *J. Trauma Acute Care Surg.* **2023**, *94*, 30–35. [CrossRef]
66. Vernikos, P.; Kampolis, C.F.; Konstantopoulos, K.; Armaganidis, A.; Karakitsos, P. The role of bronchoscopic findings and bronchoalveolar lavage fluid cytology in early diagnosis of ventilator-associated pneumonia. *Respir. Care* **2016**, *61*, 658–667. [CrossRef] [PubMed]
67. Hellyer, T.P.; McAuley, D.F.; Walsh, T.S.; Anderson, N.; Conway Morris, A.; Singh, S.; Dark, P.; Roy, A.I.; Perkins, G.D.; McMullan, R.; et al. Biomarker-guided antibiotic stewardship in suspected ventilator-associated pneumonia (VAPrapid2): A randomised controlled trial and process evaluation. *Lancet Respir. Med.* **2020**, *8*, 182–191. [CrossRef] [PubMed]
68. Patterson, T.F.; Thompson, G.R.; Denning, D.W.; Fishman, J.A.; Hadley, S.; Herbrecht, R.; Kontoyiannis, D.P.; Marr, K.A.; Morrison, V.A.; Nguyen, M.H.; et al. Practice Guidelines for the Diagnosis and Management of Aspergillosis: 2016 Update by the Infectious Diseases Society of America. *Clin. Infect. Dis.* **2016**, *63*, e1–e60. [CrossRef] [PubMed]
69. Garnacho-Montero, J.; Barrero-García, I.; León-Moya, C. Fungal infections in immunocompromised critically ill patients. *J. Intensive Med.* **2024**, *4*, 299–306. [CrossRef]
70. Azoulay, E.; Schellongowski, P.; Darmon, M. The Intensive Care Medicine research agenda on critically ill oncology and hematology patients. *Intensive Care Med.* **2017**, *43*, 1366–1382. [CrossRef]
71. Bassetti, M.; Bouza, E. Invasive mould infections in the ICU setting: Complexities and solutions. *Oxf. Acad. Press* **2017**, *72*, i39–i47. [CrossRef]
72. Al-Qadi, M.O.; Cartin-Ceba, R.; Kashyap, R.; Kaur, S.; Peters, S.G. The diagnostic yield, safety, and impact of flexible bronchoscopy in non-HIV immunocompromised critically ill patients in the intensive care unit. *Lung* **2018**, *196*, 729–736. [CrossRef]
73. Hummel, M.; Rudert, S.; Hof, H.; Hehlmann, R.; Buchheidt, D. Diagnostic yield of bronchoscopy with bronchoalveolar lavage in febrile patients with hematologic malignancies and pulmonary infiltrates. *Ann. Hematol.* **2008**, *87*, 291–297. [CrossRef]
74. Rabbat, A.; Chaoui, D.; Lefebvre, A.; Roche, N.; Legrand, O.; Lorut, C.; Rio, B.; Marie, J.P.; Huchon, G. Is BAL useful in patients with acute myeloid leukemia admitted in ICU for severe respiratory complications? *Leukemia* **2008**, *22*, 1361–1367. [CrossRef]
75. Lin, M.X.; Zang, D.; Liu, C.G.; Han, X.; Chen, J. Immune checkpoint inhibitor-related pneumonitis: Research advances in prediction and management. *Front. Immunol.* **2024**, *15*, 1266850. [CrossRef]
76. Gruson, D.; Hilbert, G.; Valentino, R.; Vargas, F.; Chene, G.; Bebear, C.; Allery, A.; Pigneux, A.; Gbikpi-Benissan, G.; Cardinaud, J.P. Utility of fiberoptic bronchoscopy in neutropenic patients admitted to the intensive care unit with pulmonary infiltrates. *Crit. Care Med.* **2000**, *28*, 2224–2230. [CrossRef] [PubMed]
77. Khalid, U.; Akram, M.J.; Butt, F.M.; Ashraf, M.B.; Khan, F. The diagnostic utility and clinical implications of bronchoalveolar lavage in cancer patients with febrile neutropenia and lung infiltrates. *Cureus* **2020**, *12*, e10268.
78. Mohanka, M.R.; Mehta, A.C.; Budev, M.M.; Machuzak, M.S.; Gildea, T.R. Impact of bedside bronchoscopy in critically ill lung transplant recipients. *J. Bronchol. Interv. Pulmonol.* **2014**, *21*, 199–207. [CrossRef] [PubMed]
79. Stéphan, F.; Zarrouki, Y.; Mougeot, C.; Imbert, A.; Kortchinsky, T.; Pilorge, C.; Rézaiguia-Delclaux, S. Non-ventilator ICU-acquired pneumonia after cardiothoracic surgery: Accuracy of diagnostic tools and outcomes. *Respir. Care* **2016**, *61*, 324–332. [PubMed]
80. van der Poll, T.; Shankar-Hari, M.; Wiersinga, W. The Immunology of Sepsis. *Immunity* **2021**, *54*, 2450–2464. [PubMed]

81. Bassetti, M.; Giacobbe, D.; Agvald-Ohman, C.; Akova, M.; Alastruey-Izquierdo, A.; Arikan-Akdagli, S.; Azoulay, E.; Blot, S.; Cornely, O.; Cuenca-Estrella, M.; et al. Invasive Fungal Diseases in Adult Patients in Intensive Care Unit (FUNDICU): 2024 consensus definitions from ESGCIP, EFISG, ESICM, ECMM, MSGERC, ISAC, and ISHAM. *Intensive Care Med.* **2024**, *50*, 502–515.
82. Taccone, F.; Van den Abeele, A.; Bulpa, P.; Misset, B.; Meersseman, W.; Cardoso, T.; Paiva, J.; Blasco-Navalpotro, M.; De Laere, E.; Dimopoulos, G.; et al. Epidemiology of invasive aspergillosis in critically ill patients: Clinical presentation, underlying conditions, and outcomes. *Crit. Care* **2015**, *19*, 7.
83. Zhang, X.; Shang, X.; Zhang, Y.; Li, X.; Yang, K.; Wang, Y.; Guo, K. Diagnostic accuracy of galactomannan and lateral flow assay in invasive aspergillosis: A diagnostic meta-analysis. *Heliyon* **2024**, *14*, e34569. [CrossRef]
84. Sahar Farghly Youssif, E.A.H.; Moharram, A.M.; Farhan, M.A.; Badary, D.M.; Hasan, A.A.A. Is bronchoscopic view a reliable method in diagnosis of tracheobronchial aspergillosis in critically ill non-neutropenic patients? *Clin. Respir. J.* **2020**, *14*, 956–964.
85. Wahidi, M.M.; Shojaee, S.; Lamb, C.R.; Ost, D.; Maldonado, F.; Eapen, G.; Caroff, D.A.; Stevens, M.P.; Ouellette, D.R.; Lilly, C.; et al. The use of bronchoscopy during the Coronavirus disease 2019 pandemic: CHEST/AABIP guideline and expert panel report. *Chest* **2020**, *158*, 1268–1281. [CrossRef]
86. Luo, F.; Darwiche, K.; Singh, S.; Torrego, A.; Steinfort, D.P.; Gasparini, S.; Liu, D.; Zhang, W.; Fernandez-Bussy, S.; Herth, F.J.F.; et al. Performing bronchoscopy in times of the COVID-19 pandemic: Practice statement from an international expert panel. *Respiration* **2020**, *99*, 417–422. [PubMed]
87. Steinfort, D.; Herth, F.; Irving, L.; Nguyen, P. Safe performance of diagnostic bronchoscopy/EBUS during the SARS-CoV-2 pandemic. *Respirology* **2020**, *7*, 703–708.
88. Arenas-De Larriva, M.; Martín-DeLeon, R.; Urrutia Royo, B.; Fernández-Navamuel, I.; Gimenez Velando, A.; Nuñez García, L.; Centeno Clemente, C.; Andreo García, F.; Rafecas Codern, A.; Fernández-Arias, C.; et al. The role of bronchoscopy in patients with SARS-CoV-2 pneumonia. *ERJ Open Res.* **2021**, *7*, 00165–02021. [PubMed]
89. Serra Mitjà, P.; Centeno, C.; Garcia-Olivé, I.; Antuori, A.; Casadellà, M.; Tazi, R.; Armestar, F.; Fernández, E.; Andreo, F.; Rosell, A. Bronchoscopy in critically ill COVID-19 patients. *J. Bronchol. Interv. Pulmonol.* **2022**, *29*, 186–190.
90. Demarzo, S.E.; Melo, J.B.C.; Carranza, M.X.M.; Oliveira, F.N.D.; Ferreira, A.d.P.; Palomino, A.L.M.; Figueiredo, V.R.; Jacomelli, M. Bronchoscopy in COVID-19 inpatients: Experience of a university hospital in the first outbreak of the disease in Brazil. *Einstein* **2022**, *20*, eAO6858.
91. Adzic-Vukicevic, T.; Mladenovic, M.; Jovanovic, S.; Soldatović, I.; Radovanovic-Spurnic, A. Invasive fungal disease in COVID-19 patients: A single-center prospective observational study. *Front. Med.* **2023**, *10*, 1084666.
92. Koehler, P.; Cornely, O.A.; Kochanek, M. Bronchoscopy safety precautions for diagnosing COVID-19 associated pulmonary aspergillosis—A simulation study. *Mycoses* **2021**, *64*, 55–59.
93. Estella, Á.; Martín-Loeches, I.; Núñez, M.R.; García, C.G.; Pesaresi, L.M.; Escors, A.A.; Prieto, M.D.L.; Calvo, J.M.S. Microbiological diagnosis of pulmonary invasive aspergillosis in critically ill patients with severe SARS-CoV-2 pneumonia: A bronchoalveolar study. *Ann. Clin. Microbiol. Antimicrob.* **2023**, *22*, 90.
94. Zhou, X.; Wu, X.; Chen, Z.; Cui, X.; Cai, Y.; Liu, Y.; Weng, B.; Zhan, Q.; Huang, L. Risk factors and the value of microbiological examinations of COVID-19 associated pulmonary aspergillosis in critically ill patients in intensive care unit: The appropriate microbiological examinations are crucial for the timely diagnosis of CAPA. *Front. Cell. Infect. Microbiol.* **2023**, *13*, 1287496.
95. Román-Montes, C.M.; Bojorges-Aguilar, S.; Díaz-Lomelí, P.; Cervantes-Sánchez, A.; Rangel-Cordero, A.; Martínez-Gamboa, A.; Sifuentes-Osornio, J.; Ponce-de León, A.; González-Lara, M.F. Tracheal aspirate galactomannan testing in COVID-19-associated pulmonary aspergillosis. *Front. Fungal Biol.* **2022**, *3*, 855914.
96. Sulaiman, I.; Chung, M.; Angel, L.; Tsay, J.C.J.; Wu, B.G.; Yeung, S.T.; Krolikowski, K.; Li, Y.; Duerr, R.; Schluger, R.; et al. Microbial signatures in the lower airways of mechanically ventilated COVID-19 patients associated with poor clinical outcome. *Nat. Microbiol.* **2021**, *6*, 1245–1258. [PubMed]
97. Kullberg, R.F.J.; de Brabander, J.; Boers, L.S.; Biemond, J.J.; Nossent, E.J.; Heunks, L.M.A.; Vlaar, A.P.J.; Bonta, P.I.; van der Poll, T.; Duitman, J.; et al. Lung Microbiota of critically ill patients with COVID-19 are associated with nonresolving acute respiratory distress syndrome. *Am. J. Respir. Crit. Care Med.* **2022**, *206*, 846–856. [PubMed]
98. Luyt, C.E.; Burrel, S.; Mokrani, D.; Pineton de Chambrun, M.; Luyt, D.; Chommeloux, J.; Guiraud, V.; Bréchot, N.; Schmidt, M.; Hekimian, G.; et al. Herpesviridae lung reactivation and infection in patients with severe COVID-19 or influenza virus pneumonia: A comparative study. *Ann. Intensive Care* **2022**, *12*, 87. [PubMed]
99. Vanbelinghen, M.C.; Atasever, B.; van der Spoel, H.J.I.; Bouman, C.C.S.; Altenburg, J.; van Dijk, K. Mini-bronchoalveolar lavage for diagnosing Coronavirus disease 2019-associated invasive pulmonary aspergillosis. *Crit. Care Explor.* **2021**, *3*, e0601. [CrossRef]
100. Wu, X.; Lu, W.; Sang, X.; Xu, Y.; Wang, T.; Zhan, X.; Hao, J.; Ren, R.; Zeng, H.; Li, S. Timing of bronchoscopy and application of scoring tools in children with severe pneumonia. *Ital. J. Pediatr.* **2023**, *49*, 44.
101. Mackanjee, H.R.; Naidoo, L.; Ramkaran, P.; Sartorius, B.; Chuturgoon, A.A. Neonatal bronchoscopy: Role in respiratory disease of the newborn-A 7 year experience. *Pediatr. Pulmonol.* **2019**, *54*, 415–420.
102. Sachdev, A.; Chugh, K.; Sethi, M.; Gupta, D.; Wattal, C.; Menon, G. Diagnosis of ventilator-associated pneumonia in children in resource-limited setting: A comparative study of bronchoscopic and nonbronchoscopic methods. *Pediatr. Crit. Care Med.* **2010**, *11*, 258–266.
103. Kebbe, J.; Abdo, T. Interstitial lung disease: The diagnostic role of bronchoscopy. *J. Thorac. Dis.* **2017**, *9*, S996–S1010.

104. Du Rand, I.A.; Blaikley, J.; Booton, R.; Chaudhuri, N.; Gupta, V.; Khalid, S.; Mandal, S.; Martin, J.; Mills, J.; Navani, N.; et al. British Thoracic Society guideline for diagnostic flexible bronchoscopy in adults: Accredited by NICE. *Thorax* **2013**, *68* (Suppl. 1), i1–i44.
105. Nandagopal, L.; Veeraputhiran, M.; Jain, T.; Soubani, A.O.; Schiffer, C.A. Bronchoscopy can be done safely in patients with thrombocytopenia. *Transfusion* **2016**, *56*, 344–348.
106. Kalil, A.C.; Metersky, M.L.; Klompas, M.; Muscedere, J.; Sweeney, D.A.; Palmer, L.B.; Napolitano, L.M.; O'Grady, N.P.; Bartlett, J.G.; Carratalà, J.; et al. Management of adults with hospital-acquired and ventilator-associated pneumonia: 2016 clinical practice guidelines by the infectious diseases society of America and the American thoracic society. *Clin. Infect. Dis.* **2016**, *63*, e61–e111.

Disclaimer/Publisher's Note: The statements, opinions and data contained in all publications are solely those of the individual author(s) and contributor(s) and not of MDPI and/or the editor(s). MDPI and/or the editor(s) disclaim responsibility for any injury to people or property resulting from any ideas, methods, instructions or products referred to in the content.

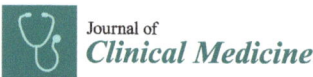 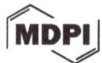

Review

Diagnostic Approach to Pneumonia in Immunocompromised Hosts

Nadir Ullah [1,†], Ludovica Fusco [2,3,†], Luigi Ametrano [2,3,†], Claudia Bartalucci [1,2], Daniele Roberto Giacobbe [1,2,*], Antonio Vena [1,2], Malgorzata Mikulska [1,2] and Matteo Bassetti [1,2]

[1] Department of Health Sciences (DISSAL), University of Genoa, 16126 Genoa, Italy; nadir.ullah@uvas.edu.pk (N.U.); bartalucciclaudia@gmail.com (C.B.); anton.vena@gmail.com (A.V.); m.mikulska@unige.it (M.M.); matteo.bassetti@hsanmartino.it (M.B.)

[2] UO Clinica Malattie Infettive, IRCCS Ospedale Policlinico San Martino, 16126 Genoa, Italy; ludo940f@gmail.com (L.F.); luigi.ametrano@outlook.com (L.A.)

[3] Department of Clinical Medicine and Surgery, University of Naples Federico II, 80138 Naples, Italy

* Correspondence: danieleroberto.giacobbe@unige.it; Tel.: +39-010-555-4654

† These authors contributed equally to this work.

Abstract: In immunocompromised patients, pneumonia presents a diagnostic challenge due to diverse etiologies, nonspecific symptoms, overlapping radiological presentation, frequent co-infections, and the potential for rapid progression to severe disease. Thus, timely and accurate diagnosis of all pathogens is crucial. This narrative review explores the latest advancements in microbiological diagnostic techniques for pneumonia in immunocompromised patients. It covers major available microbiological tools for diagnosing both community-acquired and hospital-acquired pneumonia, encompassing a wide spectrum of pathogens including bacterial, viral, fungal, and parasitic. While traditional culture methods remain pivotal in identifying many pneumonia-causing etiologies, their limitations in sensitivity and time to results have led to the rise of non-invasive antigen tests and molecular diagnostics. These are increasingly employed alongside cultures and microscopy for more efficient diagnosis, mainly in viral and fungal infections. Lastly, we report the future of pneumonia diagnostics, exploring the potential of metagenomics and CRISPR/Cas13a for more precise and rapid pathogen detection in immunocompromised populations.

Keywords: immunocompromised patients; pneumonia; microbiological diagnosis; culture; antigenic tests; polymerase chain reaction

1. Introduction

Pneumonia is an acute infection of the lung parenchyma caused by different pathogens. [1]. The clinical presentation of pneumonia could be severe leading to intensive care unit (ICU) admission, especially in immunocompromised patients who are at high risk for hypoxemic acute respiratory failure and sepsis [2].

The American Thoracic Society (ATS) provides a clear definition and diagnostic criteria for immunocompromised host pneumonia (ICHP) [3]. ICHP is defined as infectious pneumonia occurring in individuals with a quantitative or functional impairment of host immune defenses. The diagnostic criteria for ICHP include clinical suspicion of a lung infection, with or without compatible clinical signs and symptoms, accompanied by radiographic evidence of a new or worsening pulmonary infiltrate [3].

While immunocompromised states can be innate, acquired immunodeficiency is currently becoming more prevalent due to recent advances in cancer chemotherapy, solid organ transplants (SOTs), hematopoietic cell transplantation (HCT), the use of immunomodulatory drugs, and the acquired immune deficiency syndrome (AIDS) [4]. Patients with immunosuppressive conditions are at higher risk of pneumonia, which may account for 75% of all pulmonary complications [4]. Various pathogens, including bacteria, viruses, fungi, and parasites, could be responsible for pneumonia in immunocompromised patients, although bacteria represent the leading cause followed by viruses [5,6].

Patient's risk for infection with specific pathogens is influenced by the nature of their underlying immune defect (e.g., the increased susceptibility to encapsulated bacterial infections caused by *Streptococcus pneumoniae* or *Haemophilus influenzae* in patients with humoral immunity defects), but mixed immune defects (e.g., occurring in HCT recipients) should always be considered. Moreover, specific risk factors associated with the underling disease or its treatment can lead to an increased incidence in fungal, mycobacterial, and viral infections [5].

International guidelines for managing lung disease in critically ill immunocompromised patients emphasize the importance of obtaining valid diagnostic samples with invasive and non-invasive investigations [7]. Various microbiological methods can be used to diagnose bacterial pneumonia. Culture methods of samples such as blood, sputum, and bronchoalveolar lavage fluid (BALF) should be employed, although diagnostic performance of these tests could be affected by the quality of the sampling, the specific pathogen involved (e.g., atypical respiratory pathogens), and prior antibiotic use [8,9]. Therefore, important diagnostic methods also include antigen and molecular testing, especially for viral infections in which polymerase chain reaction (PCR) is actually the reference standard diagnostic method [10]. Indeed, multiple respiratory viral and bacterial infections can be diagnosed simultaneously within 2–3 h using PCR-based diagnostic panels [11]. Regarding fungal pneumonia, cultures have low sensitivity, and the fungal growth can be slow. For these reasons, antigen-based diagnostics (in blood, BAL, and serum) is the cornerstone of diagnosis in immunocompromised patients, in addition to specific radiological findings, with molecular methods slowly gaining importance [12].

The purpose of this narrative review is to discuss microbiological diagnostic methods used in pneumonia in immunocompromised patients. This review article is organized as follows: (i) diagnostics methods for community-acquired bacterial pneumoniae (CABP) and hospital-acquired bacterial pneumonia (HABP), including ventilator-associated bacterial pneumonia (VABP); (ii) diagnostic methods for viral pneumonia; (iii) diagnostic methods for fungal pneumonia; (iv) potential future approaches to the diagnosis of pneumonia; (v) conclusions.

2. Diagnostic Methods for Bacterial Pneumonia

2.1. Community-Acquired Bacterial Pneumoniae

Among the most frequent bacterial pathogens responsible for community-acquired bacterial pneumonia (CABP) in immunocompromised patients are *Streptococcus pneumoniae*, *Staphylococcus aureus*, *Hemophilus influenzae*, *Klebsiella pneumoniae*, *Mycoplasma pneumoniae*, *Chlamydia pneumoniae*, and *Legionella pneumophila* [13].

Patients with severe-CABP (defined according to ERS/ESICM/ESCMID/ALAT guidelines as a CAP that require intensive care unit admission and might require organ support, encompassing almost 5% of patient with CAP) [14], require an extensive diagnostic approach, and different microbiological tests are available including traditional culture-based methods, microscopy, antigenic testing (e.g., on urine for *Streptococcus pneumoniae* and

Legionella pneumophila), and molecular methods [15,16]. Blood cultures are recommended in the diagnostic work-up for severe-CABP and can be useful for achieving etiological diagnosis (except for atypical respiratory pathogens), although their sensitivity remains suboptimal. Thus, the diagnosis of pneumonia should not rely on blood cultures only, and their use should be carefully examined, especially with rising healthcare costs [17,18].

The diagnostic performance of various tests for CABP has been investigated across several studies. A Gram strain performed on respiratory specimens (mainly sputum) could be a rapid and useful tool to evaluate a bacterial cause of pneumonia. Its sensitivity could vary depending on the pathogen involved, reaching 62.5% for *Streptococcus pneumoniae*, 60.9% for *Haemophilus influenzae*, and just 9.1% for staphylococcal pneumonia, while reported specificity was 100% for staphylococcal pneumonia, 95.1% for *Haemophilus influenzae*, and 91.5% for *Streptococcus pneumoniae* in a prospective study conducted by Fukuyama and colleagues [19]. For instance, in a recent study, different traditional culturing methods (sputum Gram staining, BALF Gram staining, and sputum culture) were evaluated for diagnosis of a single bacterial pathogen among 287 children with CAP. Using a BALF culture as reference, the sensitivity and specificity for these methods were as follows: sputum Gram staining: sensitivity 70% and specificity 23%, sputum culture: sensitivity 64% and specificity 70%, and BALF Gram staining: sensitivity 60% and specificity 71% [20].

Respiratory specimen cultures remain crucial for performing phenotypical susceptibility testing and for the identification of etiological agents not detected by molecular methods, such as rapid direct respiratory panels. However, some important limitations should be acknowledged, such as low sensitivity and long turnaround time, while reduced sensitivity in the case of prior antibiotics can also affect the diagnostic accuracy of this method [8]. Specifically, for pneumococcal pneumonia, the sensitivity of sputum cultures has been reported to vary widely, from 29% to 94% [15].

Regarding antigenic testing, Sordé and colleagues evaluated the urinary pneumococcal antigen test in hospitalized patients with CABP, 20.3% of whom were immunocompromised, reporting a sensitivity of 70.5% and a specificity of 96% [21]. A meta-analysis of UAT performance in streptococcal pneumonia yielded similar results, with pooled sensitivities of 66% [95% confidence interval [CI], 62–71] for inpatients and 67% [95% CI 56–76] for mixed populations and specificities of 89% [95% CI 82–93] and 90% [95% CI 79–96], respectively. However, specificity was generally lower in studies involving immunocompromised patients [22]. On the other hand, a possible advantage of this test is the minimal impact of prior antibiotic use on diagnostic performance compared to respiratory cultures, as showed by Said and colleagues in a metanalysis [23].

Immunocompromised patients are particularly vulnerable to *Legionella pneumophila*, especially when cell-mediated immunity is compromised [24]. Certain clinical signs, such as diarrhea, elevated transaminases, hyponatremia, and increased LDH levels, along with environmental exposure, should raise suspicion for *Legionella* pneumonia, though symptoms are often nonspecific but rapidly progressive [25,26]. The diagnostic approach should include a urinary antigen test (that showed a pooled sensitivity and specificity of 79% [95% CI 71–85] and 100% [95% CI 99–100], respectively, in a meta-analysis), with additional tests such as respiratory PCR, when possible, since the urinary antigen test detects only *Legionella pneumophila* serotype 1 [27,28].

Regarding serological tests, they have been classically used for the etiological diagnosis of *Mycoplasma pneumoniae* CABP, although lower sensitivity than more recent molecular methods has been suggested [29]. Overall, molecular approaches can increase pathogen detection rates, as showed by an observational study including 323 patients with

CABP in which the achieved pathogen detection rate was 87% with molecular methods compared to 39% [127/323 patients] with culture-based methods, helping in the antibiotic de-escalation approach after the results [30]. However, it is important to note that molecular testing includes a limited number of targets; thus, clinicians should always consider that some organisms (depending on the employed panel) cannot be detected, or the detected microorganism can also represent a respiratory tract colonization [30].

Diagnosis of opportunistic pathogens such as *Nocardia* spp. requires high suspicion and high pre-test probability, because the culture should be performed on dedicated media and have a longer turnaround time [31]. In this setting, molecular methods such as *Nocardia* spp.-specific PCR could be useful in establishing the diagnosis. A multicenter study evaluated a PCR-based assay for nocardiosis, reporting a sensitivity of 88% and a specificity of 74% [35/47 patients] in respiratory samples [32].

Finally, the risk of active tuberculosis is increased in patients with immune impairments including HIV, diabetes, cancer, hematological malignancies (HMs) or SOT, and those receiving systemic steroids or TNFα inhibitors, and a specific diagnostic workup should be considered in a high-risk patient with a compatible clinical pattern [33]. The microbiological diagnosis of pulmonary tuberculosis is based on detecting mycobacteria through acid-fast staining, cultures, and molecular assays from induced sputum samples (three samples for both smears and cultures should be collected) or from a single lower-respiratory tract specimen in the presence of lung lesions. Indeed, the performance of these tests depends also on the form of pulmonary tuberculosis, with miliary TB having no connection with the bronchial system and thus exhibiting very low sensitivity in sputum or even BALF samples, as opposed to the cavitary form, with possible high load of mycobacteria. A meta-analysis of 27 studies reported the performance of PCR in sputum samples (culture as a reference test), with an overall sensitivity of 89% (95% CI, 85–92) and specificity of 99% (95% CI, 98–92), with higher sensitivity in the case of smear-positive vs. smear-negative samples: 98% (95% CI, 97–99) vs. 67% (95% CI, 60–74) of samples [34]. A higher sensitivity of 80% (95% CI 52–96) was also reported [35]. Nontuberculous mycobacteria (NTM) are species of mycobacteria other than *Mycobacterium tuberculosis* and *Mycobacterium leprae* who share similar risk factors for disseminated disease as those for tuberculosis, including HIV infection, steroid use, TNF-α inhibitors, diabetes, cancer, and SOT. Since NTM are environmental organisms, their presence in nonsterile respiratory specimens does not necessarily indicate a pathogenic role in lung disease, unlike in the case of tuberculosis [36]. According to the American Thoracic Society (ATS) and the Infectious Disease Society of America (IDSA), the diagnostic criteria for NTM lung disease include pulmonary symptoms, compatible radiographic findings, and either two positive sputum cultures, one positive BALF sample, or a positive lung biopsy culture with suggestive histological features [36]. In cases of disseminated disease, blood cultures on special media should be performed and maintained in incubation for at least 6 weeks. Bone marrow, fluid, or tissue samples from suspected sites should be sent for culture and histological examination with specific stains [36].

2.2. Hospital-Acquired Bacterial Pneumonia and Ventilator-Associated Bacterial Pneumonia

Conventional tests for diagnosing HABP and VABP include a Gram stain, blood culture, and culture of respiratory specimens [37]. Blood cultures are strongly recommended in all HABP and VABP episodes, although only a few cases are bacteremic, with reported low sensitivity (5–15%) across several studies [38–40], thus showing a suboptimal performance as a standalone diagnostic test [41].

Regarding cultures of respiratory specimens, a sputum culture should be performed in HABP if an adequate sample, characterized by a Gram stain showing few or no squamous epithelial cells, can be obtained [41]. In immunocompromised patients, however, lower respiratory tract specimens (e.g., collection of BALF fluid) are generally recommended for diagnosing HABP and VABP. A prospective study assessing the diagnostic performance of BALF cultures in HABP patients found that BALF cultures successfully identified 18 of 23 cases (78%), with infections defined by colony counts of at least 10^4 CFU/mL [42].

Molecular methods, particularly multiplex polymerase chain reaction (mPCR) syndromic panels, are increasingly utilized for the etiological diagnosis of HABP and VABP. A prospective study by Peiffer-Smadja and colleagues evaluated the diagnostic performance of mPCR on BAL and plugged telescoping catheter (PLC) samples from ICU patients with HABP/VABP. The mPCR panel used (Unyvero panel) demonstrated a specificity of 99% [95% CI 99–100] and sensitivity of 80% [95% CI 73–88], with higher sensitivity for Gram-negative bacteria (90% compared to 62% for Gram-positive cocci) [43]. Similar studies using the same panel reported sensitivities ranging from 73% [95% CI 59–84] to 88.8% and specificities between 94.9% and 97.9% [95% CI 95–99], using conventional culture methods as the reference standard [44,45]. A diagnostic meta-analysis found that, for the etiological diagnosis of methicillin-resistant *Staphylococcus aureus* (MRSA) in patients with HABP and CABP, the pooled sensitivity and specificity of PCR were 85% [95% CI 60–96] and 92.1% [95% CI 82–97], respectively. For MRSA VABP, the specificity was 93.7% [95% CI 77–98], but sensitivity was significantly lower at 40.3% [95% CI 17–68] [46]. Moreover, a PCR/electrospray ionization-mass spectrometry (PCR/ESI-MS) assay applied on BALF samples can provide quantitative data that may aid in differentiating between infection and colonization; although, this distinction should be based on the overall clinical picture, not just PCR results [47].

3. Diagnostic Methods for Viral Pneumonia

While an upper respiratory tract viral infection typically causes a self-limiting illness in an immunocompetent individual, it can lead to significant morbidity and mortality in an immunocompromised host. The severity of illness in this population is often attributed to the frequent occurrence of secondary infections with bacteria, fungi, or other viruses, as well as the potential spread of the virus to the lower respiratory tract [47].

While in the past, diagnostic methods for respiratory viruses include direct fluorescent antibody (DFA) assays, enzyme immunoassays, and viral culture, PCR is currently the most frequently used and most useful method, due to excellent sensitivity and specificity. Rapid Antigen Detection Tests (RADTs) have the advantage of lower cost, and the possibility of point-of-care use with immediate results. While their sensitivity for SARs-CoV-2 was acceptable, it is usually low for other viruses such as influenza or RSV [48,49].

A large study involving 6090 participants reported the performance of DFA and Rapid Antigen Detection Tests (RADTs) for the diagnosis of novel H1N1 influenza A virus along with other influenza subtypes. A total of 518/3789 (13.7%) positive results for all influenza A strains (seasonal H1N1, H3N2, and novel H1N1) were obtained with the RADT; 397/3271 (12.1%) with DFA tests. The sensitivity of the RADT and DFA assay for novel H1N1 were 21.2% and 47.2%, while the specificities were 99.5% for the RADT and 99.6% for the DFA assay [48]. A systematic review and meta-analysis reported the performance of the RADT for RSV virus infection, including 71 articles. The study reported a pooled sensitivity and specificity of 80% (95% CI 76–83) and 97% (95% CI 96–98), respectively; however, the sensitivity was 81% (95% CI 78–84) in children and only 29% (95 CI 11–48) in the adult population [49].

Viral cultures, although more sensitive, require several days to yield results and dedicated facilities, making them impractical for clinical use [50].

Real-time PCR (RT-PCR) can be used to detect various viruses from samples such as nasopharyngeal swabs, sputum, endotracheal aspirates, or BALF. Multiplex assays, which usually include influenza virus types A and B, respiratory syncytial virus (RSV), parainfluenza viruses (PIV), human rhinoviruses (HRV), human metapneumovirus (HMPV), and adenovirus (AdV), are highly sensitive and provide rapid diagnosis [51]. A review summarizing the diagnostic accuracies of RT-PCR for detecting influenza A and B, RSV, HMPV, and AdV reported that among the 5510 patient samples analyzed, the area under the receiver operating characteristic curve (AUROC) was 0.98 or higher for all the viruses mentioned, except for AdV, which had an AUROC of 0.89 [11]. Also, an automated nested multiplex PCR system, such as the FilmArray system, was found to detect up to 95% of viral pathogens with an average turnaround time of just 75 min [52,53]. Molecular methods are also recommended for the diagnosis of SARS-CoV-2 infection, since rapid antigen tests have lower sensitivity, especially in asymptomatic individuals [54].

Of note, if cytomegalovirus (CMV) is suspected, dedicated PCR should be performed, and in such cases, quantitative results are usually provided. Given the high sensitivity and negative predictive value, a negative CMV-DNA result in BALF can plausibly exclude CMV pneumonia, but there is no established cut-off for CMV-DNA in BALF that reliably differentiates between CMV pneumonia and pulmonary virus shedding without organ disease [55,56]. In a small prospective study involving 45 immunocompromised patients with lower respiratory tract infections, the authors assessed the incidence of CMV pneumonia and quantified plasma CMV DNA loads using a highly sensitive CMV nucleic acid amplification test [57]. A plasma CMV DNA load threshold of 2.91 $\log_{10}$ IU/mL was proposed as a potential screening tool to complement conventional methods for diagnosing CMV pneumonia in immunocompromised patients. They found a significant correlation between high plasma CMV DNA loads and elevated CMV DNA loads in BALF [57]. Indeed, blood testing for CMV and data on patient's history and immune status might provide additional help in deciding if CMV pneumonia is likely.

In addition to CMV, also in case of AdV, testing of blood samples to detect viremia is also useful. In the case of AdV, viremia may occur and lead to dysfunction in a single organ system, such as interstitial pneumonia, or to disseminated infection affecting two or more organ systems, which significantly increases the mortality rate to between 8% and 26% [58]. Detection of AdV in the blood may precede symptomatic disease by 2 to 3 weeks, providing an opportunity for pre-emptive intervention in recipients of allogeneic HCT. PCR testing of blood specimens is recommended if AdV disease is suspected, as the presence of AdV DNA in the blood typically indicates disseminated infection [59]. Isolated respiratory infection can also occur, even in immunocompetent patients, and ADV pneumonia has been reported in healthy young adults. Identifying patients who could benefit from antiviral treatment remains a challenge in this setting, since the currently available anti-AdV antiviral (cidofovir) is associated with significant renal toxicity.

Finally, two aspects are important in case of viral pneumonia in immunocompromised patients. First, upper respiratory tract PCR results might already be negative in the case of viral infection that progressed to the lower respiratory tract. Therefore, in the case of clinical suspicion, PCR should be performed in BALF. Second, co-infections with different pathogens are very frequent in immunocompromised patients with pneumonia, and radiological patterns might be overlapping (e.g., tree-in-bud lesions). Therefore, comprehensive testing for the most frequent viral, bacterial, and fungal pathogens should be performed in BALF, and interpretation of the clinical impact of single pathogens might be challenging.

Last but not least, severe viral pneumonia, mainly due to influenza and SARS-CoV-2, was recognized as a significant risk factor for fungal pulmonary infection, mainly invasive aspergillosis.

4. Diagnostic Methods for Fungal Pneumonia

Among the fungi responsible for pneumonia in immunocompromised patients are molds (e.g., *Aspergillus* spp. and Mucorales), *Pneumocystis jirovecii*, and *Cryptococcus* spp. [31,60]. They are all airborne pathogens, and their spores can be inhaled from the air [31,61]. An invasive fungal disease (IFD) in immunocompromised patients can be classified as proven, probable, or possible according to the EORTC/MSGERC criteria [62]. Various microbiological diagnostic methods are available to help achieve a probable (and sometimes proven) diagnosis of fungal pneumonia in immunocompromised patients, including non-culture- and culture-based methods.

4.1. Microscopy, Culture, and Histology

Culture and microscopy are employed within the diagnostic algorithms for invasive pulmonary aspergillosis (IPA) and cryptococcal pneumonia, while *Pneumocystis jirovecii* cannot be cultured [63–65]. The reference standard for the proven diagnosis of *Pneumocystis jirovecii* pneumonia (PJP) involves microscopic examination of respiratory samples using dedicated staining methods [66,67].

For IPA, the identifications of *Aspergillus* spp. in a BALF culture defines a mycological criterion for the diagnosis of probable invasive aspergillosis, while a proven diagnosis can only be achieved through histology or positive culture from a sterile site, e.g., through lung biopsy [62,68]. Regarding proven diagnosis, due to bleeding risk or respiratory insufficiency, a lung biopsy is rarely performed in severely immunocompromised patients, such as those with hematological malignancies or HCT recipients. Therefore, diagnosis of IPA is more frequently documented as probable based on a culture of BALF or antigen tests, rather than proven. Regarding cultures, although their sensitivity is only around 50% for IPA, the isolation of *Aspergillus* spp., or any other filamentous fungus, from BALF culture provides important information on species identification and antifungal susceptibility [69–71]. For the diagnosis of PJP, *Pneumocystis jirovecii* cannot be cultured as reported above, so the proven diagnosis is defined through microscopy with specific staining methods, e.g., Grocott–Gomori methenamine silver stain (highest sensitivity reported), modified Papanicolaou, Wright–Giemsa, or Gram–Weigert stains [66]. It should also be considered that the fungal load may be different in different types of populations. For example, in the case of HIV-positive patients, the fungus load is usually high; whereas in HIV-negative patients, the fungus load is usually lower; thus, diagnostic accuracy could also be affected by these differences [72]. The induced sputum test with hypertonic saline is less invasive than BAL and has been successfully used in high-fungal-load infections but does not have a high sensitivity (reported between 55% and 90%) [73,74]. In fact, it has been reported that induced sputum samples had higher sensitivity in HIV-positive patients compared to HIV-negative patients [75–77]. A recent prospective study reported [9/18 patients] 50% sensitivity for microscopy by Grocott–Gomori methenamine silver staining for diagnosing PJP pneumonia in immunocompromised patients [78]. Overall, the major drawbacks of microscopic methods for diagnosing PJP are low sensitivity, dependence on the expertise of the mycologist, and the fact that they may be time-consuming for the laboratory.

Cryptococcal pneumonia is diagnosed through microscopy or cultures of blood and sputum or BALF, and *Cryptococcus* spp. typically grows within 2–3 days after specimen collection [31,79,80]. While susceptibility testing can be performed for *Cryptococcus* spp., its routine use is not recommended due to the limited evidence linking minimum inhibitory concentrations (MICs) with clinical outcomes [81].

Microscopy (both direct and as histopathology) and cultures of BALF or pulmonary biopsy samples are the cornerstones for the diagnosis of pulmonary mucormycosis [31,82,83]. Regarding culture methods, *Mucorales* spp. can grow within 1 to 7 days on fungal culture media, though cultures may only be positive in 50% of cases [83].

4.2. Antigen Testing

Antigen testing, such as serum and BALF galactomannan (GM) tests, is a cornerstone of the diagnosis of probable IPA and has been included for decades as a mycological criterion in the dedicated guidelines [84]. A single-center retrospective study reported 78.9% [95% CI 58–71] sensitivity of serum GM and 78.6% [95% CI 55–100] sensitivity of BALF GM for probable/proven IPA [85]; another retrospective study reported 93.2% [95% CI 86–97] sensitivity and 86.8% [95% CI 83–87] specificity for the BALF GM test for diagnosing proven/probable IPA [86]. The meta-analyses from Pfeiffer and colleagues and from Leeflang and colleagues reported 70–78% pooled sensitivity of serum GM for the diagnosis of invasive aspergillosis in hematological malignancy patients [87,88]. Another meta-analyses reported 89% [95% CI 83–93] sensitivity of BALF GM for IPA diagnosis in immunocompromised patients [89].

The sensitivity of GM is affected by the type of the tested population, with significantly higher sensitivity of serum GM in neutropenic patients. On the contrary, in SOT recipients the sensitivity of serum GM was reported to be as low as 22% [95% CI 3–60] [87], and limited data are available on the diagnostic performance of BALF in SOT. Another study reported a 100% sensitivity for BALF GM in diagnosing IPA in SOT recipients, whereas serum GM had a sensitivity of 25% [90]. However, it is important to note that the number of IPA patients in the study was very low (n = 5) [90].

Several causes of false positive GM results have been reported, with treatment with piperacillin/tazobactam being one of the most important [91]. Indeed, in a retrospective study that examined the relationship between three β-lactam antibiotics and the occurrence of false-positive GM test results in patients with HM, positive serum GM occurred in the case of treatment with 27 out of 39 batches of β-lactam antibiotics, and GM test results remained positive for up to 5 days after the termination of antibiotic treatment [92]. Nonetheless, although some residual GM might still be present in some piperacillin/tazobactam, the currently available formulations of piperacillin/tazobactam no longer appear to be responsible for false-positive GM results [93]. Interestingly, infections due to other fungi, such as *Fusarium* spp., *Penicillium* spp., or even *Histoplasma* spp., can also result in positive GM testing.

Another fungal biomarker, 1, 3 beta-d-glucan (BDG), is present in the cell wall of many pathogenic fungi (except for *Mucorales* spp. and cryptococci), and for this reason is not specific for invasive aspergillosis [31,94]. A systematic review on the comparison of PCR with serum BDG and GM from 2015, reported 76.9% [95% CI 66.7–84.8] and 89.4% [95% CI 87–91] sensitivity and specificity for serum BDG for IA diagnosis [95], with poor sensitivity of BDG in SOT recipients [96]. However, serum BDG was shown to be much more useful as a supporting diagnostic tool for PJP. A study reported that serum BDG in AIDS/HIV patients with pneumonia showed a sensitivity of 92.8% [95% CI 87–97] for PJP [97]. A meta-analysis conducted by Karageorgopoulos and colleagues reported 94.8% [95% CI 91–97] sensitivity for the diagnosis of PJP in immunocompromised patients [98]. Another meta-analysis reported no differences in the specificity of the test while sensitivity was higher for HIV-positive patients and lower for HIV-negative patients [99].

The antigen method is a rapid method for the diagnosis of cryptococcal pneumonia. Serum, sputum, and BALF may be tested for the cryptococcal antigen. Oshima and colleagues assessed the diagnostic performance of cryptococcal glucuronoxylomannan antigen tests in BALF and serum in HIV-negative patients. They reported a BALF sensitivity of 82.6%, while the serum showed 73.9% sensitivity for diagnosing cryptococcal pneumonia in 23 confirmed cases [100]. Similarly to microscopy, it was reported that the serum cryptococcal antigen assay was less sensitive in HIV-negative immunocompromised patients with cryptococcal pneumonia than in HIV-positive patients with cryptococcal pneumonia, possibly due to lower fungal burden. More in detail, a sensitivity of 56–83% was reported in HIV-negative immunocompromised patients with cryptococcal pneumonia [79,101]. Indeed, while several studies reported very good diagnostic performance of the cryptococcal antigen test in HIV-positive patients with cryptococcal meningitis, the diagnostic performance of the cryptococcal antigen test in serum and BALF of patients with pulmonary cryptococcosis remains less clear [102].

Neither BDG nor GM are present in *Mucorales*; thus, negative results from these tests, in combination with lung computed tomography (CT) findings consistent with invasive fungal infection, may suggest mucormycosis and the need for dedicated diagnostic procedures such as a culture of BALF or lung samples [103]. Currently, there is no specific antigen test available for the diagnosis of *Mucorales* pneumonia, although some are under investigation, and molecular methods have been introduced [104,105].

4.3. Molecular Methods

PCR is a molecular non-culture test increasingly available for the diagnosis of various types of pulmonary fungal infections in immunocompromised patients [64]. With the development of new commercial assays and advancements in PCR standardization, the last EORTC/MSGERC definitions recognized PCR as a mycological criterion for probable IPA [64]. A meta-analysis by Han and colleagues analyzed the diagnostic performance of BALF PCR in immunocompromised high-risk patients, reporting an overall pooled specificity and sensitivity of 94% [95% CI 90–96] and 75% [95% CI 67–81], respectively, while for proven IPA, the specificity and sensitivity were 80% [95% CI 68–98] and 91% [95% CI 74–85] across 14 studies involving 2061 patients [106]. Another meta-analysis evaluated the diagnostic performance of PCR from whole blood or serum. When a single positive serum PCR result was required to diagnose IPA, the sensitivity and specificity were 80.5% [95% CI 73–86] and 78.5% [95% CI 68–86], respectively. However, when two consecutive positive PCR results were required, the specificity increased to 96.2% [95% CI, 90–99], while the sensitivity decreased to 58% [95% CI, 37–77] [107]. BALF PCR had high sensitivity but a possible lack of ability to differentiate airway colonization from infection, which is one of the limitations of PCR [64].

In addition to qualitative conventional PCR, nested PCR and quantitative real-time PCR (qPCR) are also available for diagnosing PJP. The performance of respiratory PCR assays for diagnosing PJP in high-risk patients, including HIV-positive and HIV-negative patients, was reported in a bivariate meta-analysis, with a pooled specificity and sensitivity for the overall population of 90% [95% CI 87–93] and 99% [95% CI 96–100], respectively [108]. Another meta-analysis reported the diagnostic performance of BALF PCR for the diagnosis of PJP in both HIV-positive and HIV-negative patients, with a pooled specificity and sensitivity of 91% [95% CI 83–96] and 98.3% [95% CI 91–99.7], respectively [109]. Since conventional PCR cannot differentiate airway colonization from true fungal infection [110], real-time PCR is more often recommended since its quantitative nature may help distinguish between airway colonization and true fungal infection; although, a clear cut-off still needs to be defined and standardized and may vary in different populations of immunocompromised patients [111,112]. Interestingly, in a prospective study of 86 HIV-positive patients with subacute respiratory symptoms who were suspected of having PJP, a qPCR based on the mtSSU gene from induced sputum samples was apparently able to potentially differentiate three groups (one group with PJP, one without PJP, and the third with colonized patients) based on quantification cycle (Cq) values; although, further external validation and standardization are warranted [113].

Molecular diagnostic tools have also been investigated for the diagnosis of cryptococcal pneumonia. A study utilized multiplex real-time PCR to detect *Cryptococcus* DNA in samples from AIDS patients with opportunistic pneumonia, including BALF, blood, biopsy, and other samples [114]. Multiplex Real-Time PCR was tested in 24 clinical strains and 43 clinical samples from 40 patients infected with HIV/AIDS having proven fungal infections. The in vitro sensitivity was 100% for clinical strains and 90.5% in clinical samples with positive results for 92.5% of patients, yielding positive results in four out of five cryptococcosis samples [114]. Additionally, PCR can distinguish *Cryptococcus* species by targeting the STR1F and STR1R genes [115].

For mucormycosis, molecular methods are particularly interesting since there are no antigenic methods available, and some studies have analyzed the identification of mucormycosis through PCR in serum and blood; although, this topic deserves further investigation [116]. In a small study, four cases of suspected pulmonary mucormycosis in patients with HM were successfully diagnosed using PCR on peripheral blood samples [117]. Another study employed qPCR for the early detection of mucormycosis in immunocompromised patients, detecting free DNA in the serum of 9 out of 10 patients earlier than the confirmed diagnosis through histopathological examination and positive culture, with the detection occurring between 3 and 68 days earlier [118].

4.4. Point-of-Care-Tests [POCTs] for Invasive Aspergillosis (IA)

Two main POCTs are now available for the diagnosis of IA, such as the *Aspergillus* Galactomannan lateral flow assay (GM-LFA) and *Aspergillus*-specific lateral flow device (AspLFD), while others are in development, and a body of evidence is growing rapidly [119]. Seven studies were published between 2020 and 2024: five [120–124] assessed the diagnostic performance of LFA, and two studies [125,126] covered AspLFD for IA diagnosis. The five studies on the LFA test reported 384 proven/probable/possible or chronic/probable IFD cases. Four of them used *Aspergillus* Galactomannan LFA (IMMY Diagnostics, Oklahoma, USA), and one study used QuicGM™ *Aspergillus* Galactomannan LFA (Dynamiker Biotechnology [Tianjin] Co., Ltd., Tianjin, China). There were 68 proven/probable IA cases reported in two studies using the CE-marked AspLFD test.

4.4.1. Aspergillus Galactomannan Later Flow Assay (LFA)

LFAs detect GM antigen in immunochromatographic tests and can provide rapid qualitative results in both serum and BALF samples. For both reported assays, quantitative results can be obtained through an automatic optical reader for the IMMY *Aspergillus* GM LFA and a fluorescence immunoassay analyzer for the Dynamiker LFA [119]. The details of these test have been recently reviewed [127].

A large multicenter study from China reported on 310 clinically suspected IA patients with various underlying conditions and evaluated the LFA assay as a screening tool in serum and BALF samples, with results interpreted through an immunoanalyzer and compared with the ELISA GM test. The sensitivity of the LFA was higher in BALF than serum samples (89% [95% CI 78–96] vs. 83% [95% CI 74–89]). Both the LFA and ELISA had similar specificity in serum and BALF samples, while the sensitivity of ELISA was higher in BALF than the LFA (93% [95% CI 82–98] vs. 89% [95% CI 78–96]). The total percent agreement between the LFA and ELISA in serum and BAL samples was 92% and 94%, while positive and negative percent agreement (PPA and NPA) for serum samples was 95% and 89%, with the discordance arising mainly due to the samples that were positive by ELISA and negative by the LFA [120].

Another prospective multicenter study from Turkey compared the performance of quantitative GM-LFA (using a cube reader for exact quantitate results) with GM-EIA in HM patients with suspected IA. Proven IA was diagnosed through sinonasal tissue culture or lung tissue biopsy. The sensitivity of the LFA test in serum samples was slightly higher in differentiating proven IA versus no IA than proven/probable IA versus no IA (83% vs. 75%), while specificity was 100%. Both GM-LFA and GM-EIA had 91% positive results in (10/11) proven/probable cases at a cut-off of 0.5, while for BALF an overall qualitative agreement of 82% between the two tests was observed [121].

Serin and colleagues compared serum GM LFA quantitative results to GM ELISA. They included 87 patients with IA: proven n = 11/87, probable n = 54/87, and possible n = 22/87. The test performance was reported for two groups (no IA = 76, and IA = 11). The LFA test demonstrated an excellent sensitivity and specificity of 91% for diagnosing proven IA, while GM ELISA had 0% sensitivity and 92% specificity, respectively [123].

Another study evaluated the performance of the GM-LFA in a cohort of mainly (82%) patients that had HM. Serum GM-LFA had a sensitivity and specificity of 97% [95% CI 94–99.5) 31/32] and 98% [95% CI 93–99.5] (98/100), respectively, in 32 patients with proven/probable or chronic IFD. When considering all samples, the sensitivity and specificity was 91%, and an overall qualitative agreement of 89% was observed between the two tests [122].

In a single-center retrospective study from the USA, 31 samples from 28 cancer patients with suspected IA were tested. The sensitivity and specificity of serum LFA-GM was 100% [95% CI 51–100] and 96% [95% CI 92–97] for proven IA, while EIA-GM had a lower sensitivity of 25% [95% CI 1.3–70] and specificity of 98% [95% CI 96–99] [124].

Mercier and colleagues reported in 2020 that empirical antifungal therapy significantly reduced the sensitivity of the LFA assay in BALF samples in patients with HM [128], while a recent multicenter study published in 2023 reported no significant difference in patients receiving antifungal prophylaxis or treatment compared to patients without treatment or prophylaxis. The sensitivity was 75% for all 83 patients with proven/probable IA, and after excluding 42 patients receiving antifungals (15 treatment and 27 prophylaxis), the sensitivity for proven/probable IA was 76% [121]. Limited data are available on the diagnostic performance of the LFA test in SOT recipients as compared to those with HM [129].

A multicenter study evaluated the performance of a CE-marked LFA test in patients with various underlying conditions. The sensitivity of the LFA test for diagnosing IA in BALF samples was excellent at 100% (10/10), while the specificity was very low, at only 17% (4/24) at a cut-off value of 0.5 for the optical density index (ODI). After increasing the cut-off value to 1.5 ODI, the specificity increased to 68%, while the sensitivity decreased to 68%, respectively [130].

The performance of the test differed by patients' population and sample types (serum and BALF). A recent review published in 2024 [127] reported that sensitivity and specificity of LFA test in ICU patients having viral-associated pulmonary aspergillosis was 76% and 80% in BALF samples, while in the same population the sensitivity of serum samples dropped to 55%, and similar results were found in other studies in these setting, and diagnostic performance of the serum LFA-GM test was higher in neutropenic patients [127].

Finally, the meta-analysis from Zhang and colleagues also reported lower pooled sensitivity for the LFA test in serum samples as compared to BALF samples (71% [95% CI 56–87] vs. 83% [95% CI 72–94]) [131].

4.4.2. Aspergillus-Specific Lateral Flow Device (AspLFD)

AspLFD is a qualitative immunochromatography test for the detection of the *Aspergillus* antigen in BALF and serum. The test uses a monoclonal antibody called JF5 to identify a glycoprotein (mannoproteins) that is generated by the *Aspergillus* species during active growth [127]. There are two recent studies on the diagnostic efficacy of CE-marked AspLFD for IA diagnosis, which included 279 patients with a wide variety of underlying conditions, including HM and other immunocompromised conditions.

One study compared the performance of the LFD to GM ELISA in 218 cancer patients (184 serum samples and 58 BALF). The overall performance of the test was excellent for diagnosing proven/probable IA vs. no IA (sensitivity 92% [95% CI 62–99.8] and specificity 95% [95% CI 91–98]). The sensitivity of the test was lower in serum samples as compared to BALF samples ([67% (95% CI 9–99] vs. 100% [95% CI 66–100]), while the specificity in serum samples was excellent at 99%. Both the LFD and GM had similar diagnostic performance in serum samples, while the LFD sensitivity was higher in BALF. Additionally, the study found that the sensitivity was higher in solid tumor patients as compared to patients with HM (100% [95% CI 69–100] vs. 50% [95% CI 1.3–99]) [125].

Another study from Hsiao and colleagues compared the performance of the LFD test with EIA GM in 91 immunocompromised patients, including 56 with HM and 35 on corticosteroids. The GM test had higher sensitivity than the LFD (90% (26/29) vs. 69% (20/29)), and a specificity of 99% [74/75] vs. 79% [59/75]; although, this finding was likely increased due to the use of the GM test for case classification. In addition, the study also found a significant difference in the discordance between LFD and GM in those who had been previously treated with AF (33%), as compared to those without such exposure (12%), using EORTC/MSGERC as the gold standard [126].

Finally, the diagnostic performance of the test can also vary based on population type and sample types. A review article from Heldt and Hoenigl evaluated the test performance in various settings, including SOT recipients, ICU patients, and other respiratory diseases patients. The review findings suggest that sensitivity is lowest in HM patients compared to the overall population (67% [36/54] vs. 73% [83/113]) [132].

The meta-analysis from Pan and colleagues from 2015 on LFD development studies reported lower pooled sensitivity for the LFD in serum samples as compared to BALF samples for diagnosing proven/probable IA in immunocompromised patients (68% [95% CI, 52–81] vs. 86% [95% CI 76–93]) [133].

A review article on POCTs reported on the diagnostic performance in BALF and serum samples for the AspLFD prototype and the CE-marked version. The sensitivity of the LFD prototype in BALF samples was high as compared to serum samples (71% [86/121] vs. 68% [30/44]), while the sensitivity of the test was lowest for patients with HM and highest for SOT recipients (69% [22/32] vs. 81% [17/21]). Interestingly, for CE-marked AspLFD, the sensitivity of the test was lower as compared to the prototype. The overall sensitivity of the CE-marked test in BALF samples and serum samples were 64% [98/152] vs. 20% [10/51] [119].

5. Parasitic Pneumonia

Due to better hygiene practices and improved socioeconomic conditions, parasitic infestations have declined in the past decade. Nonetheless, the increase in urbanization, the number of immunocompromised patients, and in international travel and global warming has led to a possible rise in the world population that is susceptible to parasitic diseases [134].

Toxoplasma gondii and *Strongyloides stercoralis* are the main parasites responsible for pulmonary infections and are associated with high mortality if left untreated in immunocompromised patients [31]. In spite of the high prevalence of parasitic diseases in tropical and developing nations, only a few cases of parasitic pneumonia have been reported in HIV-positive patients [134,135]. In the pre highly active antiviral therapy era, pulmonary toxoplasmosis accounted for only 4% of all pneumonia cases in AIDS patients, while currently it is extremely rare [136]. Also, *Strongyloides stercoralis*, which is common in tropical and subtropical areas, has been reported only occasionally as the cause of pneumonia in AIDS patients [135].

Diagnosing a parasitic infection of the airways can be challenging due to the wide range of clinical presentations, which are frequently nonspecific, and its rarity [134]. Standard microbiological methods, non-invasive antigen testing, and molecular testing can be used.

Disseminated toxoplasmosis has no specific sign or symptoms; fever is frequently present, and various organs, including lungs and central nervous system could be affected. Very few cases of isolated pulmonary involvement mimicking interstitial pneumonia, cytomegalovirus pneumonia, or PJP pneumonia were reported [31]. Diagnosis of toxoplasmosis is mainly based on the detection of protozoan parasites in the body tissue or PCR in blood and/or BALF [137]. Non-invasive methods such as serological testing are unreliable for the diagnosis of toxoplasmosis in immunocompromised transplant patients, as they document only the previous exposure and the risk of reactivation [138].

Currently, cases of *Toxoplasma* spp. pneumonia mainly involved transplant recipients; although, it is very rare. Indeed, a study involving 46 centers from 11 countries in the years 2010–2014 reported 87 toxoplasmosis cases: 58 in allogenic HCT and 29 in SOT recipients, while the average of transplant procedures per country was 1016 for allogenic HCT, 1524 for autologous HCT, and 155 for SOT recipients. Overall, 42 of 87 patients had severe manifestations including pulmonary, cerebral, and disseminated toxoplasmosis; 14 patients had mild manifestations (ocular toxoplasmosis and fever), while 31 had no clinical symptoms. Molecular, serological, culture, and imaging diagnostic method were used, and PCR was the most sensitive (89% [77/89]). In pulmonary toxoplasmosis, PCR was positive in 89% (17/19) of patients, whereas the sensitivity of the serological method (47% [9/19]) and microscopy (32% [6/19]) was lower [139]. Another prospective study included BALF samples from immunocompromised patients over a period of 2 years and compared the diagnostic performance of conventional staining and PCR for pulmonary toxoplasmosis. A total of 336 samples were collected, and two cases of pulmonary toxoplasmosis were diagnosed: one patient had lymphocytic lymphoma, and the other was admitted to the ICU due to IA that developed 7 days after the second liver transplantation [140]. Both cases were positive by PCR and conventional staining, and no other positive results were observed, demonstrating that in the hands of experienced parasitologists, properly performed conventional staining can have similar performance to PCR [140].

There are limited or no data available on the diagnostic performance of the microbiological and parasitological tests for the diagnosis of *Strongyloides stercoralis* pneumonia as the pulmonary infections are uncommon. *Strongyloides stercoralis* is an intestinal parasite, and a definitive diagnosis of pneumonia involves identifying the parasite in respiratory specimens [134,141]. A single-center retrospective study conducted over a period of 10 years (2004–2014) included 16 cases of severe *Strongyloides stercoralis* infection, and 15 of them had pulmonary manifestations. Although no formal assessment of diagnostic methods was performed, all cases were diagnosed by microscopic examinations of larvae through the Agar plate culture method and histopathology [142]. BALF and sputum can be used for the diagnosis of *Strongyloides stercoralis* hyperinfection syndrome when filariform larvae may be found in these fluids [31,143].

6. Metagenomics and CRISPR/Cas13a as a Possible Future Approach for the Diagnosis of Severe Pneumonia in Immunocompromised Patients

Metagenomics (mNGS) and metatranscriptomic techniques have emerged as promising diagnostic tools for pneumonia in immunocompromised patients. Nucleic acid (DNA or RNA) from respiratory samples is extracted first and then sequenced with or without PCR amplification, classified, and interpreted. Since mNGS is taxonomically agnostic, no matter what their phylogeny is, pathogens can be identified (bacteria, viral, fungal, and protozoal). A mNGS approach could also help identify resistance genes rapidly [3]. The host–pathogen interaction can also be studied through mNGS, but it may require further research for a correct evaluation and understanding of potential clinical application [144].

A retrospective study assessed the diagnostic performance of BALF mNGS compared with culture-based methods in 69 immunocompromised patients with suspected pneumonia [144]. Overall, mNGS showed higher sensitivity than culture-based methods for all evaluated pathogens (bacterial, viral, and fungal pathogens). Briefly, the sensitivity of mNGS was 93% [95% CI 70–100] for viruses, followed by 91% [95% CI 79–98] for fungi, and 80% (95% CI 63–92) for bacteria. In comparison, the sensitivity of conventional microbiological tests was 53% for viruses, followed by 50% for fungi, and 36% for bacteria, with significantly higher diagnostic accuracy for PJP [145].

A meta-analysis assessed mNGS diagnostic performance in immunocompromised patients with PJP, reporting 96% (95% CI 90–99) and 96% [95% CI 92–98] pooled sensitivity and specificity. Interestingly, the subgroup analysis revealed equally very good performance in BAL and blood samples: sensitivity and specificity in BALF of 94% (95% CI, 78–99) and 96% [95% CI 88–99] and in blood of 93% [95% CI 80–98] and 98% [95% CI 76–100]), respectively [146]. Another meta-analysis reported that the pathogen detection rate was higher for mNGS (80.4% [1233/1532]) than for culture-based methods (45.7% [705/1540]) in patients with severe pneumonia, with a potential favorable effect on mortality rates and length of ICU stay [147].

A turnaround time within 6 h (sample received to pathogens' identification time) has been reported for the diagnosis of bacterial respiratory tract infections by means of mNGS [148]. A similar turnaround time was also registered for the identification of mycobacterial species, including *Mycobacterium tuberculosis* [149,150]. Furthermore, a retrospective study reported that mNGS was less affected by prior antimicrobial use than the traditional culturing method [151]. Nonetheless, there are some important limitations of mNGS, like clinical enactment, which could be difficult due to of bioinformatics analysis requirements and other issues, such as the difficult differentiation between true infections and colonization, that still deserve further investigation [3,144].

CRISPR/Cas is a self-defense system in prokaryotes, such as bacteria and archaea, and is widely used as a genome editing tool, but more recently, it was applied also as a molecular diagnostic method in different clinical settings [152]. A retrospective study published in 2022 evaluated the diagnostic performance of a CRISPR/Cas13a-based method (Rapid-CasD) in BALF samples taken from patients suspected of having PJP (19 PJP and 43 non-PJP patients), and 52 patients were immunocompromised. The method achieved 79% [15/19] sensitivity and 98% [42/43] specificity for diagnosing PJP pneumonia, while all the PJP samples were positive by qPCR, with a sensitivity of 100% [19/19] and specificity of 65.1%

[28/43]. The RapidCasD methods showed excellent agreement with the clinical diagnosis of PJP as compared to qPCR and suggested the possibility of using this test to differentiate infection from colonization [153]. The CRISPR/Cas13a technique in BALF samples has been also studied for rapid diagnosis of invasive *A. fumigatus* aspergillosis [154]. Finally, another study used a PCR-CRISPR assay to evaluate the performance of CRISPR/Cas13 for the detection of carbapenem-resistant Klebsiella pneumoniae (CRKP). Sixty-one clinical isolates were collected (51 were CRKP and the remaining ten were carbapenem-sensitive, including *P. aeruginosa*, *E. coli*, and *A. baumannii*). The sensitivity and specificity of the PCR-CRISPR Cas13a assay with a fluorescence readout were 92% [47/51] and 100% [0/10] [155].

7. Conclusions

In conclusion, microbiological diagnosis of pneumonia in immunocompromised patients remains a challenging and evolving process due to the variety of potential pathogens (Table 1) and the limitations of traditional culture-based diagnostic methods. The combination of molecular methods and antigen testing allows for the early and accurate detection of pneumonia in this vulnerable population. The development of more rapid, sensitive, and cost-effective methods, as well as their validation in a variety of clinical settings, will require further research in this specific population.

Table 1. Common etiological agents of pneumonia in immunocompromised patients.

Etiological Agent	Commonly Reported Populations at Risk/Risk Factors	Tests Commonly Used for Diagnosis in Clinical Practice	References
Legionella	SOT, HIV, corticosteroid use, HCT	UAT, Culture (BALF, EA, sputum), PCR (BALF, EA, sputum)	[156,157]
Haemophilus spp.	Humoral immunosuppression	Culture (BALF, EA, sputum), PCR (BALF, EA, sputum)	[157,158]
Klebsiella pneumoniae	All types of immunosuppression	Culture (sputum, blood), PCR (blood, BALF, EA)	[158,159]
Streptococcus pneumoniae	Humoral immunosuppression, cancer, SOT, LLC, MM	UAT, culture (BALF, sputum, blood), PCR (sputum, BALF)	[160,161]
Staphylococcus aureus	SOT, chemotherapy, chronic lung disease	Culture (blood, sputum, EA, BALF), PCR (BALF, EA, sputum)	[157,159,162]
Pseudomonas aeruginosa	COPD, HM, HCT, cancer, cystic fibrosis, chronic kidney disease, HIV, SOT	Culture (sputum, EA, BALF), PCR (BALF, EA, sputum, blood)	[159,163]
Escherichia coli	HIV, cancer, SOT, COPD, diabetes mellitus	Culture (BALF, EA, sputum), PCR (BALF, EA, sputum, blood)	[157,164]
Nocardia spp.	HIV, SOT, cancer, chronic corticosteroid use, HCT	Culture (sputum, EA, blood, tissue biopsy, BALF), PCR (BALF, sputum)	[157,165,166]
Mycobacterium tuberculosis	All types of immunosuppression, particularly anti-TNF-alfa treatment, SOT	Microscopy (sputum smear), culture (BALF, sputum), PCR (sputum, BALF, lungs biopsy)	[167,168]
Cytomegalovirus	HCT, SOT, HIV, alemtuzumab, CLL	PCR (blood, BALF), histopathology	[31,169,170]
Varicella-Zoster virus	HIV, cancer, SOT, chronic corticosteroid use	PCR (BALF, sputum, blood), serology, DFA	[31,171,172]
Herpes simplex virus	SOT, neutropenia, chronic corticosteroid use, ICU patients	PCR (blood, BALF), serology	[31,173]
Influenza, Respiratory syncytial virus (RSV), Coronaviridae (SARS-CoV-2)	HCT, SOT, HM	PCR (BALF, nasopharyngeal, sputum), serology	[31,174,175]
Aspergillus spp.	HCT, SOT, neutropenia and corticosteroid therapy	Direct visualization, culture, GM (BALF, serum), PCR (BALF, sputum, blood)	[64,85,176]
Pneumocystis jirovecii	SOT, HM, HCT	Direct visualization, BDG (serum), PCR (BALF, sputum, blood)	[97,177,178]

Table 1. *Cont.*

Etiological Agent	Commonly Reported Populations at Risk/Risk Factors	Tests Commonly Used for Diagnosis in Clinical Practice	References
Cryptococcus spp.	HCT, SOT	Microscopy, culture (blood, sputum), antigen (serum, BALF, sputum), PCR (BALF, blood)	[31,64,79,179]
Mucorales spp.	HM, HCT	Microscopy, culture, histopathology, immunohistochemistry	[31,82,180]
Toxoplasma spp.	SOT, HCT, HIV	Microscopy, serological assay, PCR	[137,172,181]
Strongyloides stercoralis	SOT, HTLV-1, HIV, HM	Serological methods, and PCR	[182–184]

BALF: bronchoalveolar lavage fluid; BDG: 1, 3 beta d glucan; COPD: chronic obstructive pulmonary disease; DFA: direct fluoresce antibody; EA: endotracheal aspirate; HCT: hematopoietic cell transplant; HM: hematological malignancies; HTLV-1: human T-cell lymphotropic virus type 1; HIV: human immunodeficiency virus; LLC, chronic lymphocytic leukemia; MM, multiple myeloma; NAATs: nucleic acid amplification test; PCR: polymerase chain reaction; SOT: solid organ transplant; TA: tracheal aspirate; UAT: urine antigen test.

Author Contributions: N.U.: L.F., L.A., C.B., D.R.G., A.V., M.M. and M.B. made substantial contributions to this study's concept and design; N.U., L.F., and L.A. made substantial contributions to the first drafting of this manuscript; all authors made substantial contributions to the critical revision of this manuscript for important intellectual content. All authors have read and agreed to the published version of the manuscript.

Funding: This research received no external funding.

Data Availability Statement: No new data were generated.

Acknowledgments: A large language model (LLM)-based chatbot (ChatGPT-4o) was used to enhance the readability and conciseness of this manuscript. The initial draft (written by the authors without the support of an LLM) was submitted to ChatGPT-4o on 31 August 2024, with the following initial prompt, applied separately for the different parts of this manuscript, with the abstract included: "Could you improve in terms of readability the text of the following scientific article, without adding information, removing information, or changing the meaning of the sentences?" The text produced by ChatGPT-4o was then thoroughly reviewed by all authors to ensure the preservation of content and meaning.

Conflicts of Interest: Outside the submitted work, Matteo Bassetti has received funding for scientific advisory boards, travel, and speaker honoraria from Cidara, Gilead, Menarini, MSD, Mundipharma, Pfizer, and Shionogi. Outside the submitted work, Daniele Roberto Giacobbe reports investigator-initiated grants from Pfizer, Shionogi, BioMérieux, and Gilead Italia and speaker/advisor fees from Pfizer, Menarini, and Tillotts Pharma. The other authors have no conflicts of interest to disclose.

References

1. Mackenzie, G. The Definition and Classification of Pneumonia. *Pneumonia (Nathan)* **2016**, *8*, 14. [CrossRef]
2. Azoulay, E.; Mokart, D.; Kouatchet, A.; Demoule, A.; Lemiale, V. Acute Respiratory Failure in Immunocompromised Adults. *Lancet Respir. Med.* **2019**, *7*, 173–186. [CrossRef] [PubMed]
3. Cheng, G.-S.; Crothers, K.; Aliberti, S.; Bergeron, A.; Boeckh, M.; Chien, J.W.; Cilloniz, C.; Cohen, K.; Dean, N.; Dela Cruz, C.S.; et al. Immunocompromised Host Pneumonia: Definitions and Diagnostic Criteria: An Official American Thoracic Society Workshop Report. *Ann. ATS* **2023**, *20*, 341–353. [CrossRef] [PubMed]
4. Rosenow, E.C.; Wilson, W.R.; Cockerill, F.R. Pulmonary Disease in the Immunocompromised Host (First of Two Parts). *Mayo Clin. Proc.* **1985**, *60*, 473–487. [CrossRef] [PubMed]
5. Di Pasquale, M.F.; Sotgiu, G.; Gramegna, A.; Radovanovic, D.; Terraneo, S.; Reyes, L.F.; Rupp, J.; González Del Castillo, J.; Blasi, F.; Aliberti, S.; et al. Prevalence and Etiology of Community-Acquired Pneumonia in Immunocompromised Patients. *Clin. Infect. Dis.* **2019**, *68*, 1482–1493. [CrossRef] [PubMed]
6. Murali, S.; Marks, A.; Heeger, A.; Dako, F.; Febbo, J. Pneumonia in the Immunocompromised Host. *Semin. Roentgenol.* **2022**, *57*, 90–104. [CrossRef] [PubMed]

7. Maschmeyer, G.; Carratalà, J.; Buchheidt, D.; Hamprecht, A.; Heussel, C.P.; Kahl, C.; Lorenz, J.; Neumann, S.; Rieger, C.; Ruhnke, M.; et al. Diagnosis and Antimicrobial Therapy of Lung Infiltrates in Febrile Neutropenic Patients (Allogeneic SCT Excluded): Updated Guidelines of the Infectious Diseases Working Party (AGIHO) of the German Society of Hematology and Medical Oncology (DGHO). *Ann. Oncol.* **2015**, *26*, 21–33. [CrossRef] [PubMed]
8. Ogawa, M.; Hoshina, T.; Abushawish, A.; Kusuhara, K. Evaluation of the Usefulness of Culture of Induced Sputum and the Optimal Timing for the Collection of a Good-Quality Sputum Sample to Identify Causative Pathogen of Community-Acquired Pneumonia in Young Children: A Prospective Observational Study. *J. Microbiol. Immunol. Infect.* **2023**, *56*, 1036–1044. [CrossRef] [PubMed]
9. Harris, A.M.; Bramley, A.M.; Jain, S.; Arnold, S.R.; Ampofo, K.; Self, W.H.; Williams, D.J.; Anderson, E.J.; Grijalva, C.G.; McCullers, J.A.; et al. Influence of Antibiotics on the Detection of Bacteria by Culture-Based and Culture-Independent Diagnostic Tests in Patients Hospitalized with Community-Acquired Pneumonia. *Open Forum Infect. Dis.* **2017**, *4*, ofx014. [CrossRef] [PubMed]
10. Walter, J.M.; Wunderink, R.G. Testing for Respiratory Viruses in Adults With Severe Lower Respiratory Infection. *Chest* **2018**, *154*, 1213–1222. [CrossRef] [PubMed]
11. Huang, H.-S.; Tsai, C.-L.; Chang, J.; Hsu, T.-C.; Lin, S.; Lee, C.-C. Multiplex PCR System for the Rapid Diagnosis of Respiratory Virus Infection: Systematic Review and Meta-Analysis. *Clin. Microbiol. Infect.* **2018**, *24*, 1055–1063. [CrossRef]
12. Lease, E.D.; Alexander, B.D. Fungal Diagnostics in Pneumonia. *Semin. Respir. Crit. Care Med.* **2011**, *32*, 663–672. [CrossRef] [PubMed]
13. Anevlavis, S.; Bouros, D. Community Acquired Bacterial Pneumonia. *Expert. Opin. Pharmacother.* **2010**, *11*, 361–374. [CrossRef] [PubMed]
14. Martin-Loeches, I.; Torres, A.; Nagavci, B.; Aliberti, S.; Antonelli, M.; Bassetti, M.; Bos, L.D.; Chalmers, J.D.; Derde, L.; De Waele, J.; et al. ERS/ESICM/ESCMID/ALAT Guidelines for the Management of Severe Community-Acquired Pneumonia. *Intensive Care Med.* **2023**, *49*, 615–632. [CrossRef]
15. Song, J.Y.; Eun, B.W.; Nahm, M.H. Diagnosis of Pneumococcal Pneumonia: Current Pitfalls and the Way Forward. *Infect. Chemother.* **2013**, *45*, 351–366. [CrossRef]
16. Reller, L.B.; Weinstein, M.P.; Werno, A.M.; Murdoch, D.R. Laboratory Diagnosis of Invasive Pneumococcal Disease. *Clin. Infect. Dis.* **2008**, *46*, 926–932. [CrossRef]
17. Craven, D.E. Blood Cultures for Community-Acquired Pneumonia: Piecing Together a Mosaic for Doing Less. *Am. J. Respir. Crit. Care Med.* **2004**, *169*, 327–328. [CrossRef] [PubMed]
18. Fabre, V.; Carroll, K.C.; Cosgrove, S.E. Blood Culture Utilization in the Hospital Setting: A Call for Diagnostic Stewardship. *J. Clin. Microbiol.* **2022**, *60*, e0100521. [CrossRef] [PubMed]
19. Fukuyama, H.; Yamashiro, S.; Kinjo, K.; Tamaki, H.; Kishaba, T. Validation of Sputum Gram Stain for Treatment of Community-Acquired Pneumonia and Healthcare-Associated Pneumonia: A Prospective Observational Study. *BMC Infect. Dis.* **2014**, *14*, 534. [CrossRef] [PubMed]
20. Zhang, R.; Wu, Y.; Deng, G.; Deng, J. Value of Sputum Gram Stain, Sputum Culture, and Bronchoalveolar Lavage Fluid Gram Stain in Predicting Single Bacterial Pathogen among Children with Community-Acquired Pneumonia. *BMC Pulm. Med.* **2022**, *22*, 427. [CrossRef] [PubMed]
21. Sordé, R.; Falcó, V.; Lowak, M.; Domingo, E.; Ferrer, A.; Burgos, J.; Puig, M.; Cabral, E.; Len, O.; Pahissa, A. Current and Potential Usefulness of Pneumococcal Urinary Antigen Detection in Hospitalized Patients with Community-Acquired Pneumonia to Guide Antimicrobial Therapy. *Arch. Intern. Med.* **2011**, *171*. [CrossRef] [PubMed]
22. Yasuo, S.; Murata, M.; Nakagawa, N.; Kawasaki, T.; Yoshida, T.; Ando, K.; Okamori, S.; Okada, Y. Japanese ARDS clinical practice guideline systematic review task force Diagnostic Accuracy of Urinary Antigen Tests for Pneumococcal Pneumonia among Patients with Acute Respiratory Failure Suspected Pneumonia: A Systematic Review and Meta-Analysis. *BMJ Open* **2022**, *12*, e057216. [CrossRef]
23. Said, M.A.; Johnson, H.L.; Nonyane, B.A.S.; Deloria-Knoll, M.; O'Brien, K.L.; AGEDD Adult Pneumococcal Burden Study Team; Andreo, F.; Beovic, B.; Blanco, S.; Boersma, W.G.; et al. Estimating the Burden of Pneumococcal Pneumonia among Adults: A Systematic Review and Meta-Analysis of Diagnostic Techniques. *PLoS ONE* **2013**, *8*, e60273. [CrossRef] [PubMed]
24. Kao, A.S.; Myer, S.; Wickrama, M.; Ismail, R.; Hettiarachchi, M. Multidisciplinary Management of Legionella Disease in Immunocompromised Patients. *Cureus* **2021**, *13*, e19214. [CrossRef]
25. Sharma, L.; Losier, A.; Tolbert, T.; Dela Cruz, C.S.; Marion, C.R. Atypical Pneumonia: Updates on Legionella, Chlamydophila, and Mycoplasma Pneumonia. *Clin. Chest Med.* **2017**, *38*, 45–58. [CrossRef] [PubMed]
26. Sopena, N.; Sabrià-Leal, M.; Pedro-Botet, M.L.; Padilla, E.; Dominguez, J.; Morera, J.; Tudela, P. Comparative Study of the Clinical Presentation of Legionella Pneumonia and Other Community-Acquired Pneumonias. *Chest* **1998**, *113*, 1195–1200. [CrossRef]

27. Kawasaki, T.; Nakagawa, N.; Murata, M.; Yasuo, S.; Yoshida, T.; Ando, K.; Okamori, S.; Okada, Y. Diagnostic Accuracy of Urinary Antigen Tests for Legionellosis: A Systematic Review and Meta-Analysis. *Respir. Investig.* **2022**, *60*, 205–214. [CrossRef]
28. Viasus, D.; Gaia, V.; Manzur-Barbur, C.; Carratalà, J. Legionnaires' Disease: Update on Diagnosis and Treatment. *Infect. Dis. Ther.* **2022**, *11*, 973–986. [CrossRef]
29. Wang, L.; Feng, Z.; Zhao, M.; Yang, S.; Yan, X.; Guo, W.; Shi, Z.; Li, G. A Comparison Study between GeXP-Based Multiplex-PCR and Serology Assay for Mycoplasma Pneumoniae Detection in Children with Community Acquired Pneumonia. *BMC Infect. Dis.* **2017**, *17*, 518. [CrossRef]
30. Gadsby, N.J.; Russell, C.D.; McHugh, M.P.; Mark, H.; Conway Morris, A.; Laurenson, I.F.; Hill, A.T.; Templeton, K.E. Comprehensive Molecular Testing for Respiratory Pathogens in Community-Acquired Pneumonia. *Clin. Infect. Dis.* **2016**, *62*, 817–823. [CrossRef]
31. Azoulay, E.; Russell, L.; Van de Louw, A.; Metaxa, V.; Bauer, P.; Povoa, P.; Montero, J.G.; Loeches, I.M.; Mehta, S.; Puxty, K.; et al. Diagnosis of Severe Respiratory Infections in Immunocompromised Patients. *Intensive Care Med.* **2020**, *46*, 298–314. [CrossRef]
32. Rouzaud, C.; Rodriguez-Nava, V.; Catherinot, E.; Méchaï, F.; Bergeron, E.; Farfour, E.; Scemla, A.; Poirée, S.; Delavaud, C.; Mathieu, D.; et al. Clinical Assessment of a Nocardia PCR-Based Assay for Diagnosis of Nocardiosis. *J. Clin. Microbiol.* **2018**, *56*, e00002-18. [CrossRef] [PubMed]
33. Marques, I.D.B.; Azevedo, L.S.; Pierrotti, L.C.; Caires, R.A.; Sato, V.A.H.; Carmo, L.P.F.; Ferreira, G.F.; Gamba, C.; de Paula, F.J.; Nahas, W.C.; et al. Clinical Features and Outcomes of Tuberculosis in Kidney Transplant Recipients in Brazil: A Report of the Last Decade. *Clin. Transpl.* **2013**, *27*, E169–E176. [CrossRef]
34. Steingart, K.R.; Schiller, I.; Horne, D.J.; Pai, M.; Boehme, C.C.; Dendukuri, N. Xpert® MTB/RIF Assay for Pulmonary Tuberculosis and Rifampicin Resistance in Adults. *Cochrane Database Syst. Rev.* **2014**, *2014*, CD009593. [CrossRef] [PubMed]
35. Lodha, L.; Mudliar, S.R.; Singh, J.; Maurya, A.; Khurana, A.K.; Khadanga, S.; Singh, S. Diagnostic Performance of Multiplex PCR for Detection of Mycobacterium Tuberculosis Complex in Presumptive Pulmonary Tuberculosis Patients and Its Utility in Smear Negative Specimens. *J. Lab. Physicians* **2022**, *14*, 403–411. [CrossRef] [PubMed]
36. Griffith, D.E.; Aksamit, T.; Brown-Elliott, B.A.; Catanzaro, A.; Daley, C.; Gordin, F.; Holland, S.M.; Horsburgh, R.; Huitt, G.; Iademarco, M.F.; et al. An Official ATS/IDSA Statement: Diagnosis, Treatment, and Prevention of Nontuberculous Mycobacterial Diseases. *Am. J. Respir. Crit. Care Med.* **2007**, *175*, 367–416. [CrossRef]
37. Torres, A.; Niederman, M.S.; Chastre, J.; Ewig, S.; Fernandez-Vandellos, P.; Hanberger, H.; Kollef, M.; Li Bassi, G.; Luna, C.M.; Martin-Loeches, I.; et al. International ERS/ESICM/ESCMID/ALAT Guidelines for the Management of Hospital-Acquired Pneumonia and Ventilator-Associated Pneumonia: Guidelines for the Management of Hospital-Acquired Pneumonia (HAP)/Ventilator-Associated Pneumonia (VAP) of the European Respiratory Society (ERS), European Society of Intensive Care Medicine (ESICM), European Society of Clinical Microbiology and Infectious Diseases (ESCMID) and Asociación Latinoamericana Del Tórax (ALAT). *Eur. Respir. J.* **2017**, *50*, 1700582. [CrossRef] [PubMed]
38. Koulenti, D.; Tsigou, E.; Rello, J. Nosocomial Pneumonia in 27 ICUs in Europe: Perspectives from the EU-VAP/CAP Study. *Eur. J. Clin. Microbiol. Infect. Dis.* **2017**, *36*, 1999–2006. [CrossRef]
39. Murdoch, D.R.; O'Brien, K.L.; Scott, J.A.G.; Karron, R.A.; Bhat, N.; Driscoll, A.J.; Knoll, M.D.; Levine, O.S. Breathing New Life into Pneumonia Diagnostics. *J. Clin. Microbiol.* **2009**, *47*, 3405–3408. [CrossRef] [PubMed]
40. Ranzani, O.T.; Senussi, T.; Idone, F.; Ceccato, A.; Li Bassi, G.; Ferrer, M.; Torres, A. Invasive and Non-Invasive Diagnostic Approaches for Microbiological Diagnosis of Hospital-Acquired Pneumonia. *Crit. Care* **2019**, *23*, 51. [CrossRef]
41. Kalil, A.C.; Metersky, M.L.; Klompas, M.; Muscedere, J.; Sweeney, D.A.; Palmer, L.B.; Napolitano, L.M.; O'Grady, N.P.; Bartlett, J.G.; Carratalà, J.; et al. Management of Adults With Hospital-Acquired and Ventilator-Associated Pneumonia: 2016 Clinical Practice Guidelines by the Infectious Diseases Society of America and the American Thoracic Society. *Clin. Infect. Dis.* **2016**, *63*, e61–e111. [CrossRef] [PubMed]
42. Dalhoff, K.; Braun, J.; Lipp, R.; Wießmann, K.-J.; Hollandt, H.; Marre, R. Diagnostic Value of Bronchoalveolar Lavage in Patients with Opportunistic and Nonopportunistic Bacterial Pneumonia. *Infection* **1993**, *21*, 291–296. [CrossRef]
43. Peiffer-Smadja, N.; Bouadma, L.; Mathy, V.; Allouche, K.; Patrier, J.; Reboul, M.; Montravers, P.; Timsit, J.-F.; Armand-Lefevre, L. Performance and Impact of a Multiplex PCR in ICU Patients with Ventilator-Associated Pneumonia or Ventilated Hospital-Acquired Pneumonia. *Crit. Care* **2020**, *24*, 366. [CrossRef] [PubMed]
44. Papan, C.; Meyer-Buehn, M.; Laniado, G.; Nicolai, T.; Griese, M.; Huebner, J. Assessment of the Multiplex PCR-Based Assay Unyvero Pneumonia Application for Detection of Bacterial Pathogens and Antibiotic Resistance Genes in Children and Neonates. *Infection* **2018**, *46*, 189–196. [CrossRef] [PubMed]
45. Ozongwu, C.; Personne, Y.; Platt, G.; Jeanes, C.; Aydin, S.; Kozato, N.; Gant, V.; O'Grady, J.; Enne, V.I. The Unyvero P55 'Sample-in, Answer-out' Pneumonia Assay: A Performance Evaluation. *Biomol. Detect. Quantif.* **2017**, *13*, 1–6. [CrossRef] [PubMed]

46. Parente, D.M.; Cunha, C.B.; Mylonakis, E.; Timbrook, T.T. The Clinical Utility of Methicillin-Resistant *Staphylococcus aureus* (MRSA) Nasal Screening to Rule Out MRSA Pneumonia: A Diagnostic Meta-Analysis with Antimicrobial Stewardship Implications. *Clin. Infect. Dis.* **2018**, *67*, 1–7. [CrossRef]
47. Strålin, K.; Ehn, F.; Giske, C.G.; Ullberg, M.; Hedlund, J.; Petersson, J.; Spindler, C.; Özenci, V. The IRIDICA PCR/Electrospray Ionization-Mass Spectrometry Assay on Bronchoalveolar Lavage for Bacterial Etiology in Mechanically Ventilated Patients with Suspected Pneumonia. *PLoS ONE* **2016**, *11*, e0159694. [CrossRef] [PubMed]
48. Ginocchio, C.C.; Zhang, F.; Manji, R.; Arora, S.; Bornfreund, M.; Falk, L.; Lotlikar, M.; Kowerska, M.; Becker, G.; Korologos, D.; et al. Evaluation of Multiple Test Methods for the Detection of the Novel 2009 Influenza A (H1N1) during the New York City Outbreak. *J. Clin. Virol.* **2009**, *45*, 191–195. [CrossRef]
49. Chartrand, C.; Tremblay, N.; Renaud, C.; Papenburg, J. Diagnostic Accuracy of Rapid Antigen Detection Tests for Respiratory Syncytial Virus Infection: Systematic Review and Meta-Analysis. *J. Clin. Microbiol.* **2015**, *53*, 3738–3749. [CrossRef] [PubMed]
50. Hodinka, R.L. Point: Is the Era of Viral Culture over in the Clinical Microbiology Laboratory? *J. Clin. Microbiol.* **2013**, *51*, 2–4. [CrossRef]
51. Murali, S.; Langston, A.A.; Nolte, F.S.; Banks, G.; Martin, R.; Caliendo, A.M. Detection of Respiratory Viruses with a Multiplex Polymerase Chain Reaction Assay (MultiCode-PLx Respiratory Virus Panel) in Patients with Hematologic Malignancies. *Leuk. Lymphoma* **2009**, *50*, 619–624. [CrossRef]
52. Poritz, M.A.; Blaschke, A.J.; Byington, C.L.; Allen, L.; Nilsson, K.; Jones, D.E.; Thatcher, S.A.; Robbins, T.; Lingenfelter, B.; Amiott, E.; et al. FilmArray, an Automated Nested Multiplex PCR System for Multi-Pathogen Detection: Development and Application to Respiratory Tract Infection. *PLoS ONE* **2011**, *6*, e26047. [CrossRef]
53. Hammond, S.P.; Gagne, L.S.; Stock, S.R.; Marty, F.M.; Gelman, R.S.; Marasco, W.A.; Poritz, M.A.; Baden, L.R. Respiratory Virus Detection in Immunocompromised Patients with FilmArray Respiratory Panel Compared to Conventional Methods. *J. Clin. Microbiol.* **2012**, *50*, 3216–3221. [CrossRef]
54. Cesaro, S.; Ljungman, P.; Mikulska, M.; Hirsch, H.H.; Von Lilienfeld-Toal, M.; Cordonnier, C.; Meylan, S.; Mehra, V.; Styczynski, J.; Marchesi, F.; et al. Recommendations for the Management of COVID-19 in Patients with Haematological Malignancies or Haematopoietic Cell Transplantation, from the 2021 European Conference on Infections in Leukaemia (ECIL 9). *Leukemia* **2022**, *36*, 1467–1480. [CrossRef]
55. Fonseca Brito, L.; Brune, W.; Stahl, F.R. Cytomegalovirus (CMV) Pneumonitis: Cell Tropism, Inflammation, and Immunity. *Int. J. Mol. Sci.* **2019**, *20*, 3865. [CrossRef] [PubMed]
56. Ljungman, P.; Chemaly, R.F.; Khawaya, F.; Alain, S.; Avery, R.; Badshah, C.; Boeckh, M.; Fournier, M.; Hodowanec, A.; Komatsu, T.; et al. Consensus Definitions of Cytomegalovirus (CMV) Infection and Disease in Transplant Patients Including Resistant and Refractory CMV for Use in Clinical Trials: 2024 Update From the Transplant Associated Virus Infections Forum. *Clin. Infect. Dis.* **2024**, *79*, 787–794. [CrossRef] [PubMed]
57. Saksirisampant, G.; Kawamatawong, T.; Promsombat, K.; Sukkasem, W.; Liamsombut, S.; Pasomsub, E.; Bruminhent, J. A Prospective Study of Plasma and Bronchoalveolar Lavage Fluid CMV DNA Load Quantification for the Diagnosis and Outcome of CMV Pneumonitis in Immunocompromised Hosts. *J. Clin. Virol.* **2022**, *155*, 105243. [CrossRef]
58. Lindemans, C.A.; Leen, A.M.; Boelens, J.J. How I Treat Adenovirus in Hematopoietic Stem Cell Transplant Recipients. *Blood* **2010**, *116*, 5476–5485. [CrossRef]
59. Echavarria, M.; Forman, M.; van Tol, M.J.; Vossen, J.M.; Charache, P.; Kroes, A.C. Prediction of Severe Disseminated Adenovirus Infection by Serum PCR. *Lancet* **2001**, *358*, 384–385. [CrossRef]
60. Fishman, J.A.; Rubin, R.H. Infection in Organ-Transplant Recipients. *N. Engl. J. Med.* **1998**, *338*, 1741–1751. [CrossRef]
61. Patterson, T.F.; Thompson, G.R.; Denning, D.W.; Fishman, J.A.; Hadley, S.; Herbrecht, R.; Kontoyiannis, D.P.; Marr, K.A.; Morrison, V.A.; Nguyen, M.H.; et al. Practice Guidelines for the Diagnosis and Management of Aspergillosis: 2016 Update by the Infectious Diseases Society of America. *Clin. Infect. Dis.* **2016**, *63*, e1–e60. [CrossRef]
62. Donnelly, J.P.; Chen, S.C.; Kauffman, C.A.; Steinbach, W.J.; Baddley, J.W.; Verweij, P.E.; Clancy, C.J.; Wingard, J.R.; Lockhart, S.R.; Groll, A.H.; et al. Revision and Update of the Consensus Definitions of Invasive Fungal Disease From the European Organization for Research and Treatment of Cancer and the Mycoses Study Group Education and Research Consortium. *Clin. Infect. Dis.* **2020**, *71*, 1367–1376. [CrossRef] [PubMed]
63. Yamamura, D.; Xu, J. Update on Pulmonary Cryptococcosis. *Mycopathologia* **2021**, *186*, 717–728. [CrossRef]
64. Hage, C.A.; Carmona, E.M.; Epelbaum, O.; Evans, S.E.; Gabe, L.M.; Haydour, Q.; Knox, K.S.; Kolls, J.K.; Murad, M.H.; Wengenack, N.L.; et al. Microbiological Laboratory Testing in the Diagnosis of Fungal Infections in Pulmonary and Critical Care Practice. An Official American Thoracic Society Clinical Practice Guideline. *Am. J. Respir. Crit. Care Med.* **2019**, *200*, 535–550. [CrossRef]
65. Huang, L.; Cattamanchi, A.; Davis, J.L.; Boon, S.D.; Kovacs, J.; Meshnick, S.; Miller, R.F.; Walzer, P.D.; Worodria, W.; Masur, H.; et al. HIV-Associated Pneumocystis Pneumonia. *Proc. Am. Thorac. Soc.* **2011**, *8*, 294–300. [CrossRef] [PubMed]

66. Thomas, C.F.; Limper, A.H. Pneumocystis Pneumonia. *N. Engl. J. Med.* **2004**, *350*, 2487–2498. [CrossRef]
67. Sokulska, M.; Kicia, M.; Wesołowska, M.; Hendrich, A.B. Pneumocystis Jirovecii—From a Commensal to Pathogen: Clinical and Diagnostic Review. *Parasitol. Res.* **2015**, *114*, 3577–3585. [CrossRef]
68. Bassetti, M.; Giacobbe, D.R.; Agvald-Ohman, C.; Akova, M.; Alastruey-Izquierdo, A.; Arikan-Akdagli, S.; Azoulay, E.; Blot, S.; Cornely, O.A.; Cuenca-Estrella, M.; et al. Invasive Fungal Diseases in Adult Patients in Intensive Care Unit (FUNDICU): 2024 Consensus Definitions from ESGCIP, EFISG, ESICM, ECMM, MSGERC, ISAC, and ISHAM. *Intensive Care Med.* **2024**. [CrossRef] [PubMed]
69. Meersseman, W.; Van Wijngaerden, E. Invasive Aspergillosis in the ICU: An Emerging Disease. *Intensive Care Med.* **2007**, *33*, 1679–1681. [CrossRef]
70. Schroeder, M.; Simon, M.; Katchanov, J.; Wijaya, C.; Rohde, H.; Christner, M.; Laqmani, A.; Wichmann, D.; Fuhrmann, V.; Kluge, S. Does Galactomannan Testing Increase Diagnostic Accuracy for IPA in the ICU? A Prospective Observational Study. *Crit. Care* **2016**, *20*, 139. [CrossRef] [PubMed]
71. Horvath, J.A.; Dummer, S. The Use of Respiratory-Tract Cultures in the Diagnosis of Invasive Pulmonary Aspergillosis. *Am. J. Med.* **1996**, *100*, 171–178. [CrossRef]
72. Nasr, M.; Mohammad, A.; Hor, M.; Baradeiya, A.M.; Qasim, H. Exploring the Differences in Pneumocystis Pneumonia Infection Between HIV and Non-HIV Patients. *Cureus* **2022**, *14*, e27727. [CrossRef] [PubMed]
73. Salzer, H.J.F.; Schäfer, G.; Hoenigl, M.; Günther, G.; Hoffmann, C.; Kalsdorf, B.; Alanio, A.; Lange, C. Clinical, Diagnostic, and Treatment Disparities between HIV-Infected and Non-HIV-Infected Immunocompromised Patients with *Pneumocystis jirovecii* Pneumonia. *Respiration* **2018**, *96*, 52–65. [CrossRef] [PubMed]
74. Limper, A.H.; Offord, K.P.; Smith, T.F.; Martin, W.J. Pneumocystis Carinii Pneumonia. Differences in Lung Parasite Number and Inflammation in Patients with and without AIDS. *Am. Rev. Respir. Dis.* **1989**, *140*, 1204–1209. [CrossRef] [PubMed]
75. Kaur, R.; Wadhwa, A.; Bhalla, P.; Dhakad, M.S. Pneumocystis Pneumonia in HIV Patients: A Diagnostic Challenge till Date. *Med. Mycol.* **2015**, *53*, 587–592. [CrossRef]
76. Turner, D.; Schwarz, Y.; Yust, I. Induced Sputum for Diagnosing Pneumocystis Carinii Pneumonia in HIV Patients: New Data, New Issues. *Eur. Respir. J.* **2003**, *21*, 204–208. [CrossRef]
77. LaRocque, R.C.; Katz, J.T.; Perruzzi, P.; Baden, L.R. The Utility of Sputum Induction for Diagnosis of Pneumocystis Pneumonia in Immunocompromised Patients without Human Immunodeficiency Virus. *Clin. Infect. Dis.* **2003**, *37*, 1380–1383. [CrossRef] [PubMed]
78. Franconi, I.; Leonildi, A.; Erra, G.; Fais, R.; Falcone, M.; Ghelardi, E.; Lupetti, A. Comparison of Different Microbiological Procedures for the Diagnosis of Pneumocystis Jirovecii Pneumonia on Bronchoalveolar-Lavage Fluid. *BMC Microbiol.* **2022**, *22*, 143. [CrossRef]
79. Pappas, P.G.; Perfect, J.R.; Cloud, G.A.; Larsen, R.A.; Pankey, G.A.; Lancaster, D.J.; Henderson, H.; Kauffman, C.A.; Haas, D.W.; Saccente, M.; et al. Cryptococcosis in Human Immunodeficiency Virus-Negative Patients in the Era of Effective Azole Therapy. *Clin. Infect. Dis.* **2001**, *33*, 690–699. [CrossRef] [PubMed]
80. Howard-Jones, A.R.; Sparks, R.; Pham, D.; Halliday, C.; Beardsley, J.; Chen, S.C.-A. Pulmonary Cryptococcosis. *J. Fungi.* **2022**, *8*, 1156. [CrossRef]
81. Chang, C.C.; Hall, V.; Cooper, C.; Grigoriadis, G.; Beardsley, J.; Sorrell, T.C.; Heath, C.H.; the Australasian Antifungal Guidelines Steering Committee. Consensus Guidelines for the Diagnosis and Management of Cryptococcosis and Rare Yeast Infections in the Haematology/Oncology Setting, 2021. *Intern. Med. J.* **2021**, *51* (Suppl. S7), 118–142. [CrossRef] [PubMed]
82. Choi, S.; Song, J.S.; Kim, J.Y.; Cha, H.H.; Yun, J.H.; Park, J.W.; Jung, K.H.; Jo, K.M.; Jung, J.; Kim, M.J.; et al. Diagnostic Performance of Immunohistochemistry for the Aspergillosis and Mucormycosis. *Mycoses* **2019**, *62*, 1006–1014. [CrossRef]
83. Skiada, A.; Lass-Floerl, C.; Klimko, N.; Ibrahim, A.; Roilides, E.; Petrikkos, G. Challenges in the Diagnosis and Treatment of Mucormycosis. *Med. Mycol.* **2018**, *56*, 93–101. [CrossRef]
84. Lamoth, F.; Calandra, T. Early Diagnosis of Invasive Mould Infections and Disease. *J. Antimicrob. Chemother.* **2017**, *72*, i19–i28. [CrossRef] [PubMed]
85. Chun, J.Y.; Jeong, S.-J.; Kim, S.; Choi, S.; Lee, J.H.; Chung, H.S.; Park, S.; Lee, H.; Kim, H.Y.; Hwangbo, B.; et al. Performance of the Galactomannan Test for the Diagnosis of Invasive Pulmonary Aspergillosis Using Non-Invasive Proximal Airway Samples. *J. Infect.* **2024**, *88*, 106159. [CrossRef] [PubMed]
86. D'Haese, J.; Theunissen, K.; Vermeulen, E.; Schoemans, H.; De Vlieger, G.; Lammertijn, L.; Meersseman, P.; Meersseman, W.; Lagrou, K.; Maertens, J. Detection of Galactomannan in Bronchoalveolar Lavage Fluid Samples of Patients at Risk for Invasive Pulmonary Aspergillosis: Analytical and Clinical Validity. *J. Clin. Microbiol.* **2012**, *50*, 1258–1263. [CrossRef] [PubMed]
87. Pfeiffer, C.D.; Fine, J.P.; Safdar, N. Diagnosis of Invasive Aspergillosis Using a Galactomannan Assay: A Meta-Analysis. *Clin. Infect. Dis.* **2006**, *42*, 1417–1427. [CrossRef]

88. Leeflang, M.M.G.; Debets-Ossenkopp, Y.J.; Wang, J.; Visser, C.E.; Scholten, R.J.P.M.; Hooft, L.; Bijlmer, H.A.; Reitsma, J.B.; Zhang, M.; Bossuyt, P.M.M.; et al. Galactomannan Detection for Invasive Aspergillosis in Immunocompromised Patients. *Cochrane Database Syst. Rev.* **2015**, *2015*, CD007394. [CrossRef] [PubMed]
89. Li, C.; Sun, L.; Liu, Y.; Zhou, H.; Chen, J.; She, M.; Wang, Y. Diagnostic Value of Bronchoalveolar Lavage Fluid Galactomannan Assay for Invasive Pulmonary Aspergillosis in Adults: A Meta-Analysis. *J. Clin. Pharm. Ther.* **2022**, *47*, 1913–1922. [CrossRef] [PubMed]
90. Clancy, C.J.; Jaber, R.A.; Leather, H.L.; Wingard, J.R.; Staley, B.; Wheat, L.J.; Cline, C.L.; Rand, K.H.; Schain, D.; Baz, M.; et al. Bronchoalveolar Lavage Galactomannan in Diagnosis of Invasive Pulmonary Aspergillosis among Solid-Organ Transplant Recipients. *J. Clin. Microbiol.* **2007**, *45*, 1759–1765. [CrossRef]
91. Adam, O.; Auperin, A.; Wilquin, F.; Bourhis, J.; Gachot, B.; Chachaty, E. Treatment with Piperacillin-Tazobactam and False-Positive *Aspergillus* Galactomannan Antigen Test Results for Patients with Hematological Malignancies. *Clin. Infect. Dis.* **2004**, *38*, 917–920. [CrossRef] [PubMed]
92. Aubry, A.; Porcher, R.; Bottero, J.; Touratier, S.; Leblanc, T.; Brethon, B.; Rousselot, P.; Raffoux, E.; Menotti, J.; Derouin, F.; et al. Occurrence and Kinetics of False-Positive Aspergillus Galactomannan Test Results Following Treatment with Beta-Lactam Antibiotics in Patients with Hematological Disorders. *J. Clin. Microbiol.* **2006**, *44*, 389–394. [CrossRef]
93. Mikulska, M.; Furfaro, E.; Del Bono, V.; Raiola, A.M.; Ratto, S.; Bacigalupo, A.; Viscoli, C. Piperacillin/Tazobactam (Tazocin™) Seems to Be No Longer Responsible for False-Positive Results of the Galactomannan Assay. *J. Antimicrob. Chemother.* **2012**, *67*, 1746–1748. [CrossRef]
94. Fang, W.; Wu, J.; Cheng, M.; Zhu, X.; Du, M.; Chen, C.; Liao, W.; Zhi, K.; Pan, W. Diagnosis of Invasive Fungal Infections: Challenges and Recent Developments. *J. Biomed. Sci.* **2023**, *30*, 42. [CrossRef]
95. White, P.L.; Wingard, J.R.; Bretagne, S.; Löffler, J.; Patterson, T.F.; Slavin, M.A.; Barnes, R.A.; Pappas, P.G.; Donnelly, J.P. Aspergillus Polymerase Chain Reaction: Systematic Review of Evidence for Clinical Use in Comparison with Antigen Testing. *Clin. Infect. Dis.* **2015**, *61*, 1293–1303. [CrossRef] [PubMed]
96. Lamoth, F.; Akan, H.; Andes, D.; Cruciani, M.; Marchetti, O.; Ostrosky-Zeichner, L.; Racil, Z.; Clancy, C.J. Assessment of the Role of 1,3-β-d-Glucan Testing for the Diagnosis of Invasive Fungal Infections in Adults. *Clin. Infect. Dis.* **2021**, *72*, S102–S108. [CrossRef] [PubMed]
97. Wood, B.R.; Komarow, L.; Zolopa, A.R.; Finkelman, M.A.; Powderly, W.G.; Sax, P.E. Test Performance of Blood Beta-Glucan for Pneumocystis Jirovecii Pneumonia in Patients with AIDS and Respiratory Symptoms. *AIDS* **2013**, *27*, 967–972. [CrossRef] [PubMed]
98. Karageorgopoulos, D.E.; Qu, J.-M.; Korbila, I.P.; Zhu, Y.-G.; Vasileiou, V.A.; Falagas, M.E. Accuracy of β-D-Glucan for the Diagnosis of Pneumocystis Jirovecii Pneumonia: A Meta-Analysis. *Clin. Microbiol. Infect.* **2013**, *19*, 39–49. [CrossRef] [PubMed]
99. Del Corpo, O.; Butler-Laporte, G.; Sheppard, D.C.; Cheng, M.P.; McDonald, E.G.; Lee, T.C. Diagnostic Accuracy of Serum (1-3)-β-D-Glucan for Pneumocystis Jirovecii Pneumonia: A Systematic Review and Meta-Analysis. *Clin. Microbiol. Infect.* **2020**, *26*, 1137–1143. [CrossRef] [PubMed]
100. Oshima, K.; Takazono, T.; Saijo, T.; Tashiro, M.; Kurihara, S.; Yamamoto, K.; Imamura, Y.; Miyazaki, T.; Tsukamoto, M.; Yanagihara, K.; et al. Examination of Cryptococcal Glucuronoxylomannan Antigen in Bronchoalveolar Lavage Fluid for Diagnosing Pulmonary Cryptococcosis in HIV-Negative Patients. *Med. Mycol.* **2018**, *56*, 88–94. [CrossRef]
101. Singh, N.; Alexander, B.D.; Lortholary, O.; Dromer, F.; Gupta, K.L.; John, G.T.; del Busto, R.; Klintmalm, G.B.; Somani, J.; Lyon, G.M.; et al. Pulmonary Cryptococcosis in Solid Organ Transplant Recipients: Clinical Relevance of Serum Cryptococcal Antigen. *Clin. Infect. Dis.* **2008**, *46*, e12–e18. [CrossRef] [PubMed]
102. Liang, B.; Lin, Z.; Li, J.; Jiang, R.; Zhan, W.; Jian, X. Diagnostic Accuracy of Cryptococcal Antigen Test in Pulmonary Cryptococcosis: A Protocol for a Systematic Review and Meta-Analysis. *BMJ Open* **2023**, *13*, e070994. [CrossRef] [PubMed]
103. Cornely, O.A.; Arikan-Akdagli, S.; Dannaoui, E.; Groll, A.H.; Lagrou, K.; Chakrabarti, A.; Lanternier, F.; Pagano, L.; Skiada, A.; Akova, M.; et al. ESCMID† and ECMM‡ Joint Clinical Guidelines for the Diagnosis and Management of Mucormycosis 2013. *Clin. Microbiol. Infect.* **2014**, *20*, 5–26. [CrossRef]
104. Cornely, O.A.; Alastruey-Izquierdo, A.; Arenz, D.; Chen, S.C.A.; Dannaoui, E.; Hochhegger, B.; Hoenigl, M.; Jensen, H.E.; Lagrou, K.; Lewis, R.E.; et al. Global Guideline for the Diagnosis and Management of Mucormycosis: An Initiative of the European Confederation of Medical Mycology in Cooperation with the Mycoses Study Group Education and Research Consortium. *Lancet Infect. Dis.* **2019**, *19*, e405–e421. [CrossRef]
105. Burnham-Marusich, A.R.; Hubbard, B.; Kvam, A.J.; Gates-Hollingsworth, M.; Green, H.R.; Soukup, E.; Limper, A.H.; Kozel, T.R. Conservation of Mannan Synthesis in Fungi of the Zygomycota and Ascomycota Reveals a Broad Diagnostic Target. *mSphere* **2018**, *3*, e00094-18. [CrossRef] [PubMed]

106. Han, Y.; Wu, X.; Jiang, G.; Guo, A.; Jin, Z.; Ying, Y.; Lai, J.; Li, W.; Yan, F. Bronchoalveolar Lavage Fluid Polymerase Chain Reaction for Invasive Pulmonary Aspergillosis among High-Risk Patients: A Diagnostic Meta-Analysis. *BMC Pulm. Med.* **2023**, *23*, 58. [CrossRef]
107. Mengoli, C.; Cruciani, M.; Barnes, R.A.; Loeffler, J.; Donnelly, J.P. Use of PCR for Diagnosis of Invasive Aspergillosis: Systematic Review and Meta-Analysis. *Lancet Infect. Dis.* **2009**, *9*, 89–96. [CrossRef]
108. Lu, Y.; Ling, G.; Qiang, C.; Ming, Q.; Wu, C.; Wang, K.; Ying, Z. PCR Diagnosis of Pneumocystis Pneumonia: A Bivariate Meta-Analysis. *J. Clin. Microbiol.* **2011**, *49*, 4361–4363. [CrossRef]
109. Fan, L.-C.; Lu, H.-W.; Cheng, K.-B.; Li, H.-P.; Xu, J.-F. Evaluation of PCR in Bronchoalveolar Lavage Fluid for Diagnosis of Pneumocystis Jirovecii Pneumonia: A Bivariate Meta-Analysis and Systematic Review. *PLoS ONE* **2013**, *8*, e73099. [CrossRef] [PubMed]
110. Flori, P.; Bellete, B.; Durand, F.; Raberin, H.; Cazorla, C.; Hafid, J.; Lucht, F.; Sung, R.T.M. Comparison between Real-Time PCR, Conventional PCR and Different Staining Techniques for Diagnosing Pneumocystis Jiroveci Pneumonia from Bronchoalveolar Lavage Specimens. *J. Med. Microbiol.* **2004**, *53*, 603–607. [CrossRef] [PubMed]
111. Issa, N.; Gabriel, F.; Baulier, G.; Mourissoux, G.; Accoceberry, I.; Guisset, O.; Camou, F. Pneumocystosis and Quantitative PCR. *Med. Mal. Infect.* **2018**, *48*, 474–480. [CrossRef]
112. Maillet, M.; Maubon, D.; Brion, J.P.; François, P.; Molina, L.; Stahl, J.P.; Epaulard, O.; Bosseray, A.; Pavese, P. Pneumocystis Jirovecii (Pj) Quantitative PCR to Differentiate Pj Pneumonia from Pj Colonization in Immunocompromised Patients. *Eur. J. Clin. Microbiol. Infect. Dis.* **2014**, *33*, 331–336. [CrossRef]
113. Chagas, O.J.; Nagatomo, P.P.; Pereira-Chioccola, V.L.; Gava, R.; Buccheri, R.; Del Negro, G.M.B.; Benard, G. Performance of a Real Time PCR for Pneumocystis Jirovecii Identification in Induced Sputum of AIDS Patients: Differentiation between Pneumonia and Colonization. *J. Fungi* **2022**, *8*, 222. [CrossRef] [PubMed]
114. Gago, S.; Esteban, C.; Valero, C.; Zaragoza, O.; Puig de la Bellacasa, J.; Buitrago, M.J. A Multiplex Real-Time PCR Assay for Identification of Pneumocystis Jirovecii, Histoplasma Capsulatum, and Cryptococcus Neoformans/Cryptococcus Gattii in Samples from AIDS Patients with Opportunistic Pneumonia. *J. Clin. Microbiol.* **2014**, *52*, 1168–1176. [CrossRef]
115. Feng, X.; Fu, X.; Ling, B.; Wang, L.; Liao, W.; Yao, Z. Development of a Singleplex PCR Assay for Rapid Identification and Differentiation of Cryptococcus Neoformans Var. Grubii Cryptococcus Neoformans Var. Neoformans, Cryptococcus Gattii, and Hybrids. *J. Clin. Microbiol.* **2013**, *51*, 1920–1923. [CrossRef]
116. Kelly, B.T.; Pennington, K.M.; Limper, A.H. Advances in the Diagnosis of Fungal Pneumonias. *Expert. Rev. Respir. Med.* **2020**, *14*, 703–714. [CrossRef] [PubMed]
117. Ino, K.; Nakase, K.; Nakamura, A.; Nakamori, Y.; Sugawara, Y.; Miyazaki, K.; Monma, F.; Fujieda, A.; Sugimoto, Y.; Ohishi, K.; et al. Management of Pulmonary Mucormycosis Based on a Polymerase Chain Reaction (PCR) Diagnosis in Patients with Hematologic Malignancies: A Report of Four Cases. *Intern. Med.* **2017**, *56*, 707–711. [CrossRef] [PubMed]
118. Millon, L.; Larosa, F.; Lepiller, Q.; Legrand, F.; Rocchi, S.; Daguindau, E.; Scherer, E.; Bellanger, A.-P.; Leroy, J.; Grenouillet, F. Quantitative Polymerase Chain Reaction Detection of Circulating DNA in Serum for Early Diagnosis of Mucormycosis in Immunocompromised Patients. *Clin. Infect. Dis.* **2013**, *56*, e95–e101. [CrossRef] [PubMed]
119. Jenks, J.D.; Hoenigl, M. Point-of-Care Diagnostics for Invasive Aspergillosis: Nearing the Finish Line. *Expert. Rev. Mol. Diagn.* **2020**, *20*, 1009–1017. [CrossRef] [PubMed]
120. Guo, J.; Xiao, C.; Tian, W.; Lv, L.; Hu, L.; Ni, L.; Wang, D.; Li, W.; Qiao, D.; Wu, W. Performance of the Aspergillus Galactomannan Lateral Flow Assay with a Digital Reader for the Diagnosis of Invasive Aspergillosis: A Multicenter Study. *Eur. J. Clin. Microbiol. Infect. Dis.* **2024**, *43*, 249–257. [CrossRef] [PubMed]
121. Alhan, O.; Saba, R.; Akalin, E.H.; Ener, B.; Ture Yuce, Z.; Deveci, B.; Guncu, M.M.; Kahveci, H.N.; Yilmaz, A.F.; Odabasi, Z. Diagnostic Efficacy of Aspergillus Galactomannan Lateral Flow Assay in Patients with Hematological Malignancies: A Prospective Multicenter Study. *Mycopathologia* **2023**, *188*, 643–653. [CrossRef]
122. White, P.L.; Price, J.S.; Posso, R.; Cutlan-Vaughan, M.; Vale, L.; Backx, M. Evaluation of the Performance of the IMMY Sona Aspergillus Galactomannan Lateral Flow Assay When Testing Serum To Aid in Diagnosis of Invasive Aspergillosis. *J. Clin. Microbiol.* **2020**, *58*, e00053-20. [CrossRef] [PubMed]
123. Serin, I.; Dogu, M.H. Serum Aspergillus Galactomannan Lateral Flow Assay for the Diagnosis of Invasive Aspergillosis: A Single-Centre Study. *Mycoses* **2021**, *64*, 678–683. [CrossRef] [PubMed]
124. Jani, K.; McMillen, T.; Morjaria, S.; Babady, N.E. Performance of the Sōna Aspergillus Galactomannan Lateral Flow Assay in a Cancer Patient Population. *J. Clin. Microbiol.* **2021**, *59*, e0059821. [CrossRef] [PubMed]
125. Wan, L.; Cai, X.; Ling, M.; Kan, J.; Yin, M.; Wang, H. Evaluation of the JF5-Based Aspergillus Galactomannoprotein Lateral Flow Device for Diagnosing Invasive Aspergillosis in Cancer Patients. *Eur. J. Clin. Microbiol. Infect. Dis.* **2024**, *43*, 1221–1229. [CrossRef]

126. Hsiao, H.-H.; Liu, Y.-C.; Wang, H.-C.; Du, J.-S.; Tang, S.-H.; Yeh, T.-J.; Hsieh, C.-Y.; Gau, Y.-C.; Ke, Y.-L.; Chuang, T.-M.; et al. Comparison of a Novel Lateral-Flow Device to Galactomannan Assay at Different Time Periods for Detections of Invasive Aspergillosis. *J. Formos. Med. Assoc.* **2022**, *121*, 2123–2129. [CrossRef] [PubMed]
127. Matsuo, T.; Wurster, S.; Hoenigl, M.; Kontoyiannis, D.P. Current and Emerging Technologies to Develop Point-of-Care Diagnostics in Medical Mycology. *Expert. Rev. Mol. Diagn.* **2024**, *24*, 841–858. [CrossRef]
128. Mercier, T.; Dunbar, A.; de Kort, E.; Schauwvlieghe, A.; Reynders, M.; Guldentops, E.; Blijlevens, N.M.A.; Vonk, A.G.; Rijnders, B.; Verweij, P.E.; et al. Lateral Flow Assays for Diagnosing Invasive Pulmonary Aspergillosis in Adult Hematology Patients: A Comparative Multicenter Study. *Med. Mycol.* **2020**, *58*, 444–452. [CrossRef]
129. Jenks, J.D.; Miceli, M.H.; Prattes, J.; Mercier, T.; Hoenigl, M. The Aspergillus Lateral Flow Assay for the Diagnosis of Invasive Aspergillosis: An Update. *Curr. Fungal Infect. Rep.* **2020**, *14*, 378–383. [CrossRef]
130. Jenks, J.D.; Prattes, J.; Frank, J.; Spiess, B.; Mehta, S.R.; Boch, T.; Buchheidt, D.; Hoenigl, M. Performance of the Bronchoalveolar Lavage Fluid Aspergillus Galactomannan Lateral Flow Assay with Cube Reader for Diagnosis of Invasive Pulmonary Aspergillosis: A Multicenter Cohort Study. *Clin. Infect. Dis.* **2021**, *73*, e1737–e1744. [CrossRef]
131. Zhang, X.; Shang, X.; Zhang, Y.; Li, X.; Yang, K.; Wang, Y.; Guo, K. Diagnostic Accuracy of Galactomannan and Lateral Flow Assay in Invasive Aspergillosis: A Diagnostic Meta-Analysis. *Heliyon* **2024**, *10*, e34569. [CrossRef] [PubMed]
132. Heldt, S.; Hoenigl, M. Lateral Flow Assays for the Diagnosis of Invasive Aspergillosis: Current Status. *Curr. Fungal Infect. Rep.* **2017**, *11*, 45–51. [CrossRef] [PubMed]
133. Pan, Z.; Fu, M.; Zhang, J.; Zhou, H.; Fu, Y.; Zhou, J. Diagnostic Accuracy of a Novel Lateral-Flow Device in Invasive Aspergillosis: A Meta-Analysis. *J. Med. Microbiol.* **2015**, *64*, 702–707. [CrossRef]
134. Cheepsattayakorn, A.; Cheepsattayakorn, R. Parasitic Pneumonia and Lung Involvement. *Biomed. Res. Int.* **2014**, *2014*, 874021. [CrossRef] [PubMed]
135. Daley, C.L. Tropical Respiratory Medicine. 1. Pulmonary Infections in the Tropics: Impact of HIV Infection. *Thorax* **1994**, *49*, 370–378. [CrossRef]
136. Garg, D.; Madan, N.; Qaqish, O.; Nagarakanti, S.; Patel, V. Pulmonary Toxoplasmosis Diagnosed on Transbronchial Lung Biopsy in a Mechanically Ventilated Patient. *Case Rep. Infect. Dis.* **2020**, *2020*, 9710102. [CrossRef] [PubMed]
137. Liu, Q.; Wang, Z.-D.; Huang, S.-Y.; Zhu, X.-Q. Diagnosis of Toxoplasmosis and Typing of Toxoplasma Gondii. *Parasit. Vectors* **2015**, *8*, 292. [CrossRef]
138. La Hoz, R.M.; Morris, M.I. Infectious Diseases Community of Practice of the American Society of Transplantation Tissue and Blood Protozoa Including Toxoplasmosis, Chagas Disease, Leishmaniasis, Babesia, Acanthamoeba, Balamuthia, and Naegleria in Solid Organ Transplant Recipients- Guidelines from the American Society of Transplantation Infectious Diseases Community of Practice. *Clin. Transpl.* **2019**, *33*, e13546. [CrossRef]
139. Robert-Gangneux, F.; Meroni, V.; Dupont, D.; Botterel, F.; Garcia, J.M.A.; Brenier-Pinchart, M.-P.; Accoceberry, I.; Akan, H.; Abbate, I.; Boggian, K.; et al. Toxoplasmosis in Transplant Recipients, Europe, 2010–2014. *Emerg. Infect. Dis.* **2018**, *24*, 1497–1504. [CrossRef] [PubMed]
140. Desoubeaux, G.; Cabanne, É.; Franck-Martel, C.; Gombert, M.; Gyan, E.; Lissandre, S.; Renaud, M.; Monjanel, H.; Dartigeas, C.; Bailly, É.; et al. Pulmonary Toxoplasmosis in Immunocompromised Patients with Interstitial Pneumonia: A Single-Centre Prospective Study Assessing PCR-Based Diagnosis. *J. Clin. Pathol.* **2016**, *69*, 726–730. [CrossRef] [PubMed]
141. Gompels, M.M.; Todd, J.; Peters, B.S.; Main, J.; Pinching, A.J. Disseminated Strongyloidiasis in AIDS: Uncommon but Important. *AIDS* **1991**, *5*, 329–332. [CrossRef] [PubMed]
142. Nabeya, D.; Haranaga, S.; Parrott, G.L.; Kinjo, T.; Nahar, S.; Tanaka, T.; Hirata, T.; Hokama, A.; Tateyama, M.; Fujita, J. Pulmonary Strongyloidiasis: Assessment between Manifestation and Radiological Findings in 16 Severe Strongyloidiasis Cases. *BMC Infect. Dis.* **2017**, *17*, 320. [CrossRef]
143. Maayan, S.; Wormser, G.P.; Widerhorn, J.; Sy, E.R.; Kim, Y.H.; Ernst, J.A. Strongyloides Stercoralis Hyperinfection in a Patient with the Acquired Immune Deficiency Syndrome. *Am. J. Med.* **1987**, *83*, 945–948. [CrossRef] [PubMed]
144. Greninger, A.L. The Challenge of Diagnostic Metagenomics. *Expert. Rev. Mol. Diagn.* **2018**, *18*, 605–615. [CrossRef] [PubMed]
145. Lin, P.; Chen, Y.; Su, S.; Nan, W.; Zhou, L.; Zhou, Y.; Li, Y. Diagnostic Value of Metagenomic Next-Generation Sequencing of Bronchoalveolar Lavage Fluid for the Diagnosis of Suspected Pneumonia in Immunocompromised Patients. *BMC Infect. Dis.* **2022**, *22*, 416. [CrossRef] [PubMed]
146. Tekin, A.; Truong, H.H.; Rovati, L.; Lal, A.; Gerberi, D.J.; Gajic, O.; O'Horo, J.C. The Diagnostic Accuracy of Metagenomic Next-Generation Sequencing in Diagnosing Pneumocystis Pneumonia: A Systemic Review and Meta-Analysis. *Open Forum Infect. Dis.* **2023**, *10*, ofad442. [CrossRef]

147. Lv, M.; Zhu, C.; Zhu, C.; Yao, J.; Xie, L.; Zhang, C.; Huang, J.; Du, X.; Feng, G. Clinical Values of Metagenomic Next-Generation Sequencing in Patients with Severe Pneumonia: A Systematic Review and Meta-Analysis. *Front. Cell Infect. Microbiol.* **2023**, *13*, 1106859. [CrossRef] [PubMed]
148. Gu, W.; Deng, X.; Lee, M.; Sucu, Y.D.; Arevalo, S.; Stryke, D.; Federman, S.; Gopez, A.; Reyes, K.; Zorn, K.; et al. Rapid Pathogen Detection by Metagenomic Next-Generation Sequencing of Infected Body Fluids. *Nat. Med.* **2021**, *27*, 115–124. [CrossRef]
149. Hall, M.B.; Rabodoarivelo, M.S.; Koch, A.; Dippenaar, A.; George, S.; Grobbelaar, M.; Warren, R.; Walker, T.M.; Cox, H.; Gagneux, S.; et al. Evaluation of Nanopore Sequencing for Mycobacterium Tuberculosis Drug Susceptibility Testing and Outbreak Investigation: A Genomic Analysis. *Lancet Microbe* **2023**, *4*, e84–e92. [CrossRef]
150. Bouso, J.M.; Planet, P.J. Complete Nontuberculous Mycobacteria Whole Genomes Using an Optimized DNA Extraction Protocol for Long-Read Sequencing. *BMC Genom.* **2019**, *20*, 793. [CrossRef] [PubMed]
151. Miao, Q.; Ma, Y.; Wang, Q.; Pan, J.; Zhang, Y.; Jin, W.; Yao, Y.; Su, Y.; Huang, Y.; Wang, M.; et al. Microbiological Diagnostic Performance of Metagenomic Next-Generation Sequencing When Applied to Clinical Practice. *Clin. Infect. Dis.* **2018**, *67*, S231–S240. [CrossRef]
152. Puig-Serra, P.; Casado-Rosas, M.C.; Martinez-Lage, M.; Olalla-Sastre, B.; Alonso-Yanez, A.; Torres-Ruiz, R.; Rodriguez-Perales, S. CRISPR Approaches for the Diagnosis of Human Diseases. *IJMS* **2022**, *23*, 1757. [CrossRef] [PubMed]
153. Zhan, Y.; Gao, X.; Li, S.; Si, Y.; Li, Y.; Han, X.; Sun, W.; Li, Z.; Ye, F. Development and Evaluation of Rapid and Accurate CRISPR/Cas13-Based RNA Diagnostics for Pneumocystis Jirovecii Pneumonia. *Front. Cell Infect. Microbiol.* **2022**, *12*, 904485. [CrossRef]
154. Li, Z.; Wang, M.; Xu, T.; Zhan, Y.; Chen, F.; Lin, Y.; Li, S.; Cheng, J.; Ye, F. Development and Clinical Implications of a Novel CRISPR-Based Diagnostic Test for Pulmonary Aspergillus Fumigatus Infection. *J. Microbiol. Immunol. Infect.* **2022**, *55*, 749–756. [CrossRef] [PubMed]
155. Cao, Y.; Tian, Y.; Huang, J.; Xu, L.; Fan, Z.; Pan, Z.; Chen, S.; Gao, Y.; Wei, L.; Zheng, S.; et al. CRISPR/Cas13-Assisted Carbapenem-Resistant Klebsiella Pneumoniae Detection. *J. Microbiol. Immunol. Infect.* **2024**, *57*, 118–127. [CrossRef] [PubMed]
156. Bai, L.; Yang, W.; Li, Y. Clinical and Laboratory Diagnosis of Legionella Pneumonia. *Diagnostics* **2023**, *13*, 280. [CrossRef] [PubMed]
157. Mandell, L.A.; Wunderink, R.G.; Anzueto, A.; Bartlett, J.G.; Campbell, G.D.; Dean, N.C.; Dowell, S.F.; File, T.M.; Musher, D.M.; Niederman, M.S.; et al. Infectious Diseases Society of America/American Thoracic Society Consensus Guidelines on the Management of Community-Acquired Pneumonia in Adults. *Clin. Infect. Dis.* **2007**, *44* (Suppl. S2), S27–S72. [CrossRef]
158. Shoar, S.; Musher, D.M. Etiology of Community-Acquired Pneumonia in Adults: A Systematic Review. *Pneumonia (Nathan)* **2020**, *12*, 11. [CrossRef]
159. Metlay, J.P.; Waterer, G.W.; Long, A.C.; Anzueto, A.; Brozek, J.; Crothers, K.; Cooley, L.A.; Dean, N.C.; Fine, M.J.; Flanders, S.A.; et al. Diagnosis and Treatment of Adults with Community-Acquired Pneumonia. An Official Clinical Practice Guideline of the American Thoracic Society and Infectious Diseases Society of America. *Am. J. Respir. Crit. Care Med.* **2019**, *200*, e45–e67. [CrossRef]
160. Ochoa-Gondar, O.; Torras-Vives, V.; de Diego-Cabanes, C.; Satué-Gracia, E.M.; Vila-Rovira, A.; Forcadell-Perisa, M.J.; Ribas-Seguí, D.; Rodríguez-Casado, C.; Vila-Córcoles, A. Incidence and Risk Factors of Pneumococcal Pneumonia in Adults: A Population-Based Study. *BMC Pulm. Med.* **2023**, *23*, 200. [CrossRef]
161. Mattila, J.T.; Fine, M.J.; Limper, A.H.; Murray, P.R.; Chen, B.B.; Lin, P.L. Pneumonia. Treatment and Diagnosis. *Ann. Am. Thorac. Soc.* **2014**, *11* (Suppl. S4), S189–S192. [CrossRef]
162. De la Calle, C.; Morata, L.; Cobos-Trigueros, N.; Martinez, J.A.; Cardozo, C.; Mensa, J.; Soriano, A. *Staphylococcus aureus* Bacteremic Pneumonia. *Eur. J. Clin. Microbiol. Infect. Dis.* **2016**, *35*, 497–502. [CrossRef] [PubMed]
163. Restrepo, M.I.; Babu, B.L.; Reyes, L.F.; Chalmers, J.D.; Soni, N.J.; Sibila, O.; Faverio, P.; Cilloniz, C.; Rodriguez-Cintron, W.; Aliberti, S.; et al. Burden and Risk Factors for Pseudomonas Aeruginosa Community-Acquired Pneumonia: A Multinational Point Prevalence Study of Hospitalised Patients. *Eur. Respir. J.* **2018**, *52*, 1701190. [CrossRef]
164. Marrie, T.J.; Fine, M.J.; Obrosky, D.S.; Coley, C.; Singer, D.E.; Kapoor, W.N. Community-Acquired Pneumonia Due to *Escherichia Coli*. *Clin. Microbiol. Infect.* **1998**, *4*, 717–723. [CrossRef] [PubMed]
165. Alavi Darazam, I.; Shamaei, M.; Mobarhan, M.; Ghasemi, S.; Tabarsi, P.; Motavasseli, M.; Mansouri, D. Nocardiosis: Risk Factors, Clinical Characteristics and Outcome. *Iran. Red. Crescent Med. J.* **2013**, *15*, 436–439. [CrossRef]
166. Zhong, C.; Huang, P.; Zhan, Y.; Yao, Y.; Ye, J.; Zhou, H. Clinical Features of Pulmonary Nocardiosis in Patients with Different Underlying Diseases: A Case Series Study. *Infect. Drug Resist.* **2022**, *15*, 1167–1174. [CrossRef]
167. Ryu, Y.J. Diagnosis of Pulmonary Tuberculosis: Recent Advances and Diagnostic Algorithms. *Tuberc. Respir. Dis.* **2015**, *78*, 64–71. [CrossRef] [PubMed]

168. Rachow, A.; Ivanova, O.; Wallis, R.; Charalambous, S.; Jani, I.; Bhatt, N.; Kampmann, B.; Sutherland, J.; Ntinginya, N.E.; Evans, D.; et al. TB Sequel: Incidence, Pathogenesis and Risk Factors of Long-Term Medical and Social Sequelae of Pulmonary TB—A Study Protocol. *BMC Pulm. Med.* **2019**, *19*, 4. [CrossRef] [PubMed]
169. Lee, H.Y.; Rhee, C.K.; Choi, J.Y.; Lee, H.Y.; Lee, J.W.; Lee, D.G. Diagnosis of Cytomegalovirus Pneumonia by Quantitative Polymerase Chain Reaction Using Bronchial Washing Fluid from Patients with Hematologic Malignancies. *Oncotarget* **2017**, *8*, 39736–39745. [CrossRef]
170. Chemaly, R.F.; Torres, H.A.; Hachem, R.Y.; Nogueras, G.M.; Aguilera, E.A.; Younes, A.; Luna, M.A.; Rodriguez, G.; Tarrand, J.J.; Raad, I.I. Cytomegalovirus Pneumonia in Patients with Lymphoma. *Cancer* **2005**, *104*, 1213–1220. [CrossRef] [PubMed]
171. Laing, K.J.; Ouwendijk, W.J.D.; Koelle, D.M.; Verjans, G.M.G.M. Immunobiology of Varicella-Zoster Virus Infection. *J. Infect. Dis.* **2018**, *218*, S68–S74. [CrossRef] [PubMed]
172. Kaplan, J.E.; Benson, C.; Holmes, K.K.; Brooks, J.T.; Pau, A.; Masur, H.; Centers for Disease Control and Prevention (CDC); National Institutes of Health; HIV Medicine Association of the Infectious Diseases Society of America. Guidelines for Prevention and Treatment of Opportunistic Infections in HIV-Infected Adults and Adolescents: Recommendations from CDC, the National Institutes of Health, and the HIV Medicine Association of the Infectious Diseases Society of America. *MMWR Recomm. Rep.* **2009**, *58*, 1–207, quiz CE1-4.
173. Scheithauer, S.; Manemann, A.K.; Krüger, S.; Häusler, M.; Krüttgen, A.; Lemmen, S.W.; Ritter, K.; Kleines, M. Impact of Herpes Simplex Virus Detection in Respiratory Specimens of Patients with Suspected Viral Pneumonia. *Infection* **2010**, *38*, 401–405. [CrossRef]
174. Popow-Kraupp, T.; Aberle, J.H. Diagnosis of Respiratory Syncytial Virus Infection. *Open Microbiol. J.* **2011**, *5*, 128–134. [CrossRef]
175. Pascarella, G.; Strumia, A.; Piliego, C.; Bruno, F.; Del Buono, R.; Costa, F.; Scarlata, S.; Agrò, F.E. COVID-19 Diagnosis and Management: A Comprehensive Review. *J. Intern. Med.* **2020**, *288*, 192–206. [CrossRef] [PubMed]
176. Palmieri, F.; Koutsokera, A.; Bernasconi, E.; Junier, P.; von Garnier, C.; Ubags, N. Recent Advances in Fungal Infections: From Lung Ecology to Therapeutic Strategies With a Focus on Aspergillus Spp. *Front Med.* **2022**, *9*, 832510. [CrossRef] [PubMed]
177. Zhao, Z.; Huang, Y.; Ming, B.; Zhong, J.; Dong, L. Characterization and Associated Risk Factors of Pneumocystis Jirovecii Pneumonia in Patients with AIRD: A Retrospective Study. *Rheumatology* **2022**, *61*, 3766–3776. [CrossRef] [PubMed]
178. Maertens, J.; Cesaro, S.; Maschmeyer, G.; Einsele, H.; Donnelly, J.P.; Alanio, A.; Hauser, P.M.; Lagrou, K.; Melchers, W.J.G.; Helweg-Larsen, J.; et al. ECIL Guidelines for Preventing Pneumocystis Jirovecii Pneumonia in Patients with Haematological Malignancies and Stem Cell Transplant Recipients. *J. Antimicrob. Chemother.* **2016**, *71*, 2397–2404. [CrossRef]
179. Pergam, S.A. Fungal Pneumonia in Patients with Hematologic Malignancies and Hematopoietic Cell Transplantation. *Clin. Chest Med.* **2017**, *38*, 279–294. [CrossRef] [PubMed]
180. Brousse, X.; Imbert, S.; Issa, N.; Forcade, E.; Faure, M.; Chambord, J.; Ramaroson, H.; Kaminski, H.; Dumas, P.-Y.; Blanchard, E. Performance of Mucorales Spp. qPCR in Bronchoalveolar Lavage Fluid for the Diagnosis of Pulmonary Mucormycosis. *Med. Mycol.* **2024**, *62*, myae006. [CrossRef] [PubMed]
181. Montoya, J.G. Laboratory Diagnosis of Toxoplasma Gondii Infection and Toxoplasmosis. *J. Infect. Dis.* **2002**, *185* (Suppl. S1), S73–S82. [CrossRef] [PubMed]
182. Siddiqui, A.A.; Berk, S.L. Diagnosis of Strongyloides Stercoralis Infection. *Clin. Infect. Dis.* **2001**, *33*, 1040–1047. [CrossRef] [PubMed]
183. Requena-Méndez, A.; Chiodini, P.; Bisoffi, Z.; Buonfrate, D.; Gotuzzo, E.; Muñoz, J. The Laboratory Diagnosis and Follow up of Strongyloidiasis: A Systematic Review. *PLoS Negl. Trop. Dis.* **2013**, *7*, e2002. [CrossRef] [PubMed]
184. Luvira, V.; Watthanakulpanich, D.; Pittisuttithum, P. Management of Strongyloides Stercoralis: A Puzzling Parasite. *Int. Health* **2014**, *6*, 273–281. [CrossRef]

Disclaimer/Publisher's Note: The statements, opinions and data contained in all publications are solely those of the individual author(s) and contributor(s) and not of MDPI and/or the editor(s). MDPI and/or the editor(s) disclaim responsibility for any injury to people or property resulting from any ideas, methods, instructions or products referred to in the content.

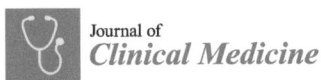

Article

Epidemiology and Clinical Relevance of *Pneumocystis jirovecii* in Non-Human Immunodeficiency Virus Patients at a Tertiary Care Center in Central Europe: A 3-Year Retrospective Study

Ágnes Jakab [1,2,†], Andrea Harmath [1,3,†], Zoltán Tóth [1,2], László Majoros [1,2], József Kónya [1,2] and Renátó Kovács [1,2,*]

[1] Department of Medical Microbiology, Faculty of Medicine, University of Debrecen, Nagyerdei krt. 98., 4032 Debrecen, Hungary; jakab.agnes@med.unideb.hu (Á.J.); harmath.andrea@med.unideb.hu (A.H.); toth.zoltan@med.unideb.hu (Z.T.); major@med.unideb.hu (L.M.); konya@med.unideb.hu (J.K.)
[2] Medical Microbiology, Clinical Centre, University of Debrecen, Nagyerdei krt. 98., 4032 Debrecen, Hungary
[3] Doctoral School of Pharmaceutical Sciences, University of Debrecen, Nagyerdei krt. 98., 4032 Debrecen, Hungary
* Correspondence: kovacs.renato@med.unideb.hu; Tel.: +36-52-255-425; Fax: +36-52-255-424
† These authors contributed equally to this work.

Abstract: Background/Objectives: This study examines the clinical characteristics of *Pneumocystis jirovecii* pneumonia (PjP) in non-Human immunodeficiency virus (HIV) patients in Hungary to describe its local epidemiological properties. **Methods**: Our study was conducted at a clinical center with more than 1700 beds at the University of Debrecen in Hungary. We included all patients without HIV infection for whom a diagnostic evaluation for *Pneumocystis* infection had been requested between 1 January 2022 and 31 December 2024. **Results**: In total, 21 cases of PjP were identified from 122 requests at the University of Debrecen Clinical Center between 2022 and 2024. The overall 30-day mortality rate was 43% in PjP. Admission to the intensive care unit (odds ratio [OR] 5.44, 95% confidence interval [CI] 1.87–14.09, $p = 0.001$), the need for mechanical ventilation (OR 4.09, 95% CI 1.45–12.14, $p = 0.015$) and hematological malignancies (OR 3.24, 95% CI 1.23–9.18, $p = 0.024$), were associated with *Pneumocystis* PCR positivity. Furthermore, a significant association was observed between elevated levels of C-reactive protein (OR 1.01, 95% CI 1–1.01, $p = 0.001$), 30-day mortality (OR 2.86, 95% CI 1.09–7.92, $p = 0.049$), and *Pneumocystis* PCR positivity. Regarding diagnostic platforms used, Fujifilm Wako assay detected serum (1-3)-β-D-glucan positivity (>7 pg/mL) from 352 copies/mL in non-HIV patients with probable PJP. **Conclusions**: Our study serves as a gap-filling investigation, providing an overview of *Pneumocystis* epidemiology in the Central European region.

Keywords: *Pneumocystis jirovecii*; (1-3)-β-D-glucan; HIV; epidemiology

1. Introduction

Pneumocystis jirovecii is an opportunistic fungal pathogen, classified as a medium-priority pathogen in the fungal priority list published by the World Health Organization [1]. Predisposing factors for *P. jirovecii*-related pneumonia (PjP) include transplantation, hematological malignancies, inflammatory or rheumatologic conditions, and related therapies that impair cell-mediated immunity [2–4]. PjP is no longer restricted to Human immunodeficiency virus (HIV)-positive patients but is increasingly diagnosed in non-HIV populations, posing new challenges for diagnosis and treatment [2–4]. In case of HIV-positive patients, the onset of PJP is usually gradual and insidious with limited radiologic findings, while in immunocompromised non-HIV individuals, clinical presentation tends to be more acute with rapid emergence of respiratory symptoms and with a mortality rate twice that of HIV-infected individuals, ranging from 30% to 60% [4–6].

P. jirovecii is globally distributed; however, data on its prevalence and incidence in Central and/or Eastern European populations are limited. The incidence of PjP in Central and Eastern European countries has been reported to range from 0.18 to 0.88 per 100,000 admissions [7–9]. However, these data usually pertain to HIV-infected patients, and there are no reliable data on the non-HIV population in this region.

Hence, the primary aim of this study was to retrospectively investigate the epidemiological data and the clinical characteristics of *P. jirovecii* infection among HIV-negative patients in one of the largest tertiary care centers in Hungary, thereby enhancing our understanding of *P. jirovecii* infections.

2. Materials and Methods

Our study was conducted at a clinical center with more than 1700 beds at the University of Debrecen in Hungary. We included all patients without HIV infection for whom a diagnostic evaluation for *Pneumocystis* infection had been requested between 1 January 2022 and 31 December 2024. In case of PJP diagnosis, we followed the EORTC/MSGERC revised definitions for *P. jirovecii* disease, where the triad of host factors, clinical characteristics, and mycologic tests was considered [10]. The diagnosis of PjP was based on the administration of therapeutic doses of corticosteroid therapy and $CD4^+$ lymphocyte count (where it was available); the presence of suggestive clinical criteria including fever, respiratory symptoms (e.g., cough, dyspnea, hypoxemia), bilateral or diffuse ground-glass opacity on X-ray with interstitial infiltrates; and a positive microbiological diagnostic test, including the detection of (1-3)-β-D-glucan in blood and/or a positive polymerase chain reaction (PCR) result from a bronchoalveolar lavage specimen or induced sputum [10] Notably, our laboratory does not perform microscopy-based examinations; therefore, according to the EORTC/MSGERC guideline, we can establish only probable PJP results [10]. In clinical practice, we adhere to the diagnostic algorithm for PJP as outlined in Table 1.

Table 1. Diagnostic algorithm used in our laboratory in the absence of microscopy-based investigation.

	Criteria	Interpretation
Clinical presentation	Clinical symptoms suggestive of PjP and bilateral or diffuse ground-glass opacity on X-ray with interstitial infiltrates.	Suggest possible PjP infection
PCR for *P. jirovecii*	Positive PCR result from respiratory sample	Indicates presence of *P. jirovecii* DNA
Detection of serum (1-3)-β-D-glucan	Elevated above diagnostic threshold	Suggests fungal infection, supports *P. jirovecii* PCR as adjunctive test
Final diagnosis	Clinical signs + Positive PCR (+elevated (1-3)-β-D-glucan)	Probable PJP diagnosis, further expert consultation may be needed

Demographic data, underlying medical conditions, hematological parameters, blood gas parameters, and details of antimicrobial therapy were collected from the patients' medical records. Concurrent bacteremia and/or fungaemia were defined as the isolation of potentially pathogenic microbes from blood culture samples at the time of *Pneumocystis* infection. PjP outcomes were monitored from the initial diagnosis until 30 days post-diagnosis or death. Regarding *Pneumocystis* laboratory diagnosis, copy numbers and serum (1-3)-β-D-glucan levels were obtained using the *Pneumocystis* ELITe MGB® Kit (Elitech Group SAS, Puteaux, France) and the Fujifilm Wako assay (FUJIFILM Wako Pure Chemical Corporation, Osaka, Japan), respectively. The limit of detection of polymerase chain reaction is <97 copies/mL, while the cut-off value of Fujifilm Wako assay is 7 pg/mL.

Univariable analysis was performed to reveal those factors, which are associated with PCR positivity. Categorical variables were analyzed using Fisher's exact test. In the case of continuous variables, a logistic regression model was used and based on the distribution of the data, the Mann–Whitney test was used for non-normally distributed variables. Data analysis was performed using GraphPad Prism software (version no.: 10.1.1). Results were considered significant if the *p*-value was <0.05.

3. Results

In total, 122 requests for *P. jirovecii* diagnosis were registered from non-HIV patients during the investigation period, of which 21 were probable PJP according to EORTC/MSGRC guidelines [10]. PjP diagnosis was based on bronchoalveolar lavage fluid positivity in 33% of cases (seven lavage samples were PCR-positive). In eight patients, the diagnosis was based on bronchial specimen positivity, while six patients had a positive induced sputum sample. The number of requests increased continuously, with 18, 31, and 73 registered in 2022, 2023, and 2024, respectively. Notably, the increase in the number of requests is not specific to *Pneumocystis*; it reflects a general trend across all areas of microbiology in the post-COVID-19 era at our clinical center. The demographic and clinical characteristics, treatment, and outcomes of *Pneumocystis*-positive patients, as well as the results of laboratory tests performed, are presented in Table 2.

Table 2. Microbiological characteristics and clinical variables for *Pneumocystis jirovecii* pneumoniae in HIV-negative patients.

Variables	Total	*Pneumocystis* PCR Positive	*Pneumocystis* PCR Negative	Odds Ratio	95% Confidence Intervals (CI)	*p*-Value
	122 (100%)	21 (17%)	101 (83%)			
Demographic						
Age						
≤50 years	33 (27%)	6 (29%)	27 (27%)	1.1	0.38–3.05	>0.999
>50 years	89 (73%)	15 (71%)	74 (73%)	0.91	0.33–2.62	>0.999
Gender						
Female	43 (35%)	7 (33%)	36 (36%)	0.90	0.35–2.36	>0.999
Male	79 (65%)	14 (67%)	65 (64%)	1.11	0.42–2.84	>0.999
Clinical presentation						
Healthcare-associated risk factors						
Intensive Care Unit	28 (23%)	11 (52%)	17 (17%)	5.44	1.87–14.09	0.001 [1]
Days in Intensive Care Unit (median and range)	0 (0–58)	3 (0–33)	0 (0–58)	1.02	0.99–1.06	0.253
Invasive mechanical ventilation	18 (15%)	7 (33%)	11 (11%)	4.09	1.45–12.14	0.015 [1]
Underlying comorbidities						
Autoimmune disease	9 (7%)	2 (10%)	7 (7%)	1.41	0.28–7.48	0.652
Diabetes mellitus	22 (18%)	1 (5%)	21 (21%)	0.19	0.02–1.27	0.118
Renal failure	15 (12%)	2 (10%)	13 (13%)	0.71	0.15–3.34	>0.999
Hematological malignancy	28 (23%)	9 (43%)	19 (19%)	3.24	1.23–9.18	0.024 [1]
Solid malignancy	28 (23%)	5 (24%)	23 (23%)	1.06	0.39–3.19	>0.999
Chronic obstructive airway disease (COPD)	13 (11%)	3 (14%)	10 (10%)	1.52	0.41–5.27	0.696
Co-infections						
Bacteriaemia	13 (11%)	5 (24%)	8 (8%)	3.63	1.15–11.5	0.047 [1]

Table 2. Cont.

Variables	Total	Pneumocystis PCR Positive	Pneumocystis PCR Negative	Odds Ratio	95% Confidence Intervals (CI)	p-Value
Fungaemia	3 (2%)	1 (5%)	2 (2%)	2.48	0.16–21.86	0.436
Adenovirus infection	4 (3%)	1 (5%)	3 (3%)	1.63	0.12–11.38	0.535
Cytomegalovirus infection	4 (3%)	2 (10%)	2 (2%)	5.21	0.76–34.13	0.137
Epstein–Barr virus infection	5 (4%)	1 (5%)	4 (4%)	1.21	0.09–8.06	>0.999
Treatment						
Corticosteroid therapy	77 (63%)	20 (95%)	57 (56%)	15.44	2.49–164.2	0.0004 [1]
Prednisone therapy ($\geq$0.3 mg/kg)	70 (57%)	16 (76%)	54 (53%)	2.79	0.99–7.3	0.088
Receipt of systemic antibiotics	64 (52%)	18 (86%)	46 (46%)	7.14	2.05–23.86	0.0007 [1]
Sulfamethoxazole/Trimethoprim	34 (28%)	17 (81%)	17 (17%)	21	6.12–61	<0.0001 [1]
Receipt of systemic antifungal	37 (30%)	8 (38%)	29 (29%)	1.53	0.56–4.01	0.438
Chemotherapeutic drugs	58 (48%)	16 (76%)	42 (42%)	4.5	1.59–11.75	0.007 [1]
Monoclonal antibodies	11 (9%)	6 (29%)	5 (5%)	7.68	2.12–26.13	0.0034 [1]
Mortality						
30-day mortality	30 (25%)	9 (43%)	21 (21%)	2.86	1.09–7.92	0.049 [1]
Laboratory results						
Blood parameters (mean with range)						
White blood cell count (giga/L)	10.2 (0.1–44.4)	10.2 (0.1–32.5)	10.2 (0.6–44.4)	1	0.94–1.07	0.99
Neutrophil granulocyte count (giga/l)	8.1 (0.3–40.6)	7 (0.3–16.8)	8.4 (0.6–40.6)	0.96	0.87–1.05	0.371
Lymphocyte count (giga/L)	1.8 (0.1–29.5)	2.7 (0.1–29.2)	1.5 (0.2–29.5)	1.12	0.94–1.35	0.213
Creatinine (μM/L)	100 (4–766)	115 (27–766)	96 (4–479)	1	1–1.01	0.448
C-reactive protein (mg/L)	89.5 (0.5–507)	156 (1.8–507)	72.9 (0.5–277.2)	1.01	1–1.01	0.001 [1]
Lactate dehydrogenase (U/L)	296 (2–4863)	369 (37–913)	267 (2–4863)	1	1–1	0.502
Blood gas parameters (mean with range)						
Partial pressure of carbon dioxide (pCO$_2$) (Hgmm)	41.6 (2.3–66)	36 (2.3–58)	48.2 (26–66)	0.948	0.89–1.01	0.097
Partial pressure of oxygen (pO$_2$) (Hgmm)	54.2 (2.3–90)	52.8 (2.3–89)	55.9 (29–90)	0.995	0.96–1.03	0.775
Bicarbonate (HCO$_3$) (mmol/L)	27 (16–41.2)	27.1 (16.7–40.3)	26.9 (16–41.2)	1	0.89–1.13	0.929
Base excess in blood (BE) (mmol/L)	1.8 (−13–16.6)	2.2 (−13–14.2)	1.2 (−8.7–16.6)	1.02	0.91–1.15	0.744

[1] Significant.

Intensive care unit admission, invasive mechanical ventilation, and hematological malignancy were observed in 52%, 33%, and 43% of patients with positive *Pneumocystis* PCR results, respectively. The majority of patients (79 out of 122 [65%]) were male, and the median age was 61 years (range: 3 to 98 years). Based on the results of univariable analysis, intensive care unit admission (OR 5.44, 95% CI 1.87–14.09, p = 0.001), invasive mechanical ventilation (OR 4.09, 95% CI 1.45–12.14, p = 0.015), hematological malignancy (OR 3.24, 95% CI 1.23–9.18, p = 0.024), and 30-day mortality (OR 2.86, 95% CI 1.09–7.92, p = 0.049) were significantly associated with *Pneumocystis* PCR positivity (Table 1).

Focusing on the applied therapies, the use of glucocorticoids, chemotherapeutic agents, and monoclonal antibodies has been shown to significantly increase the risk of PJP [11]. In our study, corticosteroid therapy (OR 15.44, 95% CI 2.49–164.2, p = 0.0004), intravenous antibiotic use (OR 7.14, 95% CI 2.05–23.86, p = 0.0007), sulfamethoxazole/trimethoprim therapy (OR 21.00, 95% CI 6.12–61.00, p < 0.0001), chemotherapeutic agents (OR 4.50, 95% CI 1.59–11.75, p = 0.007), and monoclonal antibody treatment (OR 7.68, 95% CI 2.12–26.13, p = 0.0034) were significantly associated with positive *Pneumocystis* PCR results (Table 2).

Among PCR-positive cases, 12 patients (57%) presented with fever, although its presence and severity may have been influenced by concurrent therapies. Furthermore, all PCR-positive patients exhibited bilateral or diffuse ground-glass opacities with interstitial infiltrates on chest X-ray. Notably, none of the *Pneumocystis*-positive patients had undergone solid organ or hematopoietic stem cell transplantation. CD4$^+$ cell count data were available for 11 PCR-positive patients (52%), of whom four died. The mean CD4$^+$ cell count was 1005 $\pm$ 491 cells/mm^3, with a range of 120 to 1740 cells/mm^3.

Bacterial and/or fungal bloodstream co-infections were reported in 13 (11%) cases and 3 (2%) cases, respectively. It is noteworthy that concomitant bacteraemia (OR 3.63, 95% CI 1.15–11.5, $p = 0.047$) was associated with positive *Pneumocystis* PCR results (Table 2). Bacterial and/or fungal respiratory co-infections were present in 38% of PjP cases, including *Escherichia coli* (two cases), *Staphylococcus aureus* (three cases), *Klebsiella pneumoniae* (three cases), and *Pseudomonas aeruginosa* (one case). Among the laboratory parameters examined, C-reactive protein was significantly elevated in PCR-positive cases compared to PCR-negative cases ($p = 0.001$) (Table 2). Regarding microbiological diagnosis, the median of quantitative PCR copy numbers 195 copies/mL, ranging from 97 to 684,201. Positive serum (1–3)-β-D-glucan levels were detected in 7 of the 21 cases.

4. Discussion

Based on large-scale national epidemiological data, there has been a significant increase in the prevalence and incidence of PjP in non-HIV patients [2–4,6,12]. This concerning trend is attributed to the extensive use of corticosteroids and the increased implementation of organ and stem cell transplantation [2–4,6,12]. In line with previously published studies, the most common immunocompromising conditions observed in our study were hematological and solid malignancies, which is consistent with findings in hospitalized patients with PjP in general [2,13]. In addition, hematological malignancies showed a significant relationship with *Pneumocystis* PCR positivity. In this study, 95% of patients had received corticosteroid therapy—a well-known predisposing factor for PjP [2–4]—which, along with chemotherapeutic drugs, was associated with *Pneumocystis* PCR positivity. Notably, the observed 30-day mortality was significantly higher (43%) compared to the HIV-infected population (approximately 10–15%) [5–10] and demonstrated a clear correlation with PCR positivity. Focusing on additional risk factors in *Pneumocystis* PCR-positive patients, only 2 of the 11 available $CD4^+$ cell count values were below 200. A previously published systematic reviews concluded that a $CD4^+$ cell count of less than 200 was a reliable biomarker of "high risk" category in immunocompromised non-HIV patients [14,15]. Nevertheless, higher $CD4^+$ cell number does not exclude the possibility of PJP as described by Koifman et al. [16].

In this study, 23% of the patients required admission to the intensive care unit, while 15% received invasive mechanical ventilation. Notably, both factors were significantly more common among patients showing *Pneumocystis* PCR positivity. Schmidt et al. [17] reported that more than 40% of patients required intensive care unit admission, with 36% needing invasive mechanical ventilation. According to previous data, 16% of HIV-positive and 50% to 60% of non-HIV patients require mechanical ventilation during PjP hospitalization [18,19]. Monnet et al. [20] reported a 62% mortality rate among patients who required mechanical ventilation. These previously published findings are consistent with our results.

Although diagnostic tests have improved over the last decade, several laboratory parameters can further support diagnosis. These parameters may differ between HIV-negative and HIV-positive individuals. In our study, C-reactive protein was elevated and was significantly higher among patients who showed a positive *Pneumocystis* PCR result; however, the degree of elevation is generally lower compared to that observed in bacterial infections [21]. Sage et al. [21] demonstrated that HIV-infected patients with PjP showed a significant association between elevated C-reactive protein levels, disease severity, and poor outcomes.

Based on EORTC/MSGERC guideline, the diagnosis of proven PJP is based on clinical and radiological criteria with microscopic visualization of *P. jirovecii* in respiratory specimens [10]. Although, PCR-based platforms are more sensitive than microscopic examination for the detection of *P. jirovecii*, their sensitivity does not support the differentiation between proven PJP and colonization with *P. jirovecii*. In addition, in the HIV-negative immunocompromised population, the differentiation between *P. jirovecii* colonization and active PjP remains further challenging, especially in the intensive care unit where PCR-based diagnostics are commonly used. Previous studies have shown that a significant proportion of PCR-positive cases in these patients may show colonization rather than true infection [22,23]. A multicenter retrospective study involving intensive care unit patients with severe pneumonia described that nearly 40% of those who showed *Pneumocystis* PCR positivity were classified as colonized, not infected. In case of these cases, lower lymphocyte counts and higher rates of viral co-infections (e.g., Cytomegalovirus and Epstein–Barr virus) were observed compared with patients with confirmed PjP [24]. Another major finding of this study was that *P. jirovecii* colonization was an independent predisposing factor for increased 28-day mortality, suggesting the clinical significance of the presence of *P. jirovecii* without active infection [24]. According to EORTC/MSGERC, all nucleic acid amplification tests should be validated in the appropriate clinical context (e.g., non-HIV patients vs. HIV patients) to define the thresholds of colonization and definitive PJP [10]. Quantitative PCR combined with serum (1-3)-β-D-glucan determination may aid in distinguishing disease from colonization. However, because of methodological variability, there is no universally accepted cut-off value to differentiate between the two [3].

In our study, the measured copy numbers could suggest either colonization or infection. Generally, the *P. jirovecii* load is significantly lower in non-HIV patients. Previous studies indicate that positive PCR values below 1450 copies/mL may be associated with both colonization and infection in the HIV-negative population, and patients with low pathogen densities (85 copies/mL) may still have PjP [22,23]. Serum (1-3)-β-D-glucan determination has good sensitivity and a high negative predictive value in HIV-positive patients with PjP. However, its cut-off values are not well defined, and its sensitivity in HIV-positive patients was higher than those without HIV (94% vs. 86%) with similar specificity [25,26]. Jiang et al. (2025) [24] shows that the serum (1-3)-β-D-glucan concentration in patients colonized with *P jirovecii* is lower than in patients with PjP. However, data from several patients with *P jirovecii* colonization were higher than normal values.

In light of these considerations, the differentiation between *Pneumocystis* colonization and active infection remains a significant diagnostic challenge in the present study; nonetheless, the combination of quantitative PCR and serum (1-3)-β-D-glucan determination may result in superior diagnostic performance. In our study, Fujifilm Wako assay detected serum (1-3)-β-D-glucan positivity (>7 pg/mL) from 352 copies/mL in non-HIV patients with probable PJP. As we wrote above, our laboratory did not perform microscopy-based examination during the observation period; therefore, we could not establish a proven diagnosis of *P. jirovecii* infection. Based on our local diagnostic algorithm, real-time PCR is recommended as the principal microbiological diagnostic test for PjP, while serum (1-3)-β-D-glucan testing may be performed as an adjunctive test. A positive real-time PCR result with compatible clinical course and chest X-ray or computer tomography findings is indicative of the definitive diagnosis of PjP. Furthermore, our local algorithm recommends consultation with an infectious disease specialist to differentiate true infection from colonization.

For the sake of completeness, some limitations of this study should be highlighted. First, the analysis was conducted at a single center; therefore, the number of *Pneumocystis*-positive patients was relatively small, limiting the depth of statistical analysis. Second, our laboratory does not perform microscopy-based examination; therefore, according to the

EORTC/MSGERC guideline, we can provide only probable PJP results [10]. Furthermore, this guideline wrote that CD4$^+$ cell count of less than 200 was a sensitive biomarker of "high risk" in immunocompromised patients without HIV [10]; however, here we could receive this data only from the 52% of involved PCR positive patients, which may undermine the uniformity of case definition. Despite these limitations, this study serves as a gap-filling investigation, providing an overview of *Pneumocystis* epidemiology in the Central European region.

Author Contributions: Conceptualization, Á.J., A.H. and R.K.; methodology, Á.J., A.H. and R.K.; software, R.K.; validation, R.K.; formal analysis, R.K.; investigation, Á.J., A.H. and R.K.; resources, J.K. and L.M.; data curation, R.K.; writing—original draft preparation, Á.J., A.H. and R.K.; writing—review and editing, R.K. and L.M.; visualization, R.K.; supervision, R.K.; project administration, Á.J., A.H. and R.K.; funding acquisition, A.H., R.K. and Z.T. All authors have read and agreed to the published version of the manuscript.

Funding: A.H. was supported by the EKÖP-24-0 University Research Scholarship Program of the Ministry for Culture and Innovation from the source of the National Research, Development and Innovation Fund. R.K. was supported by the Janos Bolyai Research Scholarship of the Hungarian Academy of Sciences (BO/00127/21/8). This research was supported by the Hungarian National Research, Development and Innovation Office (NKFIH FK138462 and Starting 150834).

Institutional Review Board Statement: This study was approved by the institutional ethics committee at the University of Debrecen, Regional and Institutional Research Ethics Committee (DE RKEB/IKEB) (permission number 6968-2024). The approval date is 30 October 2024.

Informed Consent Statement: According to local ethics committee's decision, no specific informed consent from patients was required for this study. Based on the published data, the identification of given patients is not possible.

Data Availability Statement: The original contributions presented in this study are included in the article material. Further inquiries can be directed to the corresponding author(s).

Conflicts of Interest: The authors declare no conflicts of interest.

Abbreviations

The following abbreviations are used in this manuscript:

PjP	*Pneumocystis jirovecii* pneumonia
HIV	Human Immunodeficiency Virus
EORTC/MSGERC	European Organization for Research and Treatment of Cancer/Invasive Fungal Infections Cooperative Group/Mycoses Study Group Education and Research Consortium
PCR	Polymerase chain reaction

References

1. WHO Fungal Priority Pathogens Report. 2022. Available online: https://www.who.int/publications/i/item/9789240060241 (accessed on 25 October 2022).
2. Fillatre, P.; Decaux, O.; Jouneau, S.; Revest, M.; Gacouin, A.; Robert-Gangneux, F.; Fresnel, A.; Guiguen, C.; Le Tulzo, Y.; Jégo, P.; et al. Incidence of *Pneumocystis jirovecii* pneumonia among groups at risk in HIV-negative patients. *Am. J. Med.* **2014**, *127*, 1242.e11–1242.e17. [CrossRef] [PubMed]
3. US Department of Health and Human Services. AIDS Info: Guidelines for the Prevention and Treatment of Opportunistic Infections in Adults and Adolescents with HIV—Pneumocystis Pneumonia. 2023. Available online: https://clinicalinfo.hiv.gov/en/guidelines/hiv-clinical-guidelines-adult-and-adolescent-opportunistic-infections/pneumocystis-0?view=full (accessed on 16 September 2024).

4. Quigley, N.; d'Amours, L.; Gervais, P.; Dion, G. Epidemiology, Risk Factors, and Prophylaxis Use for *Pneumocystis jirovecii* Pneumonia in the Non-HIV Population: A Retrospective Study in Québec, Canada. *Open Forum Infect. Dis.* **2023**, *11*, ofad639. [CrossRef] [PubMed]
5. KIofteridis, D.P.; Valachis, A.; Velegraki, M.; Antoniou, M.; Christofaki, M.; Vrentzos, G.E.; Andrianaki, A.M.; Samonis, G. Predisposing factors, clinical characteristics and outcome of *Pneumonocystis jirovecii* pneumonia in HIV-negative patients. *Kansenshogaku Zasshi.* **2014**, *88*, 21–25. [CrossRef]
6. Mundo, W.; Morales-Shnaider, L.; Tewahade, S.; Wagner, E.; Archuleta, S.; Bandali, M.; Chadalawada, S.; Johnson, S.C.; Franco-Paredes, C.; Shapiro, L.; et al. Lower Mortality Associated With Adjuvant Corticosteroid Therapy in Non-HIV-Infected Patients With *Pneumocystis jirovecii* Pneumonia: A Single-Institution Retrospective US Cohort Study. *Open Forum Infect. Dis.* **2020**, *7*, ofaa354. [CrossRef]
7. Mareș, M.; Moroti-Constantinescu, V.R.; Denning, D.W. The Burden of Fungal Diseases in Romania. *J. Fungi* **2018**, *4*, 31. [CrossRef] [PubMed]
8. Arsenijević, V.A.; Denning, D.W. Estimated Burden of Serious Fungal Diseases in Serbia. *J. Fungi* **2018**, *4*, 76. [CrossRef]
9. Chrdle, A.; Mallátová, N.; Vašáková, M.; Haber, J.; Denning, D.W. Burden of serious fungal infections in the Czech Republic. *Mycoses* **2015**, *58*, 6–14. [CrossRef]
10. Lagrou, K.; Chen, S.; Masur, H.; Viscoli, C.; Decker, C.F.; Pagano, L.; Groll, A.H. *Pneumocystis jirovecii* Disease: Basis for the Revised EORTC/MSGERC Invasive Fungal Disease Definitions in Individuals Without Human Immunodeficiency Virus. *Clin. Infect. Dis.* **2021**, *72*, S114–S120. [CrossRef]
11. Lee, R.; Huh, K.; Kang, C.K.; Kim, Y.C.; Kim, J.H.; Kim, H.; Park, J.S.; Park, J.Y.; Sung, H.; Jung, J.; et al. Diagnosis of *Pneumocystis jirovecii* Pneumonia in Non-HIV Immunocompromised Patient in Korea: A Review and Algorithm Proposed by Expert Consensus Group. *Infect. Chemother.* **2025**, *57*, 45–62. [CrossRef]
12. Bienvenu, A.L.; Traore, K.; Plekhanova, I.; Bouchrik, M.; Bossard, C.; Picot, S. Pneumocystis pneumonia suspected cases in 604 non-HIV and HIV patients. *Int. J. Infect. Dis.* **2016**, *46*, 11–17. [CrossRef]
13. Kamel, T.; Janssen-Langenstein, R.; Quelven, Q.; Chelly, J.; Valette, X.; Le, M.P.; Bourenne, J.; Garot, D.; Fillatre, P.; Labruyere, M.; et al. Pneumocystis pneumonia in intensive care: Clinical spectrum, prophylaxis patterns, antibiotic treatment delay impact, and role of corticosteroids. A French multicentre prospective cohort study. *Intensive Care Med.* **2024**, *50*, 1228–1239. [CrossRef] [PubMed]
14. Messiaen, P.E.; Cuyx, S.; Dejagere, T.; van der Hilst, J.C. The role of CD4 cell count as discriminatory measure to guide chemoprophylaxis against *Pneumocystis jirovecii* pneumonia in human immunodeficiency virus-negative immunocompromised patients: A systematic review. *Transpl. Infect. Dis.* **2017**, *19*, e12651. [CrossRef] [PubMed]
15. Giacobbe, D.R.; Dettori, S.; Di Pilato, V.; Asperges, E.; Ball, L.; Berti, E.; Blennow, O.; Bruzzone, B.; Calvet, L.; Capra Marzani, F.; et al. *Pneumocystis jirovecii* pneumonia in intensive care units: Amulticenter study by, E.S.G.C.I.P.; EFISG. *Crit. Care* **2023**, *27*, 323. [CrossRef] [PubMed]
16. Koifman, M.; Vachhani, B.; Haridasan, K.S.; Mansur, M. *Pneumocystis jirovecii* Pneumonia in a Patient With Newly Diagnosed HIV and a High CD4 Count. *Cureus* **2023**, *15*, e46680. [CrossRef]
17. Schmidt, J.J.; Lueck, C.; Ziesing, S.; Stoll, M.; Haller, H.; Gottlieb, J.; Eder, M.; Welte, T.; Hoeper, M.M.; Scherag, A.; et al. Clinical course, treatment and outcome of *Pneumocystis* pneumonia in immunocompromised adults: A retrospective analysis over 17 years. *Crit. Care* **2018**, *22*, 307. [CrossRef]
18. Kim, S.J.; Lee, J.; Cho, Y.J.; Park, Y.S.; Lee, C.H.; Yoon, H.I.; Lee, S.M.; Yim, J.J.; Lee, J.H.; Yoo, C.G.; et al. Prognostic factors of *Pneumocystis jirovecii* pneumonia in patients without HIV infection. *J. Infect.* **2014**, *69*, 88–95. [CrossRef]
19. Wan, R.; Bai, L.; Yan, Y.; Li, J.; Luo, Q.; Huang, H.; Huang, L.; Xiang, Z.; Luo, Q.; Gu, Z.; et al. A Clinically Applicable Nomogram for Predicting the Risk of Invasive Mechanical Ventilation in *Pneumocystis jirovecii* Pneumonia. *Front. Cell Infect. Microbiol.* **2022**, *12*, 850741. [CrossRef]
20. Monnet, X.; Vidal-Petiot, E.; Osman, D.; Hamzaoui, O.; Durrbach, A.; Goujard, C.; Miceli, C.; Bourée, P.; Richard, C. Critical care management and outcome of severe *Pneumocystis* pneumonia in patients with and without HIV infection. *Crit. Care* **2008**, *12*, R28, Erratum in *Crit. Care* **2009**, *13*, 407. [CrossRef]
21. Sage, E.K.; Noursadeghi, M.; Evans, H.E.; Parker, S.J.; Copas, A.J.; Edwards, S.G.; Miller, R.F. Prognostic value of C-reactive protein in HIV-infected patients with *Pneumocystis jirovecii* pneumonia. *Int. J. STD AIDS* **2010**, *21*, 288–292. [CrossRef]
22. Alanio, A.; Hauser, P.M.; Lagrou, K.; Melchers, W.J.; Helweg-Larsen, J.; Matos, O.; Cesaro, S.; Maschmeyer, G.; Einsele, H.; Donnelly, J.P.; et al. ECIL guidelines for the diagnosis of *Pneumocystis jirovecii* pneumonia in patients with haematological malignancies stem cell transplant recipients. *J. Antimicrob. Chemother.* **2016**, *71*, 2386–2396. [CrossRef]

23. Mühlethaler, K.; Bögli-Stuber, K.; Wasmer, S.; von Garnier, C.; Dumont, P.; Rauch, A.; Mühlemann, K.; Garzoni, C. Quantitative PCR to diagnose Pneumocystis pneumonia in immunocompromised non-HIV patients. *Eur. Respir. J.* **2012**, *39*, 971–978. [CrossRef] [PubMed]
24. Jiang, Y.; Huang, X.; Zhou, H.; Wang, M.; Wang, S.; Ren, X.; He, G.; Xu, J.; Wang, Q.; Dai, M.; et al. Clinical Characteristics and Prognosis of Patients With Severe Pneumonia With *Pneumocystis jirovecii* Colonization: A Multicenter, Retrospective Study. *Chest* **2025**, *167*, 54–66. [CrossRef] [PubMed]
25. Taniguchi, J.; Nakashima, K.; Matsui, H.; Watari, T.; Otsuki, A.; Ito, H.; Otsuka, Y. Low cut-off value of serum (1,3)-beta-D-glucan for the diagnosis of Pneumocystis pneumonia in non-HIV patients: A retrospective cohort study. *BMC Infect. Dis.* **2021**, *21*, 1200. [CrossRef] [PubMed]
26. Del Corpo, O.; Butler-Laporte, G.; Sheppard, D.C.; Cheng, M.P.; McDonald, E.G.; Lee, T.C. Diagnostic accuracy of serum (1-3)-β-D-glucan for *Pneumocystis jirovecii* pneumonia: A systematic review and meta-analysis. *Clin. Microbiol. Infect.* **2020**, *26*, 1137–1143. [CrossRef]

Disclaimer/Publisher's Note: The statements, opinions and data contained in all publications are solely those of the individual author(s) and contributor(s) and not of MDPI and/or the editor(s). MDPI and/or the editor(s) disclaim responsibility for any injury to people or property resulting from any ideas, methods, instructions or products referred to in the content.

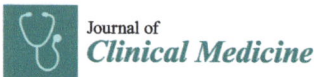 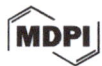

Article

Neutrophil Percentage-to-Albumin Ratio as a Prognostic Marker in Pneumonia Patients Aged 80 and Above in Intensive Care

Maside Ari [1,*], Aslı Haykir Solay [2], Tarkan Ozdemir [3], Murat Yildiz [1], Oral Mentes [4], Omer Faruk Tuten [5], Husra Tetik Manav [1], Deniz Celik [6], Melek Doganci [7], Guler Eraslan Doganay [7], Emrah Ari [8] and Eren Usul [9]

1. Department of Pulmonology, Ankara Ataturk Sanatorium Training and Research Hospital, 06290 Ankara, Türkiye; drmuratyildiz85@gmail.com (M.Y.); hsratetik@gmail.com (H.T.M.)
2. Department of Infectious Diseases and Microbiology, Ankara Etlik City Hospital, 06170 Ankara, Türkiye; aahaykir@hotmail.com
3. Department of Pulmonology, Konya Farabi Hospital, 42090 Konya, Türkiye; tarkanozdemir78@gmail.com
4. Clinic of Intensive Care Unit, Ankara Gulhane Training and Research Hospital, 06010 Ankara, Türkiye; omentes@live.com
5. Department of Pulmonology, Ankara University Health Practise and Research Hospitals, 06050 Ankara, Türkiye; omertuten@gmail.com
6. Department of Pulmonology, Alanya Alaaddin Keykubat University Education and Research Hospital, 07450 Antalya, Türkiye; drdenizcelik@hotmail.com
7. Clinic of Anesthesiology and Reanimation, Ankara Ataturk Sanatorium Training and Research Hospital, 06290 Ankara, Türkiye; melekdidik@hotmail.com (M.D.); gulerdoganay@hotmail.com.tr (G.E.D.)
8. Department of Emergency Medicine, Mamak Public Hospital, 06270 Ankara, Türkiye; dremrahari25@gmail.com
9. Department of Emergency Medicine, Ankara Etlik City Hospital, 06170 Ankara, Türkiye; usuleren7@hotmail.com
* Correspondence: masidetuten@icloud.com

Abstract: Background/Objectives: In recent years, inflammatory markers have been increasingly utilized to predict disease prognosis. The neutrophil percentage-to-albumin ratio (NPAR) has emerged as a novel biomarker reflecting inflammation and systemic response. This study was conducted to evaluate the prognostic value of NPAR in pneumonia patients aged 80 years and older hospitalized in intensive care. **Methods:** Patients aged 80 years and older who were followed up in the intensive care unit with a diagnosis of pneumonia between 1 October 2022, and 31 May 2024, were retrospectively reviewed. Demographic characteristics, laboratory data, disease severity scores (APACHE II, SOFA), intensive care interventions, and variables associated with mortality were analyzed. NPAR was calculated by dividing the neutrophil percentage by the serum albumin level. The prognostic value of NPAR was assessed using Kaplan–Meier survival analysis, receiver operating characteristic (ROC) curve analysis, and Cox regression analysis. **Results:** A total of 135 patients were included in the study. Patients with NPAR > 0.286 had significantly higher SOFA ($p = 0.002$) and APACHE II ($p = 0.007$) scores. The high NPAR group was at significantly greater risk for requiring invasive mechanical ventilation ($p = 0.003$), vasopressor support ($p = 0.042$), and developing sepsis ($p = 0.035$). Elevated NPAR was strongly associated with mortality ($p < 0.001$) and was identified as an independent predictor of mortality in the Cox regression analysis (HR = 2.488, 95% CI: 1.167–5.302, $p = 0.018$). **Conclusions:** NPAR may serve as an effective biomarker for predicting disease severity and mortality risk in pneumonia patients aged 80 years and older. Due to its simplicity and accessibility, it can be considered a practical parameter for integration into clinical practice. However, large-scale, multicenter, and prospective studies are needed to validate these findings.

Keywords: oldest old; mortality; NPAR; pneumonia; intensive care

1. Introduction

Individuals aged 80 years and older constitute a distinct age group referred to as the "oldest old" [1]. With the global increase in life expectancy, this population is projected to triple by the year 2050 [2]. The growing elderly population places a significant burden on healthcare systems by increasing the demand for medical care. Especially in oldest old individuals, the high burden of comorbid diseases, weakened immune systems and decreased functional capacity increase the susceptibility to infections and increase the risk of complications. Pneumonia in oldest old patients is often associated with more severe clinical presentations and frequently necessitates intensive care admission in the presence of any infection [3]. Moreover, the incidence of pneumonia cases requiring intensive care among this age group has been reported to be rising [4]. Therefore, accurate prediction of disease prognosis in oldest old individuals is of great importance to ensure early and appropriate interventions.

Neutrophils are key components of the innate immune system and represent the first line of defense against infections by mounting a rapid response to invading pathogens. During infectious and inflammatory processes, both the count and percentage of neutrophils increase rapidly, reflecting the magnitude of the systemic inflammatory response. Therefore, the neutrophil percentage is considered a biological indicator of infection severity and the level of inflammation [5]. Although albumin is commonly associated with nutritional status, it also functions as a negative acute-phase reactant. In the presence of systemic inflammation, hepatic synthesis of albumin decreases, capillary permeability increases, and albumin shifts into the extravascular space, resulting in reduced serum levels. This decline may reflect not only malnutrition but also the severity of the infectious or inflammatory process [6]. Due to these characteristics, albumin serves as an important parameter in prognostic assessment of infectious diseases.

In recent years, there has been a growing focus on the use of simple, rapid, and widely accessible biomarkers to evaluate inflammatory states. In this context, the neutrophil percentage-to-albumin ratio (NPAR) has emerged as a promising parameter [7]. NPAR simultaneously reflects the acute inflammatory response mediated by neutrophils and the systemic inflammatory and nutritional status represented by albumin levels [8]. Thus, it functions as a dual-purpose biomarker, indicating both infection severity and the patient's physiological reserve. Previous studies have demonstrated that NPAR is associated with mortality and adverse clinical outcomes in various conditions such as acute kidney injury, cardiovascular diseases, stroke, and sepsis [9–12]. However, the majority of these studies have focused on the general adult population or relatively younger patient groups. Data evaluating the relationship between NPAR and clinical outcomes in the very elderly population (aged ≥ 80 years) remain scarce. In older adults, reduced physiological reserve, immunosenescence, and the presence of multiple comorbidities contribute to a variable response to infections, potentially affecting the prognostic utility of biomarkers.

In this study, we aimed to investigate the prognostic value of NPAR in elderly patients with pneumonia and to evaluate its association with disease severity and clinical outcomes. We believe that the findings of this study may contribute to clinical decision-making in the management of older patients admitted to the intensive care unit.

2. Materials and Methods

This study included patients aged 80 years and older who were followed in the intensive care units of Ankara Atatürk Sanatorium Training and Research Hospital between 1 October 2022, and 31 May 2024. Data from patients diagnosed with community-acquired pneumonia were retrospectively reviewed using the hospital information system and patient medical records. Figure 1 shows a flowchart detailing the patients included in and excluded from this study.

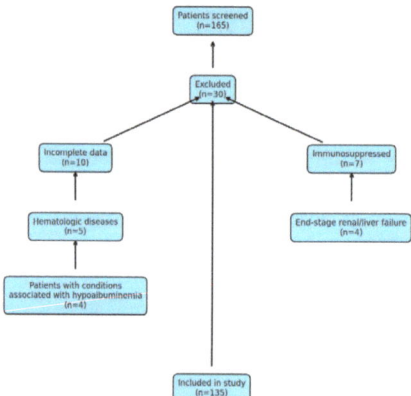

Figure 1. Flowchart of patients included in and excluded from this study.

This study was approved by the Ankara Atatürk Sanatorium Training and Research Hospital Clinical Research Ethics Committee with decision number 2839 dated 16 July 2024 and was conducted in accordance with the ethical principles stated in the Declaration of Helsinki.

The diagnosis of pneumonia was established based on the presence of the following three criteria after excluding alternative diagnoses:

1. Symptoms of lower respiratory tract infection: Fever (>38 °C), cough, purulent sputum, or a change in the character of respiratory secretions.
2. Radiographic findings consistent with pneumonia: Newly developed infiltrates on chest radiography or thoracic computed tomography.
3. Laboratory findings suggestive of infection: Leukocytosis, leukopenia, or elevated acute phase reactants.

2.1. Exclusion Criteria: Patients Who Were Not Included in the Study Were Identified Based on the Following Exclusion Criteria

Incomplete or insufficient patient data: Missing essential clinical, laboratory, or radiological data in the hospital information system or patient records.

Primary diagnoses other than pneumonia: Patients whose primary diagnosis was not pneumonia and who had alternative conditions that could mimic lower respiratory tract infections (e.g., pulmonary embolism, pulmonary edema due to congestive heart failure, interstitial lung diseases, pulmonary infiltrates due to malignancy).

Immunosuppressed patients: Patients with a history of chemotherapy, long-term corticosteroid use (>20 mg/day prednisone equivalent), immunosuppressive therapy, or solid organ/bone marrow transplantation.

Severe hematologic diseases: Patients with significant immune system impairment due to leukemia, lymphoma, or severe bone marrow failure.

End-stage renal or liver failure: Patients with end-stage chronic kidney disease (stage 5 requiring dialysis) or cirrhosis classified as Child–Pugh class C.

Diseases associated with hypoalbuminemia: Patients diagnosed with conditions that could cause hypoalbuminemia, such as chronic liver diseases or nephrotic syndrome.

2.2. Data Collection and Evaluation

Patients' comorbidities were recorded, and the most common comorbidities were identified. The impact of these comorbidities on mortality was also analyzed. Demographic data, clinical findings, complete blood count and biochemical parameters obtained within the first 24 h of intensive care unit (ICU) admission, acute phase reactants, imaging findings, administered treatments, need for respiratory and vasopressor support, requirement for renal replacement therapy, and patient outcomes were collected through the hospital information system and patient files.

The primary outcome of the study was all-cause mortality occurring within 30 days during hospitalization. Patients were followed until hospital discharge or death within the 30-day period.

The neutrophil percentage-to-albumin ratio (NPAR) was calculated using laboratory data obtained within the first 24 h of ICU admission and its association with clinical outcomes was evaluated.

Neutrophil percentage was measured using a Mindray BC-6800 automated hematology analyzer (Shenzhen Mindray Bio-medical Electronics Co., Ltd., Shenzhen, China) and recorded as a percentage. Serum albumin levels were measured in g/L using a Beckman Coulter AU680 chemistry analyzer (Beckman Coulter Inc., Brea, CA, USA). NPAR was calculated by dividing the neutrophil percentage by the serum albumin level.

2.3. Assessment of Sepsis and Disease Severity

The diagnosis of sepsis was made according to the international Sepsis-3 consensus criteria. Patients diagnosed with pneumonia and found to have a Sepsis-Related Organ Failure Assessment (SOFA) score ≥ 2 at the time of ICU admission were considered to have sepsis [13,14]. Patients who required vasopressor support to maintain a mean arterial pressure of ≥ 65 mmHg despite adequate fluid resuscitation were classified as having septic shock.

To objectively assess disease severity, the Acute Physiology and Chronic Health Evaluation II (APACHE II) score—commonly used in intensive care settings—was also calculated at the time of admission [15].

2.4. Calculation of SpO_2/FiO_2

In this study, the SpO_2/FiO_2 ratio was calculated to evaluate the patients' oxygenation status. SpO_2 values were obtained using a standard pulse oximeter, and the FiO_2 level was recorded based on the concentration of inspired oxygen. For patients receiving supplemental oxygen, FiO_2 was estimated according to the oxygen flow rate and the method of oxygen delivery. The SpO_2/FiO_2 ratio was calculated by dividing the SpO_2 value by the FiO_2 value. This calculation was performed within the first 24 h following admission to the intensive care unit. This ratio was used to classify the hypoxemic status of patients.

2.5. Patient Selection

In this study, all participants were admitted to the ICU either directly from the Emergency Department or following initial evaluation and short-term monitoring in the Department of Pulmonology. To ensure homogeneity of the study cohort and minimize variability related to the timing of clinical deterioration, only patients whose total time from initial hospital admission to ICU transfer was less than 24 h were included. This inclusion criterion was intended to capture cases of early critical illness and avoid confounding from complications developing during prolonged general ward stays.

2.6. Statistical Analysis

Statistical analyses were performed using SPSS version 27 (Statistical Package for the Social Sciences). The normality of distribution for continuous variables was assessed using the Kolmogorov–Smirnov test. Variables with normal distribution were expressed as mean ± standard deviation (Mean ± SD), while non-normally distributed variables were expressed as median and interquartile range (IQR, 25th–75th percentiles). Appropriate parametric or non-parametric tests were used to compare differences between groups. For comparisons between two independent groups, the t-test or Mann–Whitney U test was applied for continuous variables. The chi-square test (χ^2) or Fisher's exact test was used for categorical variables. The prognostic performance of NPAR in predicting mortality was evaluated using receiver operating characteristic (ROC) curve analysis. The area under the curve (AUC) was calculated for each variable, and optimal cutoff values were presented along with sensitivity and specificity. For survival analysis, Kaplan–Meier curves were generated, and differences between groups were assessed using the log-rank test. Cox regression analysis was used to identify factors associated with mortality. Initially, univariate Cox regression analysis was performed to identify candidate variables, and significant variables were then included in the multivariate model. Results of the model were reported as hazard ratios (HR) with 95% confidence intervals (CI). A p-value of <0.05 was considered statistically significant.

3. Results

A total of 135 patients were included in the study. In Table 1, demographic characteristics, clinical scores, laboratory parameters, and supportive treatment needs are compared between survivors and non-survivors. Among non-survivors, SOFA and APACHE II scores, as well as NPAR, procalcitonin, lactate, blood urea nitrogen, and creatinine levels were significantly higher, whereas albumin and platelet levels were lower. Furthermore, the need for invasive mechanical ventilation, hemodialysis, and vasopressor support was markedly higher in this group.

Table 1. Comparison of Clinical and Laboratory Parameters Between Survivors and Non-survivors.

	Survivors (N = 82, 60.8%)	Non-Survivors (N = 53, 39.2%)	p-Value
Age, years (Mean ± SD)	86.37 ± 4.90	87.64 ± 4.97	0.463
Female Sex	38 (57.6%)	28 (42.4%)	0.163
Male Sex	44 (63.8%)	25 (36.2%)	
SOFA Score	5.59 ± 2.57	8.79 ± 2.56	<0.001
APACHE-II Score	19.35 ± 5.71	28.21 ± 3.73	<0.001
Need for Hemodialysis	9 (10.9%)	24 (89.1%)	<0.001
Need for Vasopressor Support	11 (12.1%)	32 (87.9%)	<0.001
Need for Invasive Mechanical Ventilation	12 (14.6%)	48 (85.4%)	<0.001

Table 1. *Cont.*

	Survivors (N = 82, 60.8%)	Non-Survivors (N = 53, 39.2%)	p-Value
Presence of Comorbidities	63 (76.8%)	48 (90.6%)	0.042
COPD *	22 (26.8%)	24 (45.3%)	0.028
Malignancy	3 (3.7%)	7 (13.2%)	0.039
Neutrophil Percentage (%)	85 (78–90)	89 (85–92)	0.004
Albumin (g/L)	32 (27–35)	29 (24–34)	0.006
NPAR **	2.91 (2.44–21.60)	4.22 (2.98–30.92)	<0.001
Procalcitonin (ng/mL)	0.19 (0.06–0.67)	0.46 (0.21–2.63)	0.003
Lactate (mmol/L)	2.30 (1.40–3.00)	2.90 (2.40–3.40)	<0.001
Blood Urea Nitrogen (mg/dL)	51 (34–75)	82 (54–108)	<0.001
Creatinine (mg/dL)	1.13 (0.89–1.76)	1.52 (1.18–2.10)	0.010
Potassium (mmol/L)	4.00 (3.70–5.00)	4.49 (4.00–4.88)	0.102
CRP (mg/L)	32 (8–148)	62 (10–136)	0.456
Platelets ($\times 10^3/\mu L$)	223 (181–293)	169 (144–202)	<0.001

* COPD: Chronic Obstructive Pulmonary Disease ** NPAR: Neutrophil Percentage-to-Albumin Ratio.

Patients were divided into two groups, NPAR ≤ 0.286 and NPAR > 0.286, based on the cut-off value of 0.286 determined as a result of ROC analysis to evaluate the prognostic value of NPAR.

When the clinical characteristics of the patients were compared between groups, disease severity markers were found to be higher and mortality rates significantly increased in the high NPAR group. SOFA ($p = 0.002$) and APACHE II ($p = 0.007$) scores were significantly higher in patients with elevated NPAR. The need for invasive mechanical ventilation ($p = 0.003$), vasopressor therapy ($p = 0.042$), and the incidence of sepsis ($p = 0.035$) were also significantly greater in the high NPAR group. Moreover, mortality was significantly higher in patients with elevated NPAR ($p < 0.001$) (Table 2).

Table 2. Clinical Characteristics of Patients According to Neutrophil Percentage-to-Albumin Ratio Levels.

Variable	All Patients 135 (100%) N (%) Mean ± SD	NPAR ≤ 0.286 48 (35.6%) N (%) Mean ± SD *	NPAR > 0.286 87 (64.4%) N (%) Mean ± SD	p-Value
Age (years)	86.87 ± 4.95	86.65 ± 5.23	86.99 ± 4.82	0.638
Male sex	66 (48.9%)	22 (33.3%)	44 (66.7%)	0.599
SOFA score	6.84 ± 3.00	5.85 ± 2.94	7.39 ± 2.90	0.002
APACHE II score	22.83 ± 6.63	20.90 ± 7.53	23.90 ± 5.85	0.007
Renal replacement therapy	33 (24.4%)	10 (20.8%)	23 (26.4%)	0.470
Vasopressor requirement	43 (31.9%)	10 (20.8%)	33 (37.9%)	0.042

Table 2. Cont.

Variable	All Patients 135 (100%) N (%) Mean ± SD	NPAR ≤ 0.286 48 (35.6%) N (%) Mean ± SD *	NPAR > 0.286 87 (64.4%) N (%) Mean ± SD	p-Value
Invasive mechanical ventilation	60 (44.4%)	13 (27.1%)	47 (54.0%)	0.003
Requirement for high-flow nasal oxygen	82 (60.7%)	26 (54.1%)	56 (64.3%)	0.102
Requirement for noninvasive mechanical ventilation	68 (50.3%)	17 (35.4%)	51 (58.6%)	0.090
Presence of comorbidities	111 (82.2%)	47 (97.9%)	64 (73.6%)	<0.001
Cardiovascular disease	50 (37.0%)	25 (52.1%)	25 (28.7%)	0.007
Hypertension	67 (49.6%)	34 (70.8%)	33 (37.9%)	<0.001
Severity of the disease				
No sepsis	41 (30.4%)	20 (41.7%)	21 (24.1%)	0.035
Sepsis	94 (69.6%)	28 (58.3%)	66 (75.9%)	
SpO_2/FiO_2				
$SpO_2/FiO_2 > 315$	21 (15.6%)	6 (12.5%)	15 (17.2%)	0.087
$235 < SpO_2/FiO_2 \leq 315$	43 (31.9%)	21 (43.8%)	22 (25.3%)	
$148 < SpO_2/FiO_2 \leq 235$	42 (31.8%)	17 (35.4%)	25 (28.7%)	
$SpO_2/FiO_2 \leq 148$	29 (21.5%)	4 (8.3%)	25 (28.7%)	
Mortality	53 (39.3%)	9 (18.8%)	44 (50.6%)	<0.001

* NPAR: Neutrophil Percentage-to-Albumin Ratio.

When laboratory findings were compared according to NPAR levels, inflammatory and metabolic markers were found to be significantly elevated in the high NPAR group. Higher NPAR levels were associated with increased procalcitonin (p = 0.020) and lactate (p = 0.003) levels (Table 3).

Table 3. Laboratory Findings of Patients According to Neutrophil Percentage-to-Albumin Ratio (NPAR).

Laboratory Parameters	All Patients 135 (100%) Median (IQR)	NPAR ≤ 0.286 48 (35.6%) Median (IQR)	NPAR > 0.286 87 (64.4%) Median (IQR)	p-Value
Neutrophil percentage (%)	86.8 (79.6–91.8)	84.90 (75.52–90.35)	88.20 (81.40–92.20)	0.008
Albumin (g/L)	30 (36–35)	34 (32–37)	28 (25–31)	<0.001
NPAR *	0.32 (0.25–2.58)	0.24 (0.22–0.26)	2.27 (0.33–2.89)	<0.001
Procalcitonin (ng/mL)	0.30 (0.12–0.92)	0.18 (0.05–0.59)	0.36 (0.15–1.59)	0.020
Lactate	2.60 (1.62–3.10)	2.35 (1.45–2.75)	2.90 (1.90–3.30)	0.003
Blood urea nitrogen (mg/dL)	60 (36–90)	58 (33–88)	65 (48–97)	0.167

Table 3. Cont.

Laboratory Parameters	All Patients 135 (100%) Median (IQR)	NPAR ≤ 0.286 48 (35.6%) Median (IQR)	NPAR > 0.286 87 (64.4%) Median (IQR)	p-Value
Creatinine (mg/dL)	1.29 (1.0–1.95)	1.20 (0.90–1.90)	1.34 (1.06–1.97)	0.206
Potassium (mmol/L)	4.30 (3.89–4.90)	4.02 (3.70–4.80)	4.60 (4.10–5.08)	<0.001
C-reactive protein (CRP) (mg/L)	51 (9.4–141)	23 (4.9–141)	76 (39–142)	0.011
Neutrophil ($\times 10^3/\mu L$)	10.20 (7.57–14.30)	9.58 (7.74–13.04)	10.80 (7.50–15.50)	0.176
Platelet count ($\times 10^3/\mu L$)	197 (163–247)	200 (160–251)	193 (164–242)	0.811

* NPAR: Neutrophil Percentage-to-Albumin Ratio.

NPAR was calculated as 0.291 (0.244–2.16) in survivors and 0.422 (0.298–3.092) in deceased patients. This difference between the groups was statistically significant ($p < 0.001$). The AUC value calculated to evaluate the mortality prediction power of NPAR was found to be 0.692. ($p < 0.001$). The optimal cut-off value was determined as 0.286, with a sensitivity of 83%, specificity of 47.6%, positive predictive value (PPV) of 50.6%, and negative predictive value (NPV) of 81.2% (Table 4) (Figure 2).

Table 4. ROC Analysis Results of Neutrophil Percentage-to-Albumin Ratio (NPAR) for Predicting Mortality.

	AUC	95% Confidence Interval	Cut-Off Value	Sensitivity (%)	Specificity (%)	PPV (%)	NPV (%)	LR+ *	LR− **	p-Value
NPAR ***	0.692	0.599–0.784	0.286	83	47.6	50.6	81.2	1.58	0.36	<0.001

* LR+: Positive likelihood ratio; ** LR−: Negative likelihood ratio *** NPAR: Neutrophil Percentage-to-Albumin Ratio.

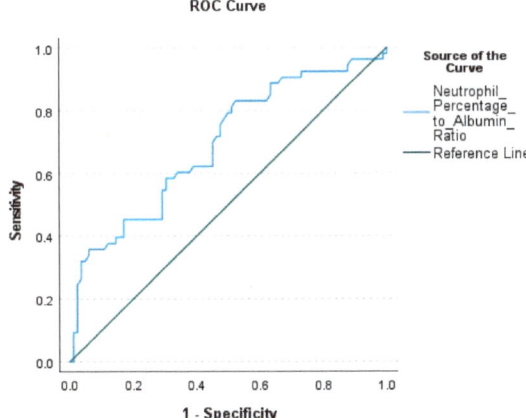

Figure 2. ROC Curve of Neutrophil Percentage-to-Albumin Ratio (NPAR) for Predicting Mortality.

In the univariate Cox regression analysis, patients with NPAR > 0.286 had a significantly increased risk of mortality (HR = 3.318, 95% CI: 1.616–6.812, $p = 0.001$). Similarly, mortality was significantly increased in patients with high APACHE-II and SOFA scores. The need for renal replacement therapy and vasopressor support were also significantly related to mortality. The strongest association was observed with the requirement for invasive mechanical ventilation (IMV); patients who required IMV had an approximately 20-fold higher risk of mortality (HR = 20.297, 95% CI: 8.019–51.374, p < 0.001). In contrast, variables such as cardiovascular disease (p = 0.524), hypertension (p = 0.172), and the presence of comorbidities (p = 0.078) were not significantly associated with mortality.

In the multivariate analysis, an NPAR level > 0.286 was identified as an independent risk factor for mortality (HR = 2.488, 95% CI: 1.167–5.302, p = 0.018). The APACHE II score remained significantly associated with increased mortality risk (HR = 1.077, 95% CI: 1.013–1.147, p = 0.019), whereas the SOFA score was not found to be an independent predictor in the multivariate model (p = 0.156). The need for renal replacement therapy was also determined to be an independent predictor of mortality (HR = 1.969, 95% CI: 1.046–3.705, p = 0.036). The requirement for invasive mechanical ventilation remained the strongest independent risk factor (Table 5).

Table 5. Cox Regression Analysis Results for Factors Associated with Mortality.

Variable	Univariate Cox Regression		Multivariate Cox Regression	
	HR (95% CI)	p-Value	HR (95% CI)	p-Value
Age	1.045 (0.989–1.104)	0.114		
Presence of comorbidities	2.290 (0.911–5.760)	0.078		
Cardiovascular disease	0.830 (0.469–1.471)	0.524		
Hypertension	0.682 (0.394–1.180)	0.172		
APACHE II score	1.163 (1.118–1.209)	**<0.001**	1.077 (1.013–1.147)	**0.019**
SOFA score	1.291 (1.193–1.398)	**<0.001**	1.100 (0.964–1.254)	0.156
NPAR * > 0.286	3.318 (1.616–6.812)	**0.001**	2.488 (1.167–5.302)	**0.018**
Need for renal replacement therapy	3.788 (2.185–6.567)	**<0.001**	1.969 (1.046–3.705)	**0.036**
Need for vasopressor therapy	4.166 (2.385–7.279)	**<0.001**	0.616 (0.311–1.220)	0.165
Need for invasive mechanical ventilation	20.297 (8.019–51.374)	**<0.001**	9.446 (3.402–26.229)	**<0.001**

* NPAR: Neutrophil Percentage-to-Albumin Ratio.

When comorbid conditions were evaluated, the rates of hypertension and cardiovascular disease were found to be higher in the low NPAR group (p < 0.001 and p = 0.007, respectively). However, when the association of comorbidities with mortality was assessed using Cox regression analysis, neither hypertension (p = 0.172) nor cardiovascular disease (p = 0.524) showed a statistically significant relationship.

According to the Kaplan–Meier survival analysis, the survival rate was significantly lower in the high NPAR group (Figure 3). The log-rank test revealed a statistically significant difference in survival times between the NPAR groups (p < 0.001).

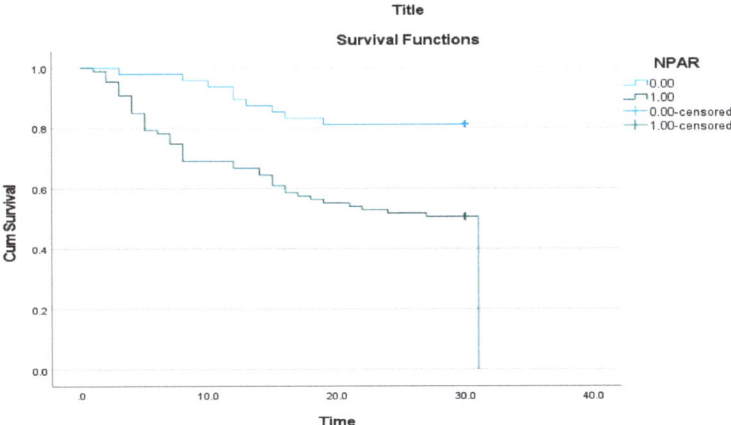

Figure 3. Kaplan–Meier Analysis of the Association Between Neutrophil Percentage-to-Albumin Ratio (NPAR) and Mortality.

4. Discussion

This study was conducted to evaluate the prognostic value of the neutrophil percentage-to-albumin ratio (NPAR) in pneumonia patients aged 80 years and older admitted to the intensive care unit. Our findings demonstrate that elevated NPAR levels are significantly associated with disease severity markers such as SOFA and APACHE II scores, and may be linked to worse clinical outcomes during the intensive care course. The results of the Kaplan–Meier survival analysis showed that higher NPAR levels were associated with significantly lower survival rates. Furthermore, in the multivariate Cox regression analysis, NPAR was identified as an independent predictor of mortality, and this association was found to be independent of other clinical variables such as comorbidities, disease severity, and organ failure. Elevated NPAR was also significantly associated with the need for invasive mechanical ventilation (IMV), vasopressor use, and the development of sepsis. This suggests that NPAR may also reflect critical clinical conditions such as hemodynamic instability and organ dysfunction. Based on these findings, NPAR—as a simple, rapid, and widely accessible laboratory parameter—may be considered a clinically useful biomarker for predicting disease severity and mortality risk in pneumonia patients aged 80 years and older. However, for a more comprehensive evaluation of this relationship, large-scale, multicenter prospective studies including different patient populations are needed.

In very elderly individuals, the immune response to infections is significantly influenced by the presence of comorbid conditions. Chronic diseases in this age group affect not only susceptibility to infections but also the severity of the clinical course and the need for intensive care. According to the literature, chronic pulmonary diseases, diabetes mellitus, cardiovascular diseases, and neurological disorders are among the most commonly reported comorbidities, and they have been associated with increased rates of sepsis and mortality [4,16]. In our study, at least one comorbid condition was present in 82.2% of the patients, with cardiovascular diseases and chronic obstructive pulmonary disease (COPD) being the most prevalent. Although the mortality rate was significantly higher among patients with comorbidities, multivariate regression analysis did not identify the presence of comorbidity as an independent predictor of mortality.

Interestingly, we observed that patients with higher NPAR values tended to have fewer comorbidities. This finding may be related to the prioritization of acute illness severity over chronic disease burden during ICU admission. Patients with fewer comorbidities but a more pronounced inflammatory response—and therefore a more severe clinical presentation—may have been more likely to be admitted to intensive care. This observation suggests that, in elderly patients, not only the presence of comorbidities but also biomarkers reflecting the degree of systemic inflammation may play a key role in patient management and risk stratification.

Serum albumin is a negative acute-phase reactant involved in inflammatory processes and exhibits antioxidant properties by interacting with bioactive lipid mediators, which are critical components of the immune response [17]. Malnutrition has previously been shown to be associated with poor clinical outcomes in patients with pneumonia [18]. It is well established that, with advancing age, nutritional deficiencies are directly related to immune system impairment. In our study, hypoalbuminemia, along with elevated NPAR, was significantly associated with increased mortality. This finding suggests that low albumin levels may influence pneumonia prognosis through mechanisms related to both inflammation and nutritional status. Therefore, in elderly patients with pneumonia, clinicians should consider not only nutritional status but also the underlying inflammatory state. When necessary, in addition to early nutritional support, interventions targeting the control of the inflammatory response should also be prioritized.

Neutrophils are key components of the systemic inflammatory response to infection and represent one of the most important cells of the innate immune system. Moreover, they are known to be closely associated with organ dysfunction in the setting of severe infections and sepsis [19]. In recent years, NPAR has been evaluated across various disease groups and has emerged as a promising prognostic biomarker. Elevated NPAR levels have been shown to be associated with mortality in patients with cerebrovascular diseases, cardiovascular diseases, and chronic obstructive pulmonary disease (COPD) [8,9,20]. In a study conducted on ICU patients diagnosed with sepsis, NPAR measured at admission was reported to be a significant predictor of 28-day mortality [21]. Although the prognostic role of NPAR has been explored in a range of clinical settings, the majority of these studies have focused on the general population or relatively younger patients. For instance, in the study by Hu et al. involving septic patients, the median age was approximately 65 years, whereas in our study, the median age was 86. Similarly, in the NHANES database analysis by Lan et al., which included a COPD population, the mean age was below 70 years [8]. While these studies have demonstrated a significant association between elevated NPAR and mortality, age-related changes such as variability in the inflammatory response, decreased serum albumin levels, and an increased burden of comorbidities may influence the prognostic performance of this parameter in older adults. Our study is among the few to evaluate the prognostic value of NPAR specifically in the very elderly population and demonstrates that NPAR is significantly associated with mortality in this age group. This finding supports the potential of NPAR as a simple and practical biomarker for early risk stratification in older patients.

A high NPAR value reflects an increased systemic inflammatory burden, resulting from an elevated neutrophil percentage, decreased serum albumin levels, or a combination of both. In patients with pneumonia, this condition simultaneously indicates a severe inflammatory response as well as compromised nutritional and physiological reserves. In elderly individuals, physiological changes such as immunosenescence, chronic low-grade inflammation, and malnutrition are common. These alterations impair immune defenses and negatively affect recovery from infections. Therefore, elevated NPAR levels in older adults may be directly associated with adverse clinical outcomes and increased mortality risk. In our study, NPAR demonstrated prognostic sensitivity comparable to that of the widely used SOFA score. Given that it is derived from only two routine laboratory parameters, NPAR may serve as a practical biomarker to support clinical decision-making in elderly patients with pneumonia.

Recent research suggests that NPAR may serve not only as a prognostic marker but also as a potential indicator for guiding therapeutic strategies. For instance, a study by Liu and Chien reported that elevated NPAR levels were significantly associated with non-alcoholic fatty liver disease and advanced liver fibrosis [7]. This finding highlights the ability of NPAR to reflect both systemic inflammation and nutritional deficits. Accordingly, early detection of elevated NPAR levels in patients with pneumonia may act as a clinical warning sign, prompting timely, targeted interventions. Specifically, early nutritional support to address hypoalbuminemia and anti-inflammatory strategies aimed at controlling neutrophil-mediated inflammation may improve outcomes in this vulnerable patient population.

According to the intensive care unit admission criteria established by the American Thoracic Society (ATS) and the Infectious Diseases Society of America (IDSA), the need for vasopressors and mechanical ventilation are considered major indicators in critically ill patients [22]. In our study, mortality was found to be higher in patients who required vasopressor support and invasive mechanical ventilation (IMV), and these factors were identified as independent predictors of mortality. Additionally, patients with elevated NPAR levels were significantly more likely to require vasopressor therapy and IMV. These findings suggest that NPAR may reflect not only inflammatory processes but also critical clinical conditions such as hemodynamic instability and respiratory failure.

The APACHE II and SOFA scores are widely used scoring systems for assessing disease severity and predicting mortality in critically ill patients [23–25]. In our study, the APACHE II score was found to be an independent prognostic predictor of mortality, whereas the SOFA score did not remain significant in the multivariate analysis. Additionally, increases in both APACHE II and SOFA scores were significantly associated with elevated NPAR levels. An NPAR level > 0.286 was shown to be an independent predictor of mortality. These findings suggest that NPAR may serve as a biomarker reflecting disease severity and could assist in the early identification of clinical deterioration (i.e., worsening physiological status, including hemodynamic instability, respiratory failure, and progression of organ dysfunction).

This study has several limitations. First, the single-center and retrospective design limits the generalizability of the findings to broader and more heterogeneous populations. The inclusion of only very elderly patients aged 80 years and older may restrict the applicability of the results to younger individuals with pneumonia. Furthermore, as all participants met ICU admission criteria, the study population may not fully represent the entire spectrum of older adults. Comorbidities were evaluated based solely on their number; validated scoring systems such as the Charlson Comorbidity Index (CCI), which could provide a more accurate assessment of their impact on mortality, were not used. Due to the retrospective nature of the study, detailed diagnostic data required for calculating the CCI were unavailable. Future studies incorporating validated comorbidity indices could enhance the accuracy of prognostic assessments.

In addition, the NPAR cutoff value used in this study was derived from a limited sample within a single center and demonstrated only moderate discriminatory performance (AUC: 0.692). Therefore, large-scale, multicenter, prospective validation studies are needed to assess the reliability and clinical applicability of this cutoff value. Although NPAR showed high sensitivity, its relatively low specificity suggests that it may not be sufficient as a standalone predictor of mortality and should be interpreted in conjunction with other clinical parameters.

Moreover, several potential confounding variables could not be evaluated due to data limitations. These include patients' objective nutritional status, timing of antibiotic initiation, timing of ICU admission, characteristics of the causative pathogens (e.g., Gram-positive/negative bacteria, viruses, fungi), and the appropriateness and duration of antibiotic therapy. These limitations, inherent to the retrospective design, should be considered when interpreting the study findings.

5. Conclusions

The findings of this study suggest that the neutrophil percentage-to-albumin ratio (NPAR) may serve as a prognostic biomarker in pneumonia patients aged 80 years and older admitted to the intensive care unit. Elevated NPAR levels were significantly associated with increased disease severity, higher mortality, and a greater need for invasive mechanical ventilation. Cox regression analysis identified NPAR as an independent predictor of mortality, supporting its potential for clinical use. Given that it is an easily calculable and widely accessible parameter, NPAR may be a useful adjunct biomarker in predicting mortality and guiding clinical decision-making in elderly patients with pneumonia. However, large-scale, multicenter, prospective studies are needed to validate these findings and further assess the role of NPAR in clinical practice.

Author Contributions: Conceptualization, M.A. and A.H.S.; methodology, T.O. and M.Y.; software, O.M. and D.C.; validation, M.D. and G.E.D.; formal analysis, E.A., H.T.M., and O.F.T.; investigation, M.A. and E.U.; resources, M.A. and A.H.S.; data curation, O.M., H.T.M., and O.F.T.; writing—original draft preparation, M.A. and A.H.S.; writing—review and editing, M.D. and G.E.D.; visualization, E.U.; supervision, D.C.; project administration, M.A. All authors have read and agreed to the published version of the manuscript.

Funding: This research received no external funding.

Institutional Review Board Statement: Ethical approval was obtained from the Clinical Research Ethics Committee of Ankara Ataturk Sanatorium Training and Research Hospital (Decision no: 2839, dated 16 July 2024).

Informed Consent Statement: Informed consent was not required due to the retrospective nature of the study.

Data Availability Statement: The original contributions presented in this study are included in the article. Further inquiries can be directed to the corresponding author.

Conflicts of Interest: The authors declare no conflicts of interest.

References

1. Cillóniz, C.; Dominedò, C.; Pericàs, J.M.; Rodriguez-Hurtado, D.; Torres, A. Community-acquired pneumonia in critically ill very old patients: A growing problem. *Eur. Respir. Rev.* **2020**, *29*, 190126. [CrossRef] [PubMed]
2. United Nations Department of Economic and Social Affairs. *Population Division: World Population Prospects 2019. Ten Key Findings*; United Nations Department of Economic and Social Affairs: New York, NY, USA, 2019.
3. Lee, S.I.; Huh, J.W.; Hong, S.B.; Koh, Y.; Lim, C.M. Age Distribution and Clinical Results of Critically Ill Patients Above 65-Year-Old in an Aging Society: A Retrospective Cohort Study. *Tuberc. Respir. Dis.* **2024**, *87*, 338–348. [CrossRef] [PubMed]
4. Laporte, L.; Hermetet, C.; Jouan, Y.; Gaborit, C.; Rouve, E.; Shea, K.M.; Si-Tahar, M.; Dequin, P.F.; Grammatico-Guillon, L.; Guillon, A. Ten-year trends in intensive care admissions for respiratory infections in the elderly. *Ann. Intensive Care* **2018**, *8*, 84. [CrossRef]
5. Othman, A.; Sekheri, M.; Filep, J.G. Roles of neutrophil granule proteins in orchestrating inflammation and immunity. *FEBS J.* **2022**, *289*, 3932–3953. [CrossRef]

6. Eckart, A.; Struja, T.; Kutz, A.; Baumgartner, A.; Baumgartner, T.; Zurfluh, S.; Neeser, O.; Huber, A.; Stanga, Z.; Mueller, B.; et al. Relationship of Nutritional Status, Inflammation, and Serum Albumin Levels During Acute Illness: A Prospective Study. *Am. J. Med.* **2020**, *133*, 713–722.e7. [CrossRef]
7. Liu, C.F.; Chien, L.W. Predictive Role of Neutrophil-Percentage-to-Albumin Ratio (NPAR) in Nonalcoholic Fatty Liver Disease and Advanced Liver Fibrosis in Nondiabetic US Adults: Evidence from NHANES 2017–2018. *Nutrients* **2023**, *15*, 1892. [CrossRef]
8. Lan, C.C.; Su, W.L.; Yang, M.C.; Chen, S.Y.; Wu, Y.K. Predictive role of neutrophil-percentage-to-albumin, neutrophil-to-lymphocyte and eosinophil-to-lymphocyte ratios for mortality in patients with COPD: Evidence from NHANES 2011–2018. *Respirology* **2023**, *28*, 1136–1146. [CrossRef]
9. Lv, X.N.; Shen, Y.Q.; Li, Z.Q.; Deng, L.; Wang, Z.J.; Cheng, J.; Hu, X.; Pu, M.J.; Yang, W.S.; Xie, P.; et al. Neutrophil percentage to albumin ratio is associated with stroke-associated pneumonia and poor outcome in patients with spontaneous intracerebral hemorrhage. *Front. Immunol.* **2023**, *14*, 1173718. [CrossRef] [PubMed]
10. Cai, J.; Li, M.; Wang, W.; Luo, R.; Zhang, Z.; Liu, H. The Relationship Between the Neutrophil Percentage-to-Albumin Ratio and Rates of 28-Day Mortality in Atrial Fibrillation Patients 80 Years of Age or Older. *J. Inflamm. Res.* **2023**, *16*, 1629–1638. [CrossRef]
11. Xu, M.; Huan, J.; Zhu, L.; Xu, J.; Song, K. The neutrophil percentage-to-albumin ratio is an independent risk factor for poor prognosis in peritoneal dialysis patients. *Ren. Fail.* **2024**, *46*, 2294149. [CrossRef]
12. Yu, Y.; Zhong, Z.; Yang, W.; Yu, J.; Li, J.; Guo, X.; Chen, J.; Mao, H.; Li, Z. Neutrophil Percentage-to-Albumin Ratio and Risk of Mortality in Patients on Peritoneal Dialysis. *J. Inflamm. Res.* **2023**, *16*, 6271–6281. [CrossRef] [PubMed]
13. Singer, M.; Deutschman, C.S.; Seymour, C.W.; Shankar-Hari, M.; Annane, D.; Bauer, M.; Bellomo, R.; Bernard, G.R.; Chiche, J.D.; Cooper-smith, C.M.; et al. The Third International Consensus Definitions for Sepsis and Septic Shock (Sepsis 3). *JAMA* **2016**, *315*, 801–810. [CrossRef] [PubMed]
14. Vincent, J.L.; Moreno, R.; Takala, J.; Willatts, S.; De Mendonça, A.; Bruining, H.; Reinhart, C.K.; Suter, P.M.; Thijs, L.G. The SOFA (Sepsis-related Organ Failure Assessment) score to describe organ dysfunction failure. On behalf of the Working Group on Sepsis-Related Problems of the European Society of Intensive Care Medicine. *Intensive Care Med.* **1996**, *22*, 707–710. [CrossRef] [PubMed]
15. Knaus, W.A.; Draper, E.A.; Wagner, D.P.; Zimmerman, J.E. APACHE II: A severity of disease classification system. *Crit. Care Med.* **1985**, *13*, 818–829. [CrossRef]
16. Montull, B.; Menéndez, R.; Torres, A.; Reyes, S.; Méndez, R.; Zalacaín, R.; Capelastegui, A.; Rajas, O.; Borderías, L.; Martin-Villasclaras, J.; et al. Predictors of Severe Sepsis among Patients Hospitalized for Community-Acquired Pneumonia. *PLoS ONE* **2016**, *11*, e0145929. [CrossRef]
17. Wiedermann, C.J. Hypoalbuminemia as Surrogate and Culprit of Infections. *Int. J. Mol. Sci.* **2021**, *22*, 4496. [CrossRef]
18. Lin, C.J.; Chang, Y.C.; Tsou, M.T.; Chan, H.L.; Chen, Y.J.; Hwang, L.C. Factors associated with hospitalization for community-acquired pneumonia in home health care patients in Taiwan. *Aging Clin. Exp. Res.* **2020**, *32*, 149–155. [CrossRef]
19. Zhang, F.; Zhang, Z.; Ma, X. Neutrophil extracellular traps and coagulation dysfunction in sepsis. *Zhonghua Wei Zhong Bing Ji Jiu Yi Xue* **2017**, *29*, 752–755.
20. Wang, X.; Zhang, Y.; Wang, Y.; Liu, J.; Xu, X.; Liu, J.; Chen, M.; Shi, L. The neutrophil percentage-to-albumin ratio is associated with all-cause mortality in patients with chronic heart failure. *BMC Cardiovasc. Disord.* **2023**, *23*, 568. [CrossRef]
21. Hu, C.; He, Y.; Li, J.; Zhang, C.; Hu, Q.; Li, W.; Hao, C. Association between neutrophil percentage-to-albumin ratio and 28-day mortality in Chinese patients with sepsis. *J. Int. Med. Res.* **2023**, *51*, 3000605231178512. [CrossRef]
22. Mandell, L.A.; Wunderink, R.G.; Anzueto, A.; Bartlett, J.G.; Campbell, G.D.; Dean, N.C.; Dowell, S.F.; File, T.M., Jr.; Musher, D.M.; Niederman, M.S.; et al. Infectious Diseases Society of America; American Thoracic Society. Infectious Diseases Society of America/American Thoracic Society consensus guidelines on the management of community-acquired pneumonia in adults. *Clin. Infect. Dis.* **2007**, *44*, S27–S72. [CrossRef] [PubMed]
23. Farajzadeh, M.; Nasrollahi, E.; Bahramvand, Y.; Mohammadkarimi, V.; Dalfardi, B.; Anushiravani, A. The use of APACHE II Scoring System for predicting clinical outcome of patients admitted to the intensive care unit: A report from a resource-limited center. *Shraz E-Med. J.* **2021**, *22*, e102858. [CrossRef]
24. Mumtaz, H.; Ejaz, M.K.; Tayyab, M.; Vohra, L.I.; Sapkota, S.; Hasan, M.; Saqib, M. APACHE scoring as an indicator of mortality rate in ICU patients: A cohort study. *Ann. Med. Surg.* **2023**, *85*, 416–421. [CrossRef] [PubMed]
25. Shafigh, N.; Hasheminik, M.; Shafigh, E.; Alipour, H.; Sayyadi, S.; Kazeminia, N.; Khoundabi, B.; Salarian, S. Prediction of mortality in ICU patients: A comparison between the SOFA score and other indicators. *Nurs. Crit. Care* **2023**, *29*, 1619–1622. [CrossRef]

Disclaimer/Publisher's Note: The statements, opinions and data contained in all publications are solely those of the individual author(s) and contributor(s) and not of MDPI and/or the editor(s). MDPI and/or the editor(s) disclaim responsibility for any injury to people or property resulting from any ideas, methods, instructions or products referred to in the content.

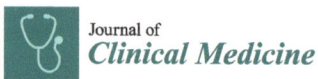

Review

Role of Respiratory Viruses in Severe Acute Respiratory Failure

David Mokrani [1] and Jean-François Timsit [1,2,*]

[1] Infectious and Intensive Care Unit, Centre Hospitalier Universitaire Bichat-Claude Bernard, Assistance Publique-Hôpitaux de Paris, 75018 Paris, France; david.mokrani@aphp.fr
[2] Infection Antimicrobials Modelling Evolution (IAME), Mixt Research Unit (UMR) 1137, INSERM, Université Paris-Cité, 75018 Paris, France
* Correspondence: jean-francois.timsit@aphp.fr

Abstract: Respiratory viruses are widespread in the community, affecting both the upper and lower respiratory tract. This review provides an updated synthesis of the epidemiology, pathophysiology, clinical impact, and management of severe respiratory viral infections in critically ill patients, with a focus on immunocompetent adults. The clinical presentation is typically nonspecific, making etiological diagnosis challenging. This limitation has been mitigated by the advent of molecular diagnostics—particularly multiplex PCR (mPCR)—which has not only improved pathogen identification at the bedside but also significantly reshaped our understanding of the epidemiology of respiratory viral infections. Routine mPCR testing has revealed that respiratory viruses are implicated in 30–40% of community-acquired pneumonia hospitalizations and are a frequent trigger of acute decompensations in patients with chronic comorbidities. While some viruses follow seasonal patterns, others circulate year-round. Influenza viruses and Pneumoviridae, including respiratory syncytial virus and human metapneumovirus, remain the principal viral pathogens associated with severe outcomes, particularly acute respiratory failure and mortality. Bacterial co-infections are also common and substantially increase both morbidity and mortality. Despite the growing contribution of respiratory viruses to the burden of critical illness, effective antiviral therapies remain limited. Neuraminidase inhibitors remain the cornerstone of treatment for severe influenza, whereas therapeutic options for other respiratory viruses are largely lacking. Optimizing early diagnosis, refining antiviral strategies, and systematically addressing bacterial co-infections are critical to improving outcomes in patients with severe viral pneumonia.

Keywords: ARDS; pneumonia; acute respiratory failure; viruses; mPCR; influenzae; pneumoviridae; respiratory syncytial virus; metapneumovirus; baloxavir; oseltamivir; emergent infections

1. Introduction

With the increasing use of molecular assays, the detection of viral pathogens in critically ill adults with respiratory illnesses has become more common. The reported prevalence rates range from 17% to 53%, depending on factors such as the study design, sample type, illness duration, and assay techniques. Viruses most frequently identified in patients with severe respiratory illnesses include influenza A and B, picornaviruses (like rhinovirus and enterovirus, e.g., enterovirus D68), human coronaviruses (229E, NL63, OC43, and HKU1), respiratory syncytial virus (RSV), human metapneumovirus (hMPV), parainfluenza virus, and adenovirus. In addition, emerging zoonotic coronaviruses—such as those causing Severe Acute Respiratory Syndrome (SARS), Middle East Respiratory Syndrome (MERS), and COVID-19—continue to be identified. However, attributing clinical illness to a specific viral pathogen remains challenging. Some viruses, such as picornaviruses, may be detected in the upper respiratory tract without causing symptoms. Conversely, upper airway samples may yield false-negative results in patients with lower respiratory tract involvement. Furthermore, the co-detection of bacterial and, less frequently, fungal pathogens is common. Nevertheless, respiratory viruses are now widely recognized as independent causes of severe disease, particularly in older adults and those with underlying comorbidities (especially the immunocompromised), and occasionally in previously healthy individuals. These infections can also exacerbate chronic conditions and increase the risk of secondary infections.

The objective of this narrative review is to provide a comprehensive synthesis of the current evidence on the management of immunocompetent adults admitted to intensive care units (ICUs) for community-acquired severe acute respiratory infections (SARIs) caused by respiratory viruses (excluding SARS-CoV-2). The review specifically focuses on viral pathogens transmitted through the respiratory route and on immunocompetent adults. Herpesviruses will not be discussed, as they are not typical respiratory pathogens, are predominantly detected in nosocomial settings, and are primarily associated with viral reactivation and relative immunosuppression in mechanically ventilated patients, rather than with true respiratory acquisition.

Literature Search Strategy

This review is based on a comprehensive literature search conducted in PubMed and Google Scholar, focusing on publications from the period following the widespread implementation of PCR testing. For each respiratory virus addressed, all relevant studies were reviewed from the time PCR testing became routinely available, with earlier publications included when essential for clinical or historical context. Search strings combined MeSH terms and free-text keywords using Boolean operators, for example: ("lower respiratory tract infection" OR "pneumonia" OR "viral pneumonia") AND ("influenza" OR "RSV" OR "respiratory syncytial virus" OR "human metapneumovirus" OR "rhinovirus" OR "adenovirus" OR "parainfluenza" OR "coronavirus"). The search was limited to English-language literature. Case reports were excluded, except for those concerning human bocavirus, due to the paucity of available clinical data. Recent and relevant peer-reviewed studies—including observational cohorts, randomized controlled trials, and meta-analyses—were prioritized. Reference lists of key articles were manually screened to ensure completeness. A total of 2897 records were initially identified through title screening. A subset was selected for abstract review, followed by the full-text evaluation of studies deemed relevant to the scope of this review.

2. Impact of Molecular Testing in Discovering Viruses in Lower Respiratory Tract Infections

The introduction of multiplex PCR (mPCR) after 2007, allowing the simultaneous detection of a broad spectrum of respiratory viruses, has profoundly transformed the epidemiological understanding of lower respiratory tract infections (LRTIs). Available platforms demonstrate a positive predictive agreement exceeding 95% when compared with gold-standard reference methods [1,2]. However, the clinical relevance of viral detection remains uncertain, ranging from true pathogenicity to incidental colonization or transient respiratory carriage. This variability likely depends on the specific virus involved, the host immune status, the timing of the specimen collection, and the anatomical sampling site.

While nasopharyngeal PCR remains the standard of care (SOC) for viral detection in most clinical settings, its relevance for diagnosing LRTIs is debated. Studies have reported both underdiagnosis—when upper airway samples yield false-negative results despite lower tract involvement—and overdiagnosis, particularly in the context of asymptomatic viral carriage or prolonged viral shedding [3]. Evidence from longitudinal nasopharyngeal sampling in U.S. households has demonstrated that a viral presence in the upper respiratory tract is common. In 108 individuals from 26 families sampled weekly, 783 viruses were recovered from nasopharyngeal PCR tests and were associated with respiratory symptoms in only 56% of cases [4]. A prolonged viral detection lasting more than 4 weeks was common for bocavirus and rhinovirus, likely reflecting either prolonged excretion or reinfections. These discrepancies highlight the limitations of relying solely on upper respiratory tract specimens for the diagnosis of severe viral pneumonia.

The use of mPCR assays that integrate both bacterial and viral targets may further influence the reported prevalence of viral infections. Among commercially available tools, the FilmArray Pneumonia Panel (FA-PP, bioMérieux™, Marcy l'Etoile, France) is currently the only mPCR platform that includes eight viral targets. Although increasing evidence supports the role of bacterial–viral co-infections in exacerbating pneumonia severity, the clinical utility of the FA-PP for their detection remains incompletely established [5–8]. The interpretation of viral epidemiology by the FA-PP is challenging due to substantial heterogeneity in study populations. Some studies focus exclusively on FA-PP-positive bacterial samples, which inherently biases the viral detection towards bacterial–viral co-infections [9–11]. Furthermore, studies often confound community- and hospital-acquired LRTIs or are limited to cohorts of SARS-CoV-2 infections, limiting conclusions about the broader role of viral detection [11,12]. Across published studies, viral detection rates using the FA-PP range from 15% to 51%, while bacterial–viral co-infections are identified in 10% to 38% of cases, depending on the population and pneumonia subtype [13–22]. In one study, the FA-PP identified nearly twice as many viral pathogens as the SOC testing, likely due to the broader scope of sputum testing compared to nasopharyngeal sampling [18]. However, in 95% of cases where the FA-PP was the only method used to detect a virus, no SOC test was performed, limiting direct comparisons and suggesting the underuse of viral diagnostics.

Collectively, these findings suggest that viral detection using mPCR pneumonia panels may provide useful clinical insight, particularly in critically ill patients. Nevertheless, the true impact of such diagnostics on clinical decision-making and patient outcomes remains to be clearly established. Further research is needed to clarify their role in pneumonia management. Table 1 summarizes the key features of currently available commercial respiratory mPCR kits.

Table 1. Commercially available respiratory mPCR kits in 2025: key features and viral targets.

	Xtag Respiratory Viral Panel FastV2	Respifinder Smart 22 Fast	Allplex Respiratory Panel Assays	Filmarray Respiratory Plus 2,1 Panel	ePlex Respiratory Pathogen 2 Panel	QIAstatDx Respiratory Panel 2
PCR	Luminex Semi quantitative	Pathofinder Final	Seegene Real time	Biofire Final	GenMark Dx Final	Qiagen Real time
Turn-around time	4 h	6 h	4 h 30 min	45 min	70 min	70 min
Targets						
Influenzae A and B	X	X	X	X	X	X
Respiratory syncytial virus	X	X	X	X	X	X
Rhinovirus/enterovirus	X	X	X	X	X	X
Human metapneumovirus	X	X	X	X	X	X
Human coronaviruses	X	X	X	X	X	X
Parainfluenza virus	X	X	X	X	X	X
Adenovirus	X	X	X	X	X	X
Bocavirus	X	X	X		X	X
Mers-Cov				X	X	
SARS-CoV-2				X	X	X

3. Physiopathology of Respiratory Viral Infections

3.1. Epithelial Tropism and Viral-Induced Cell Death

Respiratory viruses, including influenza, RSV, and hMPV, demonstrate a marked tropism for the respiratory epithelium, infecting both the upper and lower respiratory tract. Influenza primarily targets ciliated epithelial cells in the upper airways and extends to secretory cells and type I and II alveolar epithelial cells in the lower respiratory tract [23,24]. Emerging evidence indicates that α2-6 sialic acids, predominantly expressed in the upper respiratory tract, are also present in respiratory bronchioles. This enables the viral spread to the lower airways, exacerbating epithelial damage and contributing to alveolar collapse [25,26]. Similarly, RSV and hMPV compromise the epithelial barrier by disrupting tight junctions and impairing ciliary function, thereby facilitating viral dissemination throughout the respiratory tree [27,28]. Adenoviruses, although less common, exhibit a similar capacity to infect alveolar structures and cause severe pulmonary injury, even in immunocompetent hosts [29,30]. Virus-induced cell death, including apoptosis and necrosis, exacerbates this epithelial damage [31,32]. For example, influenza and RSV trigger mitochondrial dysfunction and caspase activation, which impair repair mechanisms and compromise respiratory integrity [33,34]. Advanced experimental models, such as organoids and transcriptomics, further support the ability of these viruses to infect and damage alveolar epithelial cells, highlighting their capacity to disrupt the respiratory barrier [27,35]. Collectively, these findings underscore that the pathogenesis of these viruses involves the entire respiratory tree, explaining their central role in severe LRTIs and acute respiratory failure (ARF).

3.2. Immune Dysregulation and Inflammation-Mediated Injury

Respiratory viruses trigger immune responses that are essential for viral clearance but can also drive significant immune-mediated lung injuries [36]. Influenza infection induces a strong activation of macrophages and dendritic cells, resulting in the release of cytokines such as TNF-α, IL-6, and type I interferons. While these mediators are critical for recruiting immune cells and priming adaptive immunity, the excessive release may drive a "cytokine storm", amplifying inflammation and causing diffuse alveolar damage and acute respiratory distress syndrome [37]. Similarly, RSV induces toll-like receptor activation on epithelial cells, leading to the production of chemokines, like IL-8, which recruit neutrophils and monocytes [27,38]. Although essential for pathogen clearance, these immune cells release reactive oxygen species and proteolytic enzymes that can exacerbate the epithelial injury. Respiratory viruses also alter the function of alveolar macrophages and CD8+ T cells. Macrophages, while pivotal for viral clearance, may adopt a pro-inflammatory phenotype, releasing TNF-α and IFN-γ. This overactivation contributes to epithelial disruption and lung injury. Similarly, CD8+ T cells eliminate infected epithelial cells but, when excessively activated, can cause tissue destruction and fibrosis [37]. Moreover, epithelial barrier disruption and impaired mucociliary clearance facilitate bacterial superinfections, particularly with *Streptococcus pneumoniae* and *Staphylococcus aureus*. This process is compounded by IFN-γ, which suppresses the alveolar macrophage-mediated bacterial clearance, further worsening lung injuries [39–41].

3.3. Histopathological Evidence from Human Studies

Histopathological studies demonstrate that respiratory viruses, including influenza, RSV, hMPV, and adenoviruses, cause significant injury in the lower respiratory tract. Findings from autopsy and biopsy studies reveal necrotizing bronchitis and bronchiolitis, diffuse alveolar damage with hyaline membranes, alveolar edema, and inflammatory cell infiltration as hallmarks of severe influenza infection [42]. RSV shows similar lesions, with the sloughing of the bronchiolar epithelium, mucus plugging, and neutrophilic alveolitis, contributing to airway obstruction and alveolar inflammation [43]. Adenoviruses induce necrotizing bronchopneumonia and interstitial inflammation, with severe cases reported in immunocompetent patients [44]. Although histopathological data on hMPV are scarce, the available evidence supports its potential to provoke interstitial and alveolar inflammation [45]. Across these infections, epithelial disruption facilitates secondary bacterial infections, which further exacerbate alveolar damage. The physiopathology of the respiratory viral lung injury is illustrated in Figure 1.

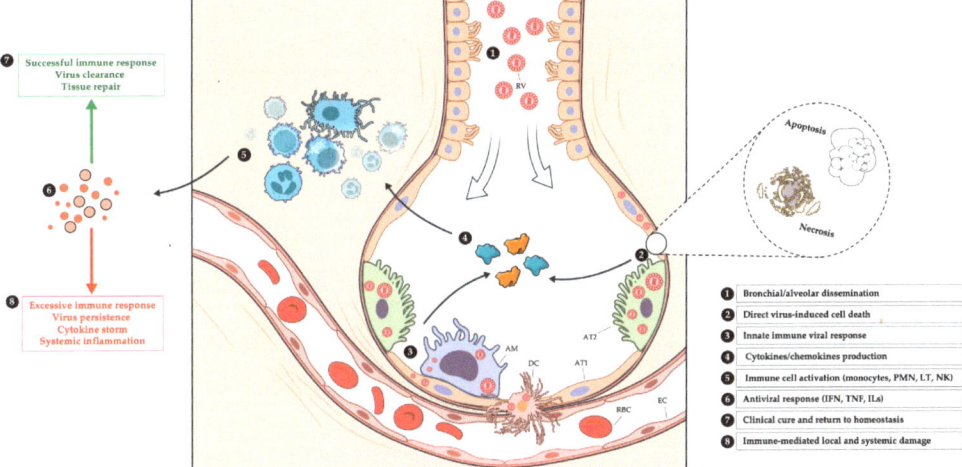

Figure 1. Pathophysiology of lung damage induced by respiratory viruses. AM: alveolar macrophages, AT1: alveolar type 1 cell, AT2: alveolar type 2 cell, DC: dendritic cell, EC: endothelial cell, IFN: interferon, ILs: interleukines, LT: T cell, NK: natural killer cell, PMN: polymorphonuclear leukocyte, RBC: red blood cell, and RV: respiratory virus. Illustrations from NIAID NIH BIOART Source Public Domain (bioart.niaid.nih.gov).

4. Clinical Consequences of Respiratory Virus in Severe Acute Respiratory Failure in ICU

Severe respiratory viral infections are a frequent cause of ICU admissions, typically presenting as ARF with or without pneumonia. Non-pneumonic ARF is often linked to exacerbations of underlying comorbidities, particularly chronic obstructive pulmonary disease (COPD) and cardiovascular conditions [46].

While the association between respiratory viruses and COPD exacerbations is well established, emerging evidence underscores their role in triggering cardiovascular complications. In a cohort of 6248 adults aged $\geq$50 years hospitalized with laboratory-confirmed RSV infections, 22.4% experienced acute cardiac events, including acute heart failure (15.8%), acute ischemic heart disease (7.5%), and hypertensive crises (1.3%) [47]. Influenza has similarly been shown to markedly increase vascular risk, with one study reporting a nearly tenfold rise in myocardial infarction risk (IRR 9.80, 95% CI 2.37–40.5) and a twelvefold increase in stroke risk (IRR 12.3, 95% CI 5.48–27.7) during the first three days post-infection [48]. These findings highlight the capacity of respiratory viruses not only to cause direct pulmonary injury but also to precipitate systemic complications.

In addition to non-pneumonic presentations, respiratory viruses are well-recognized causes of community-acquired pneumonia (CAP), with viral etiologies identified in approximately 30–40% of cases [5,49–51]. These infections typically present with systemic and respiratory symptoms, including fever, cough, myalgia, anorexia, and headache, with a median incubation period ≤ 7 days [52]. Importantly, this clinical presentation is neither specific to viral etiologies nor sufficient to distinguish between viral and bacterial causes [5,53]. Co-infections with bacterial pathogens are reported in up to 25% of viral pneumonia cases and are associated with a more severe presentation, including higher rates of sepsis and mechanical ventilation [5,54]. Thus, bacterial sampling remains crucial to guide timely antimicrobial therapy even when a viral pathogen is identified. These observations underscore the clinical heterogeneity of respiratory viral infections in ICU patients and the necessity of an integrated diagnostic approach to identify co-infections and systemic complications. Selected clinical vignettes are presented in Table 2.

Table 2. Clinical vignettes associated with major respiratory viruses.

Virus	Clinical Vignettes/Specific Data	Precautions/Prevention
Common respiratory viruses		
Influenza A and influenza B [55,56]	Short incubation (mean 2 days); viral shedding from 2 days prior to symptoms and peaks within 2–3 days afterwards. The most common cause of ICU admission either with pneumonia or with acute exacerbation of chronic or respiratory diseases. May be associated with acute myocardial infarction, myocarditis, rhabdomyolysis, acute renal failure, encephalopathy/encephalitis, and other non-pulmonary complications. New variants are associated with high transmissibility, milder diseases, and immune escape.	Droplet /Yearly vaccine
SARS-CoV-2 [57–59]	(JN.1 is the most common sublineage; KP 3.1.1 is rapidly growing). Case fatality rate is 1.9% higher in the elderly and low- and middle-income countries. Severe forms are observed in immunocompetent patients with comorbid conditions (chronic diseases, obesity, and elderly). Compared to historical variants, higher rate of cases in vaccinated people (but delay since the last dose) and shorter delay from first symptom to ICU admission (5 days). Winter season. Elderly patients with chronic respiratory or cardiac diseases.	Droplet + Airborne /Vaccine
Respiratory syncytial virus [46,60]	Immunodepression in one-third of the cases of poor prognosis. Commonly associated with exacerbation of chronic respiratory or cardiac insufficiency. Bronchospasm is common. New vaccines offer about 90% protection to adults over 65.	Contact /Vaccine
Human metapneumovirus [61]	Elderly patients with chronic respiratory or cardiac diseases. Hospital admission after a median delay of 3 days of symptoms. Half of patients present with pneumonia (interstitial). Immunodepression in one-third of the ICU cases.	Contact
Adenoviruses [62]	Usually mild symptoms, keratoconjunctivitis, and gastro-intestinal symptoms. Severe forms are rare but observed in young and middle-aged adults (median age 40 yo). ARDS is common. Some cases are associated with hepatitis. Rare cases of myocarditis, cardiomyopathy, pancreatitis, encephalitis, meningitis, and mononucleosis-like syndromes. Frequently detected in critically ill patients with severe acute respiratory infection.	Droplet + contact
Picornaviruses (rhinovirus and enterovirus)	Excretion > 2 months are common. Questionable impact on respiratory insufficiency and prognosis in immunocompetent adults.	Droplet
Human coronaviruses (229E, NL63, OC43, and HKU1) Parainfluenza (1–4)	Year-long transmissibility. May cause severe illness in the elderly, persons with comorbidities including immunosuppression. Parainfluenza: usually mild upper respiratory diseases, cases of laryngotracheobronchitis (croup) and bronchiolitis.	Contact

Table 2. Cont.

Virus	Clinical Vignettes/Specific Data	Precautions/Prevention
Uncommon and emerging viruses		
Avian influenza A/H5N1, A/H5N6, A/H7N9, and other subtypes [63]	Residence in or travel to Southeast and East Asia. Exposure to poultry or visits to poultry markets. Severe ARDS.	Airborne + contact
MERS-CoV	Severe pneumonia, gastro-intestinal symptoms. Residence in or travel to the Arabian Peninsula. Exposure to dromedary camel (in endemic areas). Nosocomial transmission risk to other patients and to healthcare workers.	Airborne + contact
Measles	Incomplete vaccination. Characteristic cutaneous rash. Progressive giant cell pneumonia.	Airborne /Vaccine
Hantaviruses (e.g., Sin Nombre and Andes)	Residence in or travel to affected areas of North, Central, or South America. Exposure to rodent excretions.	Standard

Abbreviations: ARDS, acute respiratory distress syndrome. Isolation precautions: adapted from https://www.cdc.gov/infection-control/hcp/viral-respiratory-prevention/ (accessed on 24 March 2025). NB: For all respiratory viruses: (1) Take measures to limit crowding in communal spaces, such as scheduling appointments to limit the number of patients in waiting rooms or treatment areas. (2) Encourage people with symptoms of respiratory infection to sit away from other patients. If possible, facilities may wish to place these people in a separate room while they are waiting for care. (3) During periods of increased community respiratory virus activity that results in a surge in visits, facilities could consider setting up triage stations that facilitate the rapid screening of patients for signs and symptoms of respiratory infection and separation from other patients.

5. Outcomes

Despite the clinical burden of respiratory viral infections, population-based epidemiological studies comparing outcomes remain scarce. Bajema et al. studied a retrospective cohort of 219,577 patients with a median age of 66 years from electronic health record data of non-hospitalized U.S. veterans who underwent same-day testing for SARS-CoV-2, influenza, and RSV during the autumn–winter season in 2023 and 2024 and had a single positive result (SARS-CoV-2 63%, RSV 11%, and influenzae 26%) [64]. The 30-day risk of hospitalization was similar for COVID-19 (16.2%) and influenza (16.3%), but lower for RSV (14.3%). The ICU admission rate was slightly higher for SARS-CoV-2 patients (3%) compared to RSV (1.8%) and influenza (1.5%). The 90-day risk of death was similar between the three (SARS-CoV-2: 1.8%, RSV: 1.4%, and influenzae: 1.3%).

In ICU settings, viral CAP exhibits a severity profile comparable to bacterial pneumonia, with median ventilation durations ranging from 7 to 10 days and mortality rates between 10% and 30% [5,50,65,66]. However, not all respiratory viruses carry the same prognostic weight. Among them, influenza and RSV have been consistently associated with severe outcomes in hospitalized and ICU populations. Grangier et al. reported comparable ICU lengths of stay for RSV and influenza (6–7 days), with mortality rates of 29% and 25%, respectively [65]. Similarly, Coussement et al. found no significant difference in ICU mortality between RSV (23.9%) and influenza (25.6%) [67]. hMPV, though less frequently identified, is another pathogen associated with severe disease, with ICU admission rates from 10% to 30% and early mortality between 3% and 10% [61,68,69].

By contrast, the pathogenic potential of other respiratory viruses in immunocompetent adults remains less clear. Adenoviruses, while capable of causing severe disease in immunocompromised individuals, rarely lead to severe outcomes in healthy adults. For instance, in one study involving military trainees, only 4.7% of adenovirus infections required ICU admission, and severe complications, such as ARDS, were isolated events [50,70,71]. Parainfluenza viruses, though frequently detected, are typically associated with mild disease in immunocompetent individuals, with ICU mortality rates of approximately 3% and a minimal need for mechanical ventilation [72,73]. Data on rhinovirus are more equivocal. Retrospective ICU studies estimate a mortality rate of around 30%, but these numbers are frequently confounded by co-infections or underlying conditions [74,75]. Seasonal coronaviruses, such as OC43, NL63, and 229E, are rarely implicated in severe pneumonia among immunocompetent adults, and their role as primary pathogens remains unclear [50,76,77]. Human bocavirus exhibits a similarly doubtful pathogenicity, with only sporadic reports of ARDS or ICU admission in adults [78,79].

Beyond viral etiology, bacterial co-infections represent a critical determinant of outcomes in ICU patients. Such co-infections have been reported in up to 25% of patients, depending on patient characteristics and the extent of bacterial sampling [5,46,50,51,80–83]. In ICU settings, Voiriot et al. showed that patients with mixed infections had higher mechanical ventilation rates and mortality (28.9%) compared with patients with isolated bacterial (13%) or viral (11.3%) infections [5]. These findings are supported by a meta-analysis showing a twofold increase in the mortality risk associated with mixed infections (OR 2.1, 95% CI 1.32–3.31) [51]. Furthermore, a database study involving 15,906 patients with viral respiratory infections revealed that mixed infections were associated with a threefold increase in ICU admissions (OR 2.9, 95% CI 2.3–3.6) and 30-day mortality (OR 2.6, 95% CI 1.9–3.7) [82].

Cardiovascular complications are another key factor worsening outcomes. In a large cohort of RSV-related hospitalizations, acute cardiac events were significantly associated with higher ICU admission rates (25.8% vs. 16.5%; ARR 1.54, 95% CI 1.23–1.93) and in-hospital mortality (8.1% vs. 4.0%; ARR 1.77, 95% CI 1.36–2.31) [47]. These findings underscore the critical importance of the early recognition and targeted management of cardiovascular complications in ICU patients with viral respiratory infections. Importantly, the role of respiratory viruses in precipitating COPD exacerbations has been extensively reviewed elsewhere. Clinical outcomes by virus types are summarized in Table 3.

Table 3. Prognosis of severe viral respiratory infections in immunocompetent patients.

	ICU Admission in Hospitalized Patients (%)	During ICU Stay			
		Mechanical Ventilation (%)	Bacterial Co-Infection (%)	ARDS (%)	Mortality (%)
Seasonal influenza [56,84–87]	15–20	30–65	35	25–50	15–25
Respiratory syncytial virus [46,60,67,81]	15–20	30–35	25–35	15–20	10–15
Human metapneumovirus [61,68,69]	5–10	40–50	20	10–25	20
Rhinovirus [75,88,89]	15–20	50	30	?	30
Parainfluenza viruses * [73]	25	?	30	?	20–25
Adenovirus * [70]	5	40–50	?	10–20	0–5
Seasonal coronaviruses * [90,91]	15–30	0–7	20–30	0–3	?
Bocavirus [78] *	?	Case reports	Case reports	Case reports	Case reports

Abbreviations: ARDS, acute respiratory distress syndrome. ? Missing data indicate insufficient evidence or lack of reported cases. * Data are derived from small sample sizes and should be interpreted with caution.

Population at Risk of Severe Outcome

Among immunocompetent patients, an older age and pre-existing comorbidities—especially cardiopulmonary disease—are the most consistent predictors of adverse outcomes [92,93]. RSV hospitalization rates increase significantly with age, reaching 136.9–255.6 per 100,000 in individuals aged ≥65 years, with even higher rates observed in those with COPD, coronary artery disease, or heart failure [94]. Beyond acute complications, severe infections in older adults often lead to prolonged functional decline; for instance, 33% of RSV-hospitalized patients exhibit persistent impairments six months post-discharge [95]. Similarly, influenza disproportionately affects patients with pre-existing comorbidities, substantially increasing risks of hospitalization, ICU admission, and mortality [93]. These findings underscore the importance of targeted prevention and management strategies for high-risk populations, particularly older adults and individuals with cardiopulmonary diseases, to reduce both the immediate and long-term impacts of severe respiratory viral infections. Vaccines effective against RSV and influenza are cornerstones of the prevention strategy in these populations [96].

6. Treatment of Severe Respiratory Viral Infections

6.1. Noninvasive Respiratory Support in Viral Pneumonia

The COVID-19 pandemic re-established noninvasive respiratory support as a central component of acute respiratory failure management. Observational data from large cohorts initially suggested potential benefits of alternatives to standard oxygen therapy. In the COVID-19-ICU cohort (n = 4754), high-flow nasal cannula (HFNC) was associated with a reduced risk of oxygenation failure—defined as intubation or death without intubation—compared to standard oxygen (adjusted OR 0.60; 95% CI 0.36–0.99), whereas noninvasive ventilation was associated with an increased 90-day mortality (adjusted OR 2.75; 95% CI 1.79–4.21) [97]. However, these findings were not confirmed in the COVIDI-CUS randomized trial (n = 546), which compared HFNC, CPAP, and standard oxygen in ICU patients with COVID-19. The study found no significant differences in 28-day intubation rates between HFNC and standard oxygen (HR 1.04; 95% CI 0.69–1.55), or between

CPAP and standard oxygen (HR 1.08; 95% CI 0.71–1.63), challenging the assumption that advanced noninvasive strategies are superior in this setting [98].

There are currently no randomized data specifically addressing non-COVID-19 viral pneumonia. In this context, the evidence must be extrapolated from broader populations with acute hypoxemic respiratory failure. A 2024 meta-analysis of 63 studies (n = 10,230) evaluated HFNC versus conventional oxygen therapy across various etiologies, including COVID-19 (n = 3782) and non-COVID-19 pneumonia (n = 1583). HFNC was associated with a reduced escalation to invasive ventilation (RR 0.85; 95% CI 0.76–0.95) and to noninvasive ventilation (RR 0.70; 95% CI 0.50–0.98) but had no effect on hospital mortality (RR 1.08; 95% CI 0.93–1.26). Although the population included some patients with non-COVID-19 pneumonia, no prespecified subgroup analysis was conducted.

Taken together, while HFNC appears safe and may reduce the need for intubation in selected patients, the current evidence does not support the preferential use of any specific non-invasive strategy in non-COVID-19 viral pneumonia. Outside of well-established indications—such as noninvasive ventilation in acute exacerbations of COPD or cardiogenic pulmonary edema—the choice of respiratory support remains empirical. Dedicated randomized trials are needed to evaluate ventilatory strategies in patients with confirmed viral pneumonia.

6.2. Antiviral Therapy

For severe influenza-associated pneumonia, neuraminidase inhibitors (NAIs), particularly oseltamivir, remain the cornerstone of treatment despite limited evidence in critically ill patients. Key questions persist regarding the effectiveness of antivirals on patient outcomes, the optimal duration of therapy (5 days vs. prolonged courses), and whether monotherapy or combination regimens offer superior benefits. A recent meta-analysis of eight randomized controlled trials in severe influenza reported no significant differences in mortality or ICU admissions compared to placebos, but oseltamivir and peramivir reduced hospital stays by 1.63 and 1.73 days, respectively [99]. Observational studies suggest that an extended oseltamivir therapy ($\geq$10 days) may yield better outcomes in ICU settings, with a 6.2% absolute reduction in mortality (adjusted OR: 0.53, 95% CI: 0.40–0.69), although these findings await confirmation in randomized trials [100]. Combination regimens, such as oseltamivir–zanamivir, have failed to demonstrate an added efficacy and may increase adverse effects [101]. Similarly, novel agents, like baloxavir, targeting distinct viral replication pathways, have not shown superiority in hospitalized patients. The FLAGSTONE trial confirmed that baloxavir combined with NAIs offered no clinical advantage over NAI monotherapy in severe cases [102]. Ongoing studies, including the REMAP-CAP trial (http://clinicaltrials.gov: NCT02735707), are expected to provide more clarity on the optimal antiviral strategies for critically ill patients with influenza.

RSV treatment remains a significant challenge. Ribavirin, historically considered for RSV, has demonstrated an inconsistent efficacy and potential toxicity, limiting its role, particularly in immunocompetent patients [81,103]. While prophylactic monoclonal antibodies, such as palivizumab and nirsevimab, have been explored for infants and high-risk children, their therapeutic potential in adults remains unproven and requires further investigation. Emerging agents, like zelicapavir, are currently under evaluation for older adults with cardiopulmonary comorbidities, but robust trial data are still awaited. For other respiratory viruses, effective antiviral therapies are unavailable, making supportive care, such as oxygen supplementation, advanced ventilatory strategies, and monitoring for bacterial superinfections, the primary approach. Promising investigation agents targeting viral fusion proteins and replication pathways show potential but remain in early development. Table 4 summarizes therapeutic options available in cases of severe RVI.

Table 4. Available antiviral therapies for viral pneumonia.

Treatment	Outcome	Comment
Influenza		
Oseltamivir [99,104–106] (oral)	*Outpatient population* No reduction in hospitalization risk in the general population (RR, 0.79; 95% CI, 0.48–1.29) No reduction in hospitalization risk in high-risk patients (RR, 0.65; 0.33–1.28) No reduction in hospitalization risk in patients >65 years (RR, 1.01; 95% CI, 0.21–4.90) *Hospitalized population* Modest reduction in hospital stay duration (mean difference −1.63 days, 95% CI −2.81 to −0.45) No impact on ICU admission No impact on mortality	No specific serious adverse events Reported resistance: ~1% of strains globally
Peramivir [99,107,108] (IV)	*Outpatient population (compared to oseltamivir)* No difference in time to alleviation of influenza symptoms *Hospitalized population (compared to oseltamivir)* No difference in hospital stay duration No impact on ICU admission No impact on mortality	No specific serious adverse events Rare resistance Second-line therapy: For oseltamivir resistance or when oral administration is not possible
Zanamivir [109] (inhaled, IV)	*Hospitalized population (compared to oseltamivir)* No difference in time to alleviation of influenza symptoms No impact on ICU admission No impact on mortality	No specific serious adverse events Rare resistance Second-line therapy: For oseltamivir resistance or when oral administration is not possible
Baloxavir [102,110,111] (oral)	*Outpatient population (compared to oseltamivir)* No difference in time to alleviation of influenza symptoms *Hospitalized population: baloxavir + oseltamivir compared to oseltamivir alone* No clinical benefit from adding baloxavir	Second-line therapy: For oseltamivir resistance (no cross-resistance with neuraminidase inhibitors)?
Respiratory syncytial virus		
Ribavirin [112] (oral, inhaled, IV)	Reduced mortality in LRTIs in patients with hematologic malignancies or hematopoietic stem cell transplants (aOR 0.19 [0.07, 0.51]) No indication for immunocompetent patients	Adverse events: nephrotoxicity, anemia, and rash
Adenovirus		
Cidofovir [113] (IV).	Weak evidence (mainly case reports in pediatric patients) suggesting potential effect on adenovirus clearance in immunocompromised patients	Adverse events: nephrotoxicity and leukopenia

6.3. Immunomodulation

The role of corticosteroids in viral pneumonia remains highly debated. The CAPE-COD trial demonstrated a mortality reduction with low-dose hydrocortisone in severe CAP, though subgroup analyses did not specifically address viral etiologies [114]. In influenza-associated pneumonia, observational studies and meta-analyses have consistently indicated that corticosteroid use is associated with an increased mortality (OR 3.90, 95% CI 2.31–6.60) and higher rates of hospital-acquired infections (OR 2.74, 95% CI 1.51–4.95) [115]. However, these findings must be interpreted cautiously, as the absence of high-quality RCTs and the potential for confounding by indications—given that corticosteroids are often used in the most critically ill patients—complicate definitive conclusions. Beyond influenza, data on corticosteroid use in other viral respiratory infections remain limited, and no randomized controlled trials currently provide clear guidance. A recent individual participant data meta-analysis by Smit et al., evaluating corticosteroid therapy in severe CAP, found no statistically significant heterogeneity in treatment effect based on microbiological etiology [116]. However, point estimates of mortality reduction consistently disfavored corticosteroids in viral infections: -2.6% (95% CI -7.1 to 1.5) for viral CAP, -4.0% (-9.4 to 1.0) for viral-only CAP, -3.6% (-11.5 to 4.2) for influenza, and -4.4% (-13.4 to 4.2) for influenza-only cases. These trends underscore the need for caution when considering corticosteroids in the management of viral pneumonia in the absence of robust pathogen-specific evidence.

Efforts to address these evidence gaps are ongoing. Trials such as REMAP-CAP (http://clinicaltrias.gov: NCT02735707) and RECOVERY (http://clinicaltrials.gov: NCT04381936) are investigating the efficacy of corticosteroids and other immunomodulatory agents, including tocilizumab and baricitinib, across various viral pneumonias. These trials are essential for establishing evidence-based guidelines and optimizing outcomes in critically ill patients. Until then, the decision to use immunomodulatory therapies should remain highly individualized, carefully balancing potential risks—such as delayed viral clearance and secondary infections—against plausible clinical benefits in selected cases.

7. Vaccination as a Key Strategy Against Severe Respiratory Viral Infections

While antiviral treatments have shown variable efficacy, vaccination remains the most effective strategy for preventing severe respiratory viral infections (RVIs), particularly in high-risk populations such as the elderly. Among common seasonal respiratory viruses, vaccines are currently available for influenza and RSV, in addition to SARS-CoV-2.

For influenza, vaccine effectiveness is largely dependent on the antigenic match with circulating strains during a given season [117]. The greatest benefit is observed in individuals aged $\geq$65 years. A systematic review by Demicheli et al. found that influenza vaccination reduced the risk of confirmed influenza from 6% to 2.4%, and likely decreased the incidence of influenza-like illness from 6% to 3.5% in this population [118]. Newall et al. estimated that in the United States, a 1% increase in the overall influenza vaccine uptake during the influenza season was associated with a 0.33 (95% CI: 0.20–0.47) per 100,000 population reduction in pneumonia- and influenza-related deaths [119]. Similar findings were reported in France between 2000 and 2009, where vaccination prevented 2000 deaths annually and had an estimated effectiveness of 35% against influenza-attributable mortality. In this population, approximately 2650 vaccinations were required to prevent one influenza-related death among older adults [120].

A newly approved RSV vaccine has recently become available for older adults. Real-world data from an epidemic season (October 2023–March 2024) demonstrated that in individuals aged $\geq$60 years, the RSV vaccine effectiveness was 77% (95% CI: 70–83) against

RSV-associated emergency department visits, 80% (95% CI: 71–85) against RSV-related hospitalization, and 81% (95% CI: 52–92) against ICU admission or death [121].

Finally, ensuring a high vaccine coverage against respiratory viruses that are now rare due to near-eradication remains crucial, as illustrated by the recent resurgence of measles in the United States (228 cases as of 7 March 2025) [122,123]. Measles is highly contagious (12–18 secondary cases per infected individual) and potentially fatal [124]. The current recommended two-dose vaccination strategy is highly effective, providing 90–99% protection. In infected individuals, pneumonitis is frequent but usually mild in immunocompetent patients; however, ARF requiring ICU admission occurs in about 3% of the cases [125]. In critically ill patients, the disease is much more severe. A French ICU cohort from the 2009–2011 outbreak showed that measles primarily affected young patients (median age: 29.2 years) who had not received the full two-dose vaccine regimen. The disease progression was severe, with ARDS occurring in 9 of 36 patients and mortality in 5 of 36 cases [126]. These findings collectively underscore the central role of vaccination in mitigating the burden of severe RVIs—both from currently circulating pathogens and from those re-emerging due to lapses in immunization coverage. For measles in particular, maintaining high vaccination rates is essential, as severe complications can occur even in previously healthy adults, and no specific antiviral treatment is available.

8. Future Risks

8.1. Post-Pandemic Effects

The COVID-19 pandemic has profoundly reshaped the epidemiology of respiratory pathogens. Non-pharmaceutical interventions, such as lockdowns, mask mandates, and travel restrictions, led to an unprecedented decline in pathogen circulation. Influenza transmission, for instance, was reduced by over 95%, significantly disrupting global patterns of spread [127,128]. While these measures reduced short-term transmission, they also limited natural immunity development—a phenomenon referred to as "immunity debt". Interruptions in vaccination campaigns and a reduced vaccine uptake further weakened the herd immunity, heightening the risk of severe post-pandemic outbreaks.

The case of influenza A(H3N2) illustrates the cascading consequences of these disruptions. In Australia, genetic analyses revealed that dominant H3N2 strains in 2022 (subclade 3C.2a1b.2a.2) were introduced via international travel after restrictions were lifted [129]. The antigenic drift between successive strains was linked to more intense epidemics, marked by higher transmission rates, increased adult cases, and H3N2 dominance [127,129,130]. Such examples demonstrate the enduring consequences of pandemic-related disruptions, emphasizing the importance of continuous surveillance, robust vaccination efforts, and targeted public health measures to address these evolving risks.

8.2. Emerging Threats

Beyond the established endemic respiratory viruses, emerging viral threats pose an increasing challenge to global health, driven by environmental changes, globalization, and evolving pathogen characteristics. The SARS, MERS, and COVID-19 pandemics underscore the potential for novel pathogens to cause severe outbreaks, with high mortality rates and a significant global impact [131,132]. Influenza remains a persistent concern, particularly the emergence of highly pathogenic avian strains with pandemic potential [63,133]. A(H5N1) virus spread from east Asia to west Asia and Africa is the most common. It was associated with a hospitalization rate of more than 90% and a case fatality rate of more than 50% [134]. Although few clustering cases have been reported, human to human transmission is unlikely. Beyond these known threats, arboviruses such as dengue and chikungunya are expanding geographically due to climate change and the proliferation of mosquito vectors [135,136]. This geographical shift poses a growing risk of outbreaks in previously unaffected regions, including parts of Europe. The resurgence of measles due to a decrease in vaccination coverage should also be kept in mind. These evolving dynamics highlight the urgent need for robust surveillance systems, cross-border collaboration, and innovative research to anticipate, detect, and mitigate the impact of respiratory viral emergencies. As masking is effective in reducing contamination, the situations where it should be recommended or mandated as well as the optimal filtration characteristics should be better defined [137].

9. Conclusions

Severe respiratory viral infections remain a major cause of ICU admissions, particularly in older adults and those with comorbidities. The widespread use of molecular diagnostics has improved viral detection, yet its clinical relevance, particularly in differentiating colonization from infection, remains debated. Influenza and Pneumoviridae (RSV, hMPV) are the most severe pathogens, often complicated by bacterial co-infections that worsen outcomes. While neuraminidase inhibitors are standard for severe influenza, effective antiviral options for other respiratory viruses are lacking. Future research should focus on optimizing antiviral strategies, refining the role of immunomodulation, and improving the early identification of high-risk patients to enhance clinical outcomes.

Author Contributions: Conceptualization; methodology; investigation; resources; writing—original draft preparation and review and editing, D.M. and J.-F.T.; supervision, J.-F.T. All authors have read and agreed to the published version of the manuscript.

Funding: This research received no external funding.

Conflicts of Interest: J.F.T. declares scientific board participations at Menarini, Advanz, Merck, and Biomerieux and lectures in symposia for Qiagen, Biomerieux, Merck, Pfizer, Shionogi, and Mundipharma outside of the submitted work. D.M. declares lectures in symposia for Menarini.

Abbreviations

The following abbreviations are used in this manuscript:

ARDS	acute respiratory distress syndrome
ARF	acute respiratory failure
CAP	community-acquired pneumonia
CDC	Centers for Disease Control and Prevention
CI	confidence interval
COPD	chronic obstructive pulmonary disease
COVID-19	Coronavirus Disease 2019
FA-PP	Film-Array Pneumonia Panel
HFNC	high-flow nasal cannula
hMPV	human metapneumovirus
ICU	intensive care unit
IFN	Interferon
IRR	incidence rate ratio
LRTI	lower respiratory tract infection
MERS	Middle East Respiratory Syndrome
mPCR	multiplex PCR
NAI	neuraminidase inhibitor
NPI	non-pharmaceutical intervention
OR	odds ratio
PCR	Polymerase Chain Reaction

RSV	respiratory syncytial virus	
RVI	respiratory viral infection	
SARI	severe acute respiratory infection	
SARS	Severe Acute Respiratory Syndrome	
SARS-CoV-2	Severe Acute Respiratory Syndrome Coronavirus 2	
SOC	standard of care	
TNF	tumor necrosis factor	

References

1. Leber, A.L.; Lisby, J.G.; Hansen, G.; Relich, R.F.; Schneider, U.V.; Granato, P.; Young, S.; Pareja, J.; Hannet, I. Multicenter Evaluation of the QIAstat-Dx Respiratory Panel for Detection of Viruses and Bacteria in Nasopharyngeal Swab Specimens. *J. Clin. Microbiol.* **2020**, *58*, e00155-20. [CrossRef] [PubMed]
2. Visseaux, B.; Le Hingrat, Q.; Collin, G.; Bouzid, D.; Lebourgeois, S.; Le Pluart, D.; Deconinck, L.; Lescure, F.-X.; Lucet, J.-C.; Bouadma, L.; et al. Evaluation of the QIAstat-Dx Respiratory SARS-CoV-2 Panel, the First Rapid Multiplex PCR Commercial Assay for SARS-CoV-2 Detection. *J. Clin. Microbiol.* **2020**, *58*, e00630-20. [CrossRef]
3. van Someren Gréve, F.; Juffermans, N.P.; Bos, L.D.J.; Binnekade, J.M.; Braber, A.; Cremer, O.L.; de Jonge, E.; Molenkamp, R.; Ong, D.S.Y.; Rebers, S.P.H.; et al. Respiratory Viruses in Invasively Ventilated Critically Ill Patients-A Prospective Multcenter Observational Study. *Crit. Care Med.* **2018**, *46*, 29–36. [CrossRef] [PubMed]
4. Byington, C.L.; Ampofo, K.; Stockmann, C.; Adler, F.R.; Herbener, A.; Miller, T.; Sheng, X.; Blaschke, A.J.; Crisp, R.; Pavia, A.T. Community Surveillance of Respiratory Viruses Among Families in the Utah Better Identification of Germs-Longitudinal Viral Epidemiology (BIG-LoVE) Study. *Clin. Infect. Dis.* **2015**, *61*, 1217–1224. [CrossRef]
5. Voiriot, G.; Visseaux, B.; Cohen, J.; Nguyen, L.B.L.; Neuville, M.; Morbieu, C.; Burdet, C.; Radjou, A.; Lescure, F.-X.; Smonig, R.; et al. Viral-Bacterial Coinfection Affects the Presentation and Alters the Prognosis of Severe Community-Acquired Pneumonia. *Crit. Care* **2016**, *20*, 375. [CrossRef]
6. Loubet, P.; Voiriot, G.; Houhou-Fidouh, N.; Neuville, M.; Bouadma, L.; Lescure, F.-X.; Descamps, D.; Timsit, J.-F.; Yazdanpanah, Y.; Visseaux, B. Impact of Respiratory Viruses in Hospital-Acquired Pneumonia in the Intensive Care Unit: A Single-Center Retrospective Study. *J. Clin. Virol.* **2017**, *91*, 52–57. [CrossRef] [PubMed]
7. Martin-Loeches, I.; Schultz, M.J.; Vincent, J.-L.; Alvarez-Lerma, F.; Bos, L.D.; Solé-Violán, J.; Torres, A.; Rodriguez, A. Increased Incidence of Co-Infection in Critically Ill Patients with Influenza. *Intensive Care Med.* **2017**, *43*, 48–58. [CrossRef]
8. Zilberbeg, M.D.; Khan, I.; Shorr, A.F. Respiratory Viruses in Nosocomial Pneumonia: An Evolving Paradigm. *Viruses* **2023**, *15*, 1676. [CrossRef]
9. Jitmuang, A.; Puttinad, S.; Hemvimol, S.; Pansasiri, S.; Horthongkham, N. A Multiplex Pneumonia Panel for Diagnosis of Hospital-Acquired and Ventilator-Associated Pneumonia in the Era of Emerging Antimicrobial Resistance. *Front. Cell. Infect. Microbiol.* **2022**, *12*, 977320. [CrossRef]
10. Kosai, K.; Akamatsu, N.; Ota, K.; Mitsumoto-Kaseida, F.; Sakamoto, K.; Hasegawa, H.; Izumikawa, K.; Mukae, H.; Yanagihara, K. BioFire FilmArray Pneumonia Panel Enhances Detection of Pathogens and Antimicrobial Resistance in Lower Respiratory Tract Specimens. *Ann. Clin. Microbiol. Antimicrob.* **2022**, *21*, 24. [CrossRef]
11. Molina, F.J.; Botero, L.E.; Isaza, J.P.; Cano, L.E.; López, L.; Tamayo, L.; Torres, A. Diagnostic Concordance between BioFire® FilmArray® Pneumonia Panel and Culture in Patients with COVID-19 Pneumonia Admitted to Intensive Care Units: The Experience of the Third Wave in Eight Hospitals in Colombia. *Crit. Care* **2022**, *26*, 130. [CrossRef] [PubMed]
12. Cohen, R.; Babushkin, F.; Finn, T.; Geller, K.; Alexander, H.; Datnow, C.; Uda, M.; Shapiro, M.; Paikin, S.; Lellouche, J. High Rates of Bacterial Pulmonary Co-Infections and Superinfections Identified by Multiplex PCR among Critically Ill COVID-19 Patients. *Microorganisms* **2021**, *9*, 2483. [CrossRef] [PubMed]
13. Gastli, N.; Loubinoux, J.; Daragon, M.; Lavigne, J.-P.; Saint-Sardos, P.; Pailhoriès, H.; Lemarié, C.; Benmansour, H.; d'Humières, C.; Broutin, L.; et al. Multicentric Evaluation of BioFire FilmArray Pneumonia Panel for Rapid Bacteriological Documentation of Pneumonia. *Clin. Microbiol. Infect.* **2021**, *27*, 1308–1314. [CrossRef]
14. Lee, S.H.; Ruan, S.-Y.; Pan, S.-C.; Lee, T.-F.; Chien, J.-Y.; Hsueh, P.-R. Performance of a Multiplex PCR Pneumonia Panel for the Identification of Respiratory Pathogens and the Main Determinants of Resistance from the Lower Respiratory Tract Specimens of Adult Patients in Intensive Care Units. *J. Microbiol. Immunol. Infect.* **2019**, *52*, 920–928. [CrossRef] [PubMed]
15. Gong, J.; Yang, J.; Liu, L.; Chen, X.; Yang, G.; He, Y.; Sun, R. Evaluation and Clinical Practice of Pathogens and Antimicrobial Resistance Genes of BioFire FilmArray Pneumonia Panel in Lower Respiratory Tract Infections. *Infection* **2024**, *52*, 545–555. [CrossRef]

16. Verroken, A.; Favresse, J.; Anantharajah, A.; Rodriguez-Villalobos, H.; Wittebole, X.; Laterre, P.-F. Optimized Antibiotic Management of Critically Ill Patients with Severe Pneumonia Following Multiplex Polymerase Chain Reaction Testing: A Prospective Clinical Exploratory Trial. *Antibiotics* **2024**, *13*, 67. [CrossRef]
17. Søgaard, K.K.; Hinic, V.; Goldenberger, D.; Gensch, A.; Schweitzer, M.; Bättig, V.; Siegemund, M.; Bassetti, S.; Bingisser, R.; Tamm, M.; et al. Evaluation of the Clinical Relevance of the Biofire© FilmArray Pneumonia Panel among Hospitalized Patients. *Infection* **2024**, *52*, 173–181. [CrossRef]
18. Falsey, A.R.; Branche, A.R.; Croft, D.P.; Formica, M.A.; Peasley, M.R.; Walsh, E.E. Real-Life Assessment of BioFire FilmArray Pneumonia Panel in Adults Hospitalized with Respiratory Illness. *J. Infect. Dis.* **2024**, *229*, 214–222. [CrossRef]
19. Shen, X.; Feng, B.; Shi, W.; Cheng, W.; Zhang, T. Concomitant Viral and Bacterial Pneumonia among Patients in ICU with Mechanical Respiratory Support. *J. Infect. Dev. Ctries.* **2022**, *16*, 1482–1489. [CrossRef]
20. Kamel, N.A.; Alshahrani, M.Y.; Aboshanab, K.M.; El Borhamy, M.I. Evaluation of the BioFire FilmArray Pneumonia Panel Plus to the Conventional Diagnostic Methods in Determining the Microbiological Etiology of Hospital-Acquired Pneumonia. *Biology* **2022**, *11*, 377. [CrossRef]
21. Enne, V.I.; Aydin, A.; Baldan, R.; Owen, D.R.; Richardson, H.; Ricciardi, F.; Russell, C.; Nomamiukor-Ikeji, B.O.; Swart, A.-M.; High, J.; et al. Multicentre Evaluation of Two Multiplex PCR Platforms for the Rapid Microbiological Investigation of Nosocomial Pneumonia in UK ICUs: The INHALE WP1 Study. *Thorax* **2022**, *77*, 1220–1228. [CrossRef] [PubMed]
22. Buchan, B.W.; Windham, S.; Balada-Llasat, J.-M.; Leber, A.; Harrington, A.; Relich, R.; Murphy, C.; Dien Bard, J.; Naccache, S.; Ronen, S.; et al. Practical Comparison of the BioFire FilmArray Pneumonia Panel to Routine Diagnostic Methods and Potential Impact on Antimicrobial Stewardship in Adult Hospitalized Patients with Lower Respiratory Tract Infections. *J. Clin. Microbiol.* **2020**, *58*, e00135-20. [CrossRef]
23. Matrosovich, M.N.; Matrosovich, T.Y.; Gray, T.; Roberts, N.A.; Klenk, H.-D. Human and Avian Influenza Viruses Target Different Cell Types in Cultures of Human Airway Epithelium. *Proc. Natl. Acad. Sci. USA* **2004**, *101*, 4620–4624. [CrossRef] [PubMed]
24. Fiege, J.K.; Langlois, R.A. Investigating Influenza A Virus Infection: Tools to Track Infection and Limit Tropism. *J. Virol.* **2015**, *89*, 6167–6170. [CrossRef]
25. Kumlin, U.; Olofsson, S.; Dimock, K.; Arnberg, N. Sialic Acid Tissue Distribution and Influenza Virus Tropism. *Influenza Other Respir. Viruses* **2008**, *2*, 147–154. [CrossRef] [PubMed]
26. Shinya, K.; Ebina, M.; Yamada, S.; Ono, M.; Kasai, N.; Kawaoka, Y. Influenza Virus Receptors in the Human Airway. *Nature* **2006**, *440*, 435–436. [CrossRef]
27. Nicolas de Lamballerie, C.; Pizzorno, A.; Dubois, J.; Julien, T.; Padey, B.; Bouveret, M.; Traversier, A.; Legras-Lachuer, C.; Lina, B.; Boivin, G.; et al. Characterization of Cellular Transcriptomic Signatures Induced by Different Respiratory Viruses in Human Reconstituted Airway Epithelia. *Sci. Rep.* **2019**, *9*, 11493. [CrossRef]
28. Rameix-Welti, M.-A.; Le Goffic, R.; Hervé, P.-L.; Sourimant, J.; Rémot, A.; Riffault, S.; Yu, Q.; Galloux, M.; Gault, E.; Eléouët, J.-F. Visualizing the Replication of Respiratory Syncytial Virus in Cells and in Living Mice. *Nat. Commun.* **2014**, *5*, 5104. [CrossRef]
29. Kajon, A.E.; Lu, X.; Erdman, D.D.; Louie, J.; Schnurr, D.; George, K.S.; Koopmans, M.P.; Allibhai, T.; Metzgar, D. Molecular Epidemiology and Brief History of Emerging Adenovirus 14-Associated Respiratory Disease in the United States. *J. Infect. Dis.* **2010**, *202*, 93–103. [CrossRef]
30. Dudding, B.A.; Wagner, S.C.; Zeller, J.A.; Gmelich, J.T.; French, G.R.; Top, F.H. Fatal Pneumonia Associated with Adenovirus Type 7 in Three Military Trainees. *N. Engl. J. Med.* **1972**, *286*, 1289–1292. [CrossRef]
31. Arndt, U.; Wennemuth, G.; Barth, P.; Nain, M.; Al-Abed, Y.; Meinhardt, A.; Gemsa, D.; Bacher, M. Release of Macrophage Migration Inhibitory Factor and CXCL8/Interleukin-8 from Lung Epithelial Cells Rendered Necrotic by Influenza A Virus Infection. *J. Virol.* **2002**, *76*, 9298–9306. [CrossRef] [PubMed]
32. Lam, W.Y.; Tang, J.W.; Yeung, A.C.M.; Chiu, L.C.M.; Sung, J.J.Y.; Chan, P.K.S. Avian Influenza Virus A/HK/483/97(H5N1) NS1 Protein Induces Apoptosis in Human Airway Epithelial Cells. *J. Virol.* **2008**, *82*, 2741–2751. [CrossRef] [PubMed]
33. Atkin-Smith, G.K.; Duan, M.; Chen, W.; Poon, I.K.H. The Induction and Consequences of Influenza A Virus-Induced Cell Death. *Cell Death Dis.* **2018**, *9*, 1002. [CrossRef] [PubMed]
34. Hu, M.; Schulze, K.E.; Ghildyal, R.; Henstridge, D.C.; Kolanowski, J.L.; New, E.J.; Hong, Y.; Hsu, A.C.; Hansbro, P.M.; Wark, P.A.; et al. Respiratory Syncytial Virus Co-Opts Host Mitochondrial Function to Favour Infectious Virus Production. *eLife* **2019**, *8*, e42448. [CrossRef]
35. Bui, C.H.T.; Chan, R.W.Y.; Ng, M.M.T.; Cheung, M.-C.; Ng, K.-C.; Chan, M.P.K.; Chan, L.L.Y.; Fong, J.H.M.; Nicholls, J.M.; Peiris, J.S.M.; et al. Tropism of Influenza B Viruses in Human Respiratory Tract Explants and Airway Organoids. *Eur. Respir. J.* **2019**, *54*, 1900008. [CrossRef]
36. Clementi, N.; Ghosh, S.; De Santis, M.; Castelli, M.; Criscuolo, E.; Zanoni, I.; Clementi, M.; Mancini, N. Viral Respiratory Pathogens and Lung Injury. *Clin. Microbiol. Rev.* **2021**, *34*, e00103-20. [CrossRef]

37. Newton, A.H.; Cardani, A.; Braciale, T.J. ƒcousse The Host Immune Response in Respiratory Virus Infection: Balancing Virus Clearance and Immunopathology. *Semin. Immunopathol.* **2016**, *38*, 471–482. [CrossRef]
38. Murawski, M.R.; Bowen, G.N.; Cerny, A.M.; Anderson, L.J.; Haynes, L.M.; Tripp, R.A.; Kurt-Jones, E.A.; Finberg, R.W. Respiratory Syncytial Virus Activates Innate Immunity through Toll-Like Receptor 2. *J. Virol.* **2009**, *83*, 1492–1500. [CrossRef]
39. Sun, K.; Metzger, D.W. Inhibition of Pulmonary Antibacterial Defense by Interferon-γ during Recovery from Influenza Infection. *Nat. Med.* **2008**, *14*, 558–564. [CrossRef]
40. Stark, J.M.; Stark, M.A.; Colasurdo, G.N.; LeVine, A.M. Decreased Bacterial Clearance from the Lungs of Mice Following Primary Respiratory Syncytial Virus Infection. *J. Med. Virol.* **2006**, *78*, 829–838. [CrossRef]
41. Iverson, A.R.; Boyd, K.L.; McAuley, J.L.; Plano, L.R.; Hart, M.E.; McCullers, J.A. Influenza Virus Primes Mice for Pneumonia From Staphylococcus Aureus. *J. Infect. Dis.* **2011**, *203*, 880–888. [CrossRef] [PubMed]
42. Taubenberger, J.K.; Morens, D.M. The Pathology of Influenza Virus Infections. *Annu. Rev. Pathol.* **2008**, *3*, 499–522. [CrossRef]
43. Johnson, J.E.; Gonzales, R.A.; Olson, S.J.; Wright, P.F.; Graham, B.S. The Histopathology of Fatal Untreated Human Respiratory Syncytial Virus Infection. *Mod. Pathol.* **2007**, *20*, 108–119. [CrossRef]
44. Pritt, B.S.; Aubry, M.C. Histopathology of Viral Infections of the Lung. *Semin. Diagn. Pathol.* **2017**, *34*, 510–517. [CrossRef]
45. Vargas, S.O.; Kozakewich, H.P.W.; Perez-Atayde, A.R.; McAdam, A.J. Pathology of Human Metapneumovirus Infection: Insights into the Pathogenesis of a Newly Identified Respiratory Virus. *Pediatr. Dev. Pathol.* **2004**, *7*, 478–486; discussion 421. [CrossRef] [PubMed]
46. Mokrani, D.; Le Hingrat, Q.; Thy, M.; Choquet, C.; Joly, V.; Lariven, S.; Rioux, C.; Deconinck, L.; Loubet, P.; Papo, T.; et al. Clinical Characteristics and Outcomes of Respiratory Syncytial Virus-Associated ARF in Immunocompetent Patients: A Seven-Year Experience at a Tertiary Hospital in France. *J. Infect.* **2024**, *89*, 106180. [CrossRef]
47. Woodruff, R.C.; Melgar, M.; Pham, H.; Sperling, L.S.; Loustalot, F.; Kirley, P.D.; Austin, E.; Yousey-Hindes, K.; Openo, K.P.; Ryan, P.; et al. Acute Cardiac Events in Hospitalized Older Adults with Respiratory Syncytial Virus Infection. *JAMA Intern. Med.* **2024**, *184*, 602–611. [CrossRef]
48. Warren-Gash, C.; Blackburn, R.; Whitaker, H.; McMenamin, J.; Hayward, A.C. Laboratory-Confirmed Respiratory Infections as Triggers for Acute Myocardial Infarction and Stroke: A Self-Controlled Case Series Analysis of National Linked Datasets from Scotland. *Eur. Respir. J.* **2018**, *51*, 1701794. [CrossRef] [PubMed]
49. Shorr, A.F.; Fisher, K.; Micek, S.T.; Kollef, M.H. The Burden of Viruses in Pneumonia Associated with Acute Respiratory Failure: An Underappreciated Issue. *Chest* **2018**, *154*, 84–90. [CrossRef]
50. Choi, S.-H.; Hong, S.-B.; Ko, G.-B.; Lee, Y.; Park, H.J.; Park, S.-Y.; Moon, S.M.; Cho, O.-H.; Park, K.-H.; Chong, Y.P.; et al. Viral Infection in Patients with Severe Pneumonia Requiring Intensive Care Unit Admission. *Am. J. Respir. Crit. Care Med.* **2012**, *186*, 325–332. [CrossRef]
51. Burk, M.; El-Kersh, K.; Saad, M.; Wiemken, T.; Ramirez, J.; Cavallazzi, R. Viral Infection in Community-Acquired Pneumonia: A Systematic Review and Meta-Analysis. *Eur. Respir. Rev.* **2016**, *25*, 178–188. [CrossRef] [PubMed]
52. Jennings, L.C.; Anderson, T.P.; Beynon, K.A.; Chua, A.; Laing, R.T.R.; Werno, A.M.; Young, S.A.; Chambers, S.T.; Murdoch, D.R. Incidence and Characteristics of Viral Community-Acquired Pneumonia in Adults. *Thorax* **2008**, *63*, 42–48. [CrossRef]
53. Lieberman, D.; Shimoni, A.; Shemer-Avni, Y.; Keren-Naos, A.; Shtainberg, R.; Lieberman, D. Respiratory Viruses in Adults with Community-Acquired Pneumonia. *Chest* **2010**, *138*, 811–816. [CrossRef] [PubMed]
54. Montull, B.; Menéndez, R.; Torres, A.; Reyes, S.; Méndez, R.; Zalacaín, R.; Capelastegui, A.; Rajas, O.; Borderías, L.; Martin-Villasclaras, J.; et al. Predictors of Severe Sepsis among Patients Hospitalized for Community-Acquired Pneumonia. *PLoS ONE* **2016**, *11*, e0145929. [CrossRef] [PubMed]
55. Krammer, F.; Smith, G.J.D.; Fouchier, R.A.M.; Peiris, M.; Kedzierska, K.; Doherty, P.C.; Palese, P.; Shaw, M.L.; Treanor, J.; Webster, R.G.; et al. Influenza. *Nat. Rev. Dis. Primers* **2018**, *4*, 3. [CrossRef]
56. Fartoukh, M.; Voiriot, G.; Guérin, L.; Ricard, J.D.; Combes, A.; Faure, M.; Benghanem, S.; de Montmollin, E.; Tandjaoui-Lambiotte, Y.; Vieillard-Baron, A.; et al. Seasonal Burden of Severe Influenza Virus Infection in the Critically Ill Patients, Using the Assistance Publique-Hôpitaux de Paris Clinical Data Warehouse: A Pilot Study. *Ann. Intensive Care* **2021**, *11*, 117. [CrossRef]
57. de Prost, N.; Audureau, E.; Guillon, A.; Handala, L.; Préau, S.; Guigon, A.; Uhel, F.; Le Hingrat, Q.; Delamaire, F.; Grolhier, C.; et al. Clinical Phenotypes and Outcomes Associated with SARS-CoV-2 Omicron Sublineage JN.1 in Critically Ill COVID-19 Patients: A Prospective, Multicenter Cohort Study in France, November 2022 to January 2024. *Ann. Intensive Care* **2024**, *14*, 101. [CrossRef]
58. Datadot [En Ligne]. COVID-19 Cases | WHO COVID-19 Dashboard. Available online: https://data.who.int/dashboards/covid19/cases (accessed on 21 March 2025).
59. Kaku, Y.; Uriu, K.; Okumura, K.; Genotype to Phenotype Japan (G2P-Japan) Consortium; Ito, J.; Sato, K. Virological Characteristics of the SARS-CoV-2 KP.3.1.1 Variant. *Lancet Infect. Dis.* **2024**, *24*, e609. [CrossRef]

60. Gaillet, A.; Layese, R.; Fourati, S.; Celante, H.; Pham, T.; Benghanem, S.; Mekontso Dessap, A.; de Montmollin, E.; Pirault, J.; Vieillard-Baron, A.; et al. Clinical Phenotypes and Outcomes Associated with Respiratory Syncytial Virus Infection in Critically Ill Patients: A Retrospective Multicentre Cohort Study in Great Paris Area Hospitals, 2017–2023. *J. Infect. Dis.* **2025**, jiaf129. [CrossRef]
61. Philippot, Q.; Rammaert, B.; Dauriat, G.; Daubin, C.; Schlemmer, F.; Costantini, A.; Tandjaoui-Lambiotte, Y.; Neuville, M.; Desrochettes, E.; Ferré, A.; et al. Human Metapneumovirus Infection Is Associated with a Substantial Morbidity and Mortality Burden in Adult Inpatients. *Heliyon* **2024**, *10*, e33231. [CrossRef]
62. Lin, F.; Zhou, Q.; Li, W.; Xiao, W.; Li, S.; Liu, B.; Li, H.; Cui, Y.; Lu, R.; Li, Y.; et al. A Prediction Model for Acute Respiratory Distress Syndrome in Immunocompetent Adults with Adenovirus-Associated Pneumonia: A Multicenter Retrospective Analysis. *BMC Pulm. Med.* **2023**, *23*, 431. [CrossRef]
63. Garg, S.; Reinhart, K.; Couture, A.; Kniss, K.; Davis, C.T.; Kirby, M.K.; Murray, E.L.; Zhu, S.; Kraushaar, V.; Wadford, D.A.; et al. Highly Pathogenic Avian Influenza A(H5N1) Virus Infections in Humans. *N. Engl. J. Med.* **2025**, *392*, 843–854. [CrossRef]
64. Bajema, K.L.; Bui, D.P.; Yan, L.; Li, Y.; Rajeevan, N.; Vergun, R.; Berry, K.; Huang, Y.; Lin, H.-M.; Aslan, M.; et al. Severity and Long-Term Mortality of COVID-19, Influenza, and Respiratory Syncytial Virus. *JAMA Intern. Med.* **2025**, *185*, 324–334. [CrossRef] [PubMed]
65. Grangier, B.; Vacheron, C.-H.; De Marignan, D.; Casalegno, J.-S.; Couray-Targe, S.; Bestion, A.; Ader, F.; Richard, J.-C.; Frobert, E.; Argaud, L.; et al. Comparison of Mortality and Outcomes of Four Respiratory Viruses in the Intensive Care Unit: A Multicenter Retrospective Study. *Sci. Rep.* **2024**, *14*, 6690. [CrossRef] [PubMed]
66. Cillóniz, C.; Ewig, S.; Ferrer, M.; Polverino, E.; Gabarrús, A.; Puig de la Bellacasa, J.; Mensa, J.; Torres, A. Community-Acquired Polymicrobial Pneumonia in the Intensive Care Unit: Aetiology and Prognosis. *Crit. Care* **2011**, *15*, R209. [CrossRef] [PubMed]
67. Coussement, J.; Zuber, B.; Garrigues, E.; Gros, A.; Vandueren, C.; Epaillard, N.; Voiriot, G.; Tandjaoui-Lambiotte, Y.; Lascarrou, J.-B.; Boissier, F.; et al. Characteristics and Outcomes of Patients in the ICU with Respiratory Syncytial Virus Compared with Those with Influenza Infection: A Multicenter Matched Cohort Study. *Chest* **2022**, *161*, 1475–1484. [CrossRef]
68. Choi, S.-H.; Hong, S.-B.; Huh, J.W.; Jung, J.; Kim, M.J.; Chong, Y.P.; Kim, S.-H.; Sung, H.; Koo, H.J.; Do, K.-H.; et al. Outcomes of Severe Human Metapneumovirus-Associated Community-Acquired Pneumonia in Adults. *J. Clin. Virol.* **2019**, *117*, 1–4. [CrossRef]
69. Hasvold, J.; Sjoding, M.; Pohl, K.; Cooke, C.; Hyzy, R.C. The Role of Human Metapneumovirus in the Critically Ill Adult Patient. *J. Crit. Care* **2016**, *31*, 233–237. [CrossRef]
70. Vento, T.J.; Prakash, V.; Murray, C.K.; Brosch, L.C.; Tchandja, J.B.; Cogburn, C.; Yun, H.C. Pneumonia in Military Trainees: A Comparison Study Based on Adenovirus Serotype 14 Infection. *J. Infect. Dis.* **2011**, *203*, 1388–1395. [CrossRef]
71. Wiemken, T.; Peyrani, P.; Bryant, K.; Kelley, R.R.; Summersgill, J.; Arnold, F.; Carrico, R.; McKinney, W.P.; Jonsson, C.; Carrico, K.; et al. Incidence of Respiratory Viruses in Patients with Community-Acquired Pneumonia Admitted to the Intensive Care Unit: Results from the Severe Influenza Pneumonia Surveillance (SIPS) Project. *Eur. J. Clin. Microbiol. Infect. Dis.* **2013**, *32*, 705–710. [CrossRef]
72. Zhou, F.; Wang, Y.; Liu, Y.; Liu, X.; Gu, L.; Zhang, X.; Pu, Z.; Yang, G.; Liu, B.; Nie, Q.; et al. Disease Severity and Clinical Outcomes of Community-Acquired Pneumonia Caused by Non-Influenza Respiratory Viruses in Adults: A Multicentre Prospective Registry Study from the CAP-China Network. *Eur. Respir. J.* **2019**, *54*, 1802406. [CrossRef] [PubMed]
73. Russell, E.; Yang, A.; Tardrew, S.; Ison, M.G. Parainfluenza Virus in Hospitalized Adults: A 7-Year Retrospective Study. *Clin. Infect. Dis.* **2019**, *68*, 298–305. [CrossRef] [PubMed]
74. Karhu, J.; Ala-Kokko, T.I.; Vuorinen, T.; Ohtonen, P.; Syrjälä, H. Lower Respiratory Tract Virus Findings in Mechanically Ventilated Patients with Severe Community-Acquired Pneumonia. *Clin. Infect. Dis.* **2014**, *59*, 62–70. [CrossRef]
75. Choi, S.-H.; Huh, J.W.; Hong, S.-B.; Lee, J.Y.; Kim, S.-H.; Sung, H.; Do, K.-H.; Lee, S.-O.; Kim, M.-N.; Jeong, J.-Y.; et al. Clinical Characteristics and Outcomes of Severe Rhinovirus-Associated Pneumonia Identified by Bronchoscopic Bronchoalveolar Lavage in Adults: Comparison with Severe Influenza Virus-Associated Pneumonia. *J. Clin. Virol.* **2015**, *62*, 41–47. [CrossRef] [PubMed]
76. Gaunt, E.R.; Hardie, A.; Claas, E.C.J.; Simmonds, P.; Templeton, K.E. Epidemiology and Clinical Presentations of the Four Human Coronaviruses 229E, HKU1, NL63, and OC43 Detected over 3 Years Using a Novel Multiplex Real-Time PCR Method. *J. Clin. Microbiol.* **2010**, *48*, 2940–2947. [CrossRef]
77. Chung, H.; Hong, S.-B.; Huh, J.W.; Sung, H.; Do, K.-H.; Lee, S.-O.; Lim, C.-M.; Koh, Y.; Choi, S.-H. Clinical Features and Outcomes of Severe Pneumonia Caused by Endemic Human Coronavirus in Adults. *Am. J. Respir. Crit. Care Med.* **2022**, *205*, 1116–1118. [CrossRef]
78. Choi, S.-H.; Huh, J.W.; Hong, S.-B.; Jung, J.; Kim, M.J.; Chong, Y.P.; Kim, S.-H.; Sung, H.; Chae, E.J.; Do, K.-H.; et al. Severe Human Bocavirus-Associated Pneumonia in Adults at a Referral Hospital, Seoul, South Korea. *Emerg. Infect. Dis.* **2021**, *27*, 226–228. [CrossRef]

79. Ishiguro, T.; Hirota, S.; Kobayashi, Y.; Takano, K.; Kobayashi, Y.; Shimizu, Y.; Takayanagi, N. Fatal Primary Human Bocavirus Pneumonia in an Immunocompetent Adult. *Intern. Med.* **2020**, *59*, 421–424. [CrossRef]
80. Lee, N.; Lui, G.C.Y.; Wong, K.T.; Li, T.C.M.; Tse, E.C.M.; Chan, J.Y.C.; Yu, J.; Wong, S.S.M.; Choi, K.W.; Wong, R.Y.K.; et al. High Morbidity and Mortality in Adults Hospitalized for Respiratory Syncytial Virus Infections. *Clin. Infect. Dis.* **2013**, *57*, 1069–1077. [CrossRef]
81. Celante, H.; Oubaya, N.; Fourati, S.; Beaune, S.; Khellaf, M.; Casalino, E.; Ricard, J.-D.; Vieillard-Baron, A.; Heming, N.; Mekontso Dessap, A.; et al. Prognosis of Hospitalised Adult Patients with Respiratory Syncytial Virus Infection: A Multicentre Retrospective Cohort Study. *Clin. Microbiol. Infect.* **2023**, *29*, 943.e1–943.e8. [CrossRef]
82. Liu, Y.; Ling, L.; Wong, S.H.; Wang, M.H.; Fitzgerald, J.R.; Zou, X.; Fang, S.; Liu, X.; Wang, X.; Hu, W.; et al. Outcomes of Respiratory Viral-Bacterial Co-Infection in Adult Hospitalized Patients. *eClinicalMedicine* **2021**, *37*, 100955. [CrossRef] [PubMed]
83. Loubet, P.; Fernandes, J.; de Pouvourville, G.; Sosnowiez, K.; Elong, A.; Guilmet, C.; Omichessan, H.; Bureau, I.; Fagnani, F.; Emery, C.; et al. Respiratory Syncytial Virus-Related Hospital Stays in Adults in France from 2012 to 2021: A National Hospital Database Study. *J. Clin. Virol.* **2024**, *171*, 105635. [CrossRef]
84. Ackerson, B.; Tseng, H.F.; Sy, L.S.; Solano, Z.; Slezak, J.; Luo, Y.; Fischetti, C.A.; Shinde, V. Severe Morbidity and Mortality Associated with Respiratory Syncytial Virus Versus Influenza Infection in Hospitalized Older Adults. *Clin. Infect. Dis.* **2019**, *69*, 197–203. [CrossRef] [PubMed]
85. Beumer, M.C.; Koch, R.M.; van Beuningen, D.; OudeLashof, A.M.; van de Veerdonk, F.L.; Kolwijck, E.; van der Hoeven, J.G.; Bergmans, D.C.; Hoedemaekers, C.W.E. Influenza Virus and Factors That Are Associated with ICU Admission, Pulmonary Co-Infections and ICU Mortality. *J. Crit. Care* **2019**, *50*, 59–65. [CrossRef]
86. Verdier, V.; Lilienthal, F.; Desvergez, A.; Gazaille, V.; Winer, A.; Paganin, F. Severe Forms of Influenza Infections Admitted in Intensive Care Units: Analysis of Mortality Factors. *Influenza Other Respir. Viruses* **2023**, *17*, e13168. [CrossRef] [PubMed]
87. Bonmarin, I.; Belchior, E.; Bergounioux, J.; Brun-Buisson, C.; Mégarbane, B.; Chappert, J.L.; Hubert, B.; Strat, Y.L.; Lévy-Bruhl, D. Intensive Care Unit Surveillance of Influenza Infection in France: The 2009/10 Pandemic and the Three Subsequent Seasons. *Eurosurveillance* **2015**, *20*, 30066. [CrossRef]
88. Bouzid, D.; Hadad, O.; Bertine, M.; Houhou-Fidouh, N.; Mirand, A.; Duval, X.; Bunel, V.; Borie, R.; Lucet, J.C.; Descamps, D.; et al. Rhinoviruses: Molecular Diversity and Clinical Characteristics. *Int. J. Infect. Dis.* **2022**, *118*, 144–149. [CrossRef]
89. Boon, H.; Meinders, A.-J.; van Hannen, E.J.; Tersmette, M.; Schaftenaar, E. Comparative Analysis of Mortality in Patients Admitted with an Infection with Influenza A/B Virus, Respiratory Syncytial Virus, Rhinovirus, Metapneumovirus or SARS-CoV-2. *Influenza Other Respir. Viruses* **2024**, *18*, e13237. [CrossRef]
90. Rodriguez-Nava, G.; Egoryan, G.; Dong, T.; Zhang, Q.; Hyser, E.; Poudel, B.; Yanez-Bello, M.A.; Trelles-Garcia, D.P.; Chung, C.W.; Pyakuryal, B.; et al. Comparison of Clinical Characteristics and Outcomes of Hospitalized Patients with Seasonal Coronavirus Infection and COVID-19: A Retrospective Cohort Study. *BMC Infect. Dis.* **2022**, *22*, 618. [CrossRef]
91. Lee, N.; Smith, S.; Zelyas, N.; Klarenbach, S.; Zapernick, L.; Bekking, C.; So, H.; Yip, L.; Tipples, G.; Taylor, G.; et al. Burden of Noninfluenza Respiratory Viral Infections in Adults Admitted to Hospital: Analysis of a Multiyear Canadian Surveillance Cohort from 2 Centres. *CMAJ* **2021**, *193*, E439–E446. [CrossRef]
92. Savic, M.; Penders, Y.; Shi, T.; Branche, A.; Pirçon, J.-Y. Respiratory Syncytial Virus Disease Burden in Adults Aged 60 Years and Older in High-Income Countries: A Systematic Literature Review and Meta-Analysis. *Influenza Other Respir. Viruses* **2023**, *17*, e13031. [CrossRef] [PubMed]
93. Maleki, F.; Welch, V.; Lopez, S.M.C.; Cane, A.; Langer, J.; Enstone, A.; Markus, K.; Wright, O.; Hewitt, N.; Whittle, I. Understanding the Global Burden of Influenza in Adults Aged 18–64 Years: A Systematic Literature Review from 2012 to 2022. *Adv. Ther.* **2023**, *40*, 4166–4188. [CrossRef] [PubMed]
94. Branche, A.R.; Saiman, L.; Walsh, E.E.; Falsey, A.R.; Sieling, W.D.; Greendyke, W.; Peterson, D.R.; Vargas, C.Y.; Phillips, M.; Finelli, L. Incidence of Respiratory Syncytial Virus Infection Among Hospitalized Adults, 2017-2020. *Clin. Infect. Dis.* **2022**, *74*, 1004–1011. [CrossRef] [PubMed]
95. Branche, A.R.; Saiman, L.; Walsh, E.E.; Falsey, A.R.; Jia, H.; Barrett, A.; Alba, L.; Phillips, M.; Finelli, L. Change in Functional Status Associated with Respiratory Syncytial Virus Infection in Hospitalized Older Adults. *Influenza Other Respir. Viruses* **2022**, *16*, 1151–1160. [CrossRef]
96. Bajema, K.L.; Yan, L.; Li, Y.; Argraves, S.; Rajeevan, N.; Fox, A.; Vergun, R.; Berry, K.; Bui, D.; Huang, Y.; et al. Respiratory Syncytial Virus Vaccine Effectiveness among US Veterans, September, 2023 to March, 2024: A Target Trial Emulation Study. *Lancet Infect. Dis.* **2025**. [CrossRef]
97. Schmidt, M.; Demoule, A.; Hajage, D.; Pham, T.; Combes, A.; Dres, M.; Lebbah, S.; Kimmoun, A.; Mercat, A.; Beduneau, G.; et al. Benefits and Risks of Noninvasive Oxygenation Strategy in COVID-19: A Multicenter, Prospective Cohort Study (COVID-ICU) in 137 Hospitals. *Crit. Care* **2021**, *25*, 421. [CrossRef]

98. Bouadma, L.; Mekontso-Dessap, A.; Burdet, C.; Merdji, H.; Poissy, J.; Dupuis, C.; Guitton, C.; Schwebel, C.; Cohen, Y.; Bruel, C.; et al. High-Dose Dexamethasone and Oxygen Support Strategies in Intensive Care Unit Patients with Severe COVID-19 Acute Hypoxemic Respiratory Failure: The COVIDICUS Randomized Clinical Trial. *JAMA Intern. Med.* **2022**, *182*, 906–916. [CrossRef]
99. Gao, Y.; Guyatt, G.; Uyeki, T.M.; Liu, M.; Chen, Y.; Zhao, Y.; Shen, Y.; Xu, J.; Zheng, Q.; Li, Z.; et al. Antivirals for Treatment of Severe Influenza: A Systematic Review and Network Meta-Analysis of Randomised Controlled Trials. *Lancet* **2024**, *404*, 753–763. [CrossRef]
100. Moreno, G.; Carbonell, R.; Díaz, E.; Martín-Loeches, I.; Restrepo, M.I.; Reyes, L.F.; Solé-Violán, J.; Bodí, M.; Canadell, L.; Guardiola, J.; et al. Effectiveness of Prolonged versus Standard-Course of Oseltamivir in Critically Ill Patients with Severe Influenza Infection: A Multicentre Cohort Study. *J. Med. Virol.* **2023**, *95*, e29010. [CrossRef]
101. Duval, X.; van der Werf, S.; Blanchon, T.; Mosnier, A.; Bouscambert-Duchamp, M.; Tibi, A.; Enouf, V.; Charlois-Ou, C.; Vincent, C.; Andreoletti, L.; et al. Efficacy of Oseltamivir-Zanamivir Combination Compared to Each Monotherapy for Seasonal Influenza: A Randomized Placebo-Controlled Trial. *PLoS Med.* **2010**, *7*, e1000362. [CrossRef]
102. Kumar, D.; Ison, M.G.; Mira, J.-P.; Welte, T.; Hwan Ha, J.; Hui, D.S.; Zhong, N.; Saito, T.; Katugampola, L.; Collinson, N.; et al. Combining Baloxavir Marboxil with Standard-of-Care Neuraminidase Inhibitor in Patients Hospitalised with Severe Influenza (FLAGSTONE): A Randomised, Parallel-Group, Double-Blind, Placebo-Controlled, Superiority Trial. *Lancet Infect. Dis.* **2022**, *22*, 718–730. [CrossRef]
103. Tejada, S.; Martinez-Reviejo, R.; Karakoc, H.N.; Peña-López, Y.; Manuel, O.; Rello, J. Ribavirin for Treatment of Subjects with Respiratory Syncytial Virus-Related Infection: A Systematic Review and Meta-Analysis. *Adv. Ther.* **2022**, *39*, 4037–4051. [CrossRef]
104. Hanula, R.; Bortolussi-Courval, É.; Mendel, A.; Ward, B.J.; Lee, T.C.; McDonald, E.G. Evaluation of Oseltamivir Used to Prevent Hospitalization in Outpatients with Influenza: A Systematic Review and Meta-Analysis. *JAMA Intern. Med.* **2024**, *184*, 18–27. [CrossRef] [PubMed]
105. Gubareva, L.V.; Besselaar, T.G.; Daniels, R.S.; Fry, A.; Gregory, V.; Huang, W.; Hurt, A.C.; Jorquera, P.A.; Lackenby, A.; Leang, S.-K.; et al. Global Update on the Susceptibility of Human Influenza Viruses to Neuraminidase Inhibitors, 2015–2016. *Antivir. Res.* **2017**, *146*, 12–20. [CrossRef] [PubMed]
106. Lina, B.; Boucher, C.; Osterhaus, A.; Monto, A.S.; Schutten, M.; Whitley, R.J.; Nguyen-Van-Tam, J.S. Five Years of Monitoring for the Emergence of Oseltamivir Resistance in Patients with Influenza A Infections in the Influenza Resistance Information Study. *Influenza Other Respir. Viruses* **2018**, *12*, 267–278. [CrossRef] [PubMed]
107. Kohno, S.; Yen, M.-Y.; Cheong, H.-J.; Hirotsu, N.; Ishida, T.; Kadota, J.; Mizuguchi, M.; Kida, H.; Shimada, J. S-021812 Clinical Study Group Phase III Randomized, Double-Blind Study Comparing Single-Dose Intravenous Peramivir with Oral Oseltamivir in Patients with Seasonal Influenza Virus Infection. *Antimicrob. Agents Chemother.* **2011**, *55*, 5267–5276. [CrossRef]
108. Chen, H.-D.; Wang, X.; Yu, S.-L.; Ding, Y.-H.; Wang, M.-L.; Wang, J.-N. Clinical Effectiveness of Intravenous Peramivir Compared with Oseltamivir in Patients with Severe Influenza A with Primary Viral Pneumonia: A Randomized Controlled Study. *Open Forum Infect. Dis.* **2021**, *8*, ofaa562. [CrossRef]
109. Marty, F.M.; Vidal-Puigserver, J.; Clark, C.; Gupta, S.K.; Merino, E.; Garot, D.; Chapman, M.J.; Jacobs, F.; Rodriguez-Noriega, E.; Husa, P.; et al. Intravenous Zanamivir or Oral Oseltamivir for Hospitalised Patients with Influenza: An International, Randomised, Double-Blind, Double-Dummy, Phase 3 Trial. *Lancet Respir. Med.* **2017**, *5*, 135–146. [CrossRef]
110. Hayden, F.G.; Sugaya, N.; Hirotsu, N.; Lee, N.; de Jong, M.D.; Hurt, A.C.; Ishida, T.; Sekino, H.; Yamada, K.; Portsmouth, S.; et al. Baloxavir Marboxil for Uncomplicated Influenza in Adults and Adolescents. *N. Engl. J. Med.* **2018**, *379*, 913–923. [CrossRef]
111. Ison, M.G.; Portsmouth, S.; Yoshida, Y.; Shishido, T.; Mitchener, M.; Tsuchiya, K.; Uehara, T.; Hayden, F.G. Early Treatment with Baloxavir Marboxil in High-Risk Adolescent and Adult Outpatients with Uncomplicated Influenza (CAPSTONE-2): A Randomised, Placebo-Controlled, Phase 3 Trial. *Lancet Infect. Dis.* **2020**, *20*, 1204–1214. [CrossRef]
112. Manothummetha, K.; Mongkolkaew, T.; Tovichayathamrong, P.; Boonyawairote, R.; Meejun, T.; Srisurapanont, K.; Phongkhun, K.; Sanguankeo, A.; Torvorapanit, P.; Moonla, C.; et al. Ribavirin Treatment for Respiratory Syncytial Virus Infection in Patients with Haematologic Malignancy and Haematopoietic Stem Cell Transplant Recipients: A Systematic Review and Meta-Analysis. *Clin. Microbiol. Infect.* **2023**, *29*, 1272–1279. [CrossRef] [PubMed]
113. Lindemans, C.A.; Leen, A.M.; Boelens, J.J. How I Treat Adenovirus in Hematopoietic Stem Cell Transplant Recipients. *Blood* **2010**, *116*, 5476–5485. [CrossRef] [PubMed]
114. Dequin, P.-F.; Meziani, F.; Quenot, J.-P.; Kamel, T.; Ricard, J.-D.; Badie, J.; Reignier, J.; Heming, N.; Plantefève, G.; Souweine, B.; et al. Hydrocortisone in Severe Community-Acquired Pneumonia. *N. Engl. J. Med.* **2023**, *388*, 1931–1941. [CrossRef] [PubMed]
115. Lansbury, L.E.; Rodrigo, C.; Leonardi-Bee, J.; Nguyen-Van-Tam, J.; Shen Lim, W. Corticosteroids as Adjunctive Therapy in the Treatment of Influenza: An Updated Cochrane Systematic Review and Meta-Analysis. *Crit. Care Med.* **2020**, *48*, e98–e106. [CrossRef]

116. Smit, J.M.; Van Der Zee, P.A.; Stoof, S.C.M.; Van Genderen, M.E.; Snijders, D.; Boersma, W.G.; Confalonieri, P.; Salton, F.; Confalonieri, M.; Shih, M.-C.; et al. Predicting Benefit from Adjuvant Therapy with Corticosteroids in Community-Acquired Pneumonia: A Data-Driven Analysis of Randomised Trials. *Lancet Respir. Med.* **2025**, *13*, 221–233. [CrossRef]
117. Tanner, A.R.; Dorey, R.B.; Brendish, N.J.; Clark, T.W. Influenza Vaccination: Protecting the Most Vulnerable. *Eur. Respir. Rev.* **2021**, *30*, 200258. [CrossRef]
118. Demicheli, V.; Jefferson, T.; Di Pietrantonj, C.; Ferroni, E.; Thorning, S.; Thomas, R.E.; Rivetti, A. Vaccines for Preventing Influenza in the Elderly. *Cochrane Database Syst. Rev.* **2018**, *2*, CD004876. [CrossRef]
119. Newall, A.T.; Nazareno, A.L.; Muscatello, D.J.; Boettiger, D.; Viboud, C.; Simonsen, L.; Turner, R.M. The Association between Influenza Vaccination Uptake and Influenza and Pneumonia-Associated Deaths in the United States. *Vaccine* **2024**, *42*, 2044–2050. [CrossRef]
120. Bonmarin, I.; Belchior, E.; Lévy-Bruhl, D. Impact of Influenza Vaccination on Mortality in the French Elderly Population during the 2000–2009 Period. *Vaccine* **2015**, *33*, 1099–1101. [CrossRef]
121. Payne, A.B.; Watts, J.A.; Mitchell, P.K.; Dascomb, K.; Irving, S.A.; Klein, N.P.; Grannis, S.J.; Ong, T.C.; Ball, S.W.; DeSilva, M.B.; et al. Respiratory Syncytial Virus (RSV) Vaccine Effectiveness against RSV-Associated Hospitalisations and Emergency Department Encounters among Adults Aged 60 Years and Older in the USA, October, 2023, to March, 2024: A Test-Negative Design Analysis. *Lancet* **2024**, *404*, 1547–1559. [CrossRef]
122. Dyer, O. Measles: Texas Outbreak Spreads to New Mexico. *BMJ* **2025**, *388*, r357. [CrossRef] [PubMed]
123. Kuppalli, K.; Perl, T.M. Measles in Texas: Waning Vaccination and a Stark Warning for Public Health. *Lancet Infect. Dis.* **2025**, *25*, 485–487. [CrossRef] [PubMed]
124. Hübschen, J.M.; Gouandjika-Vasilache, I.; Dina, J. Measles. *Lancet* **2022**, *399*, 678–690. [CrossRef] [PubMed]
125. Lombardo, D.; Ciampi, G.; Spicuzza, L. Severe and Fatal Measles-Associated Pneumonia during an Outbreak in Italy: Data from the Heart of the Epidemic. *Adv. Respir. Med.* **2020**, *88*, 197–203. [CrossRef]
126. Rafat, C.; Klouche, K.; Ricard, J.-D.; Messika, J.; Roch, A.; Machado, S.; Sonneville, R.; Guisset, O.; Pujol, W.; Guérin, C.; et al. Severe Measles Infection: The Spectrum of Disease in 36 Critically Ill Adult Patients. *Medicine* **2013**, *92*, 257–272. [CrossRef]
127. Chen, Z.; Tsui, J.L.-H.; Gutierrez, B.; Busch Moreno, S.; du Plessis, L.; Deng, X.; Cai, J.; Bajaj, S.; Suchard, M.A.; Pybus, O.G.; et al. COVID-19 Pandemic Interventions Reshaped the Global Dispersal of Seasonal Influenza Viruses. *Science* **2024**, *386*, eadq3003. [CrossRef]
128. Chow, E.J.; Uyeki, T.M.; Chu, H.Y. The Effects of the COVID-19 Pandemic on Community Respiratory Virus Activity. *Nat. Rev. Microbiol.* **2023**, *21*, 195–210. [CrossRef]
129. Wang, X.; Walker, G.; Kim, K.W.; Stelzer-Braid, S.; Scotch, M.; Rawlinson, W.D. The Resurgence of Influenza A/H3N2 Virus in Australia after the Relaxation of COVID-19 Restrictions during the 2022 Season. *J. Med. Virol.* **2024**, *96*, e29922. [CrossRef]
130. Perofsky, A.C.; Huddleston, J.; Hansen, C.L.; Barnes, J.R.; Rowe, T.; Xu, X.; Kondor, R.; Wentworth, D.E.; Lewis, N.; Whittaker, L.; et al. Antigenic Drift and Subtype Interference Shape A(H3N2) Epidemic Dynamics in the United States. *Elife* **2024**, *13*, RP91849. [CrossRef]
131. Rabaan, A.A.; Alenazy, M.F.; Alshehri, A.A.; Alshahrani, M.A.; Al-Subaie, M.F.; Alrasheed, H.A.; Al Kaabi, N.A.; Thakur, N.; Bouafia, N.A.; Alissa, M.; et al. An Updated Review on Pathogenic Coronaviruses (CoVs) amid the Emergence of SARS-CoV-2 Variants: A Look into the Repercussions and Possible Solutions. *J. Infect. Public Health* **2023**, *16*, 1870–1883. [CrossRef]
132. de Wit, E.; van Doremalen, N.; Falzarano, D.; Munster, V.J. SARS and MERS: Recent Insights into Emerging Coronaviruses. *Nat. Rev. Microbiol.* **2016**, *14*, 523–534. [CrossRef] [PubMed]
133. Girard, M.P.; Tam, J.S.; Assossou, O.M.; Kieny, M.P. The 2009 A (H1N1) Influenza Virus Pandemic: A Review. *Vaccine* **2010**, *28*, 4895–4902. [CrossRef] [PubMed]
134. Lai, S.; Qin, Y.; Cowling, B.J.; Ren, X.; Wardrop, N.A.; Gilbert, M.; Tsang, T.K.; Wu, P.; Feng, L.; Jiang, H.; et al. Global Epidemiology of Avian Influenza A H5N1 Virus Infection in Humans, 1997-2015: A Systematic Review of Individual Case Data. *Lancet Infect. Dis.* **2016**, *16*, e108–e118. [CrossRef] [PubMed]
135. Zatta, M.; Brichler, S.; Vindrios, W.; Melica, G.; Gallien, S. Autochthonous Dengue Outbreak, Paris Region, France, September–October 2023. *Emerg. Infect. Dis.* **2023**, *29*, 2538–2540. [CrossRef]
136. Watson, R. Chikungunya Fever Is Transmitted Locally in Europe for First Time. *BMJ* **2007**, *335*, 532–533. [CrossRef]
137. Greenhalgh, T.; MacIntyre, C.R.; Baker, M.G.; Bhattacharjee, S.; Chughtai, A.A.; Fisman, D.; Kunasekaran, M.; Kvalsvig, A.; Lupton, D.; Oliver, M.; et al. Masks and Respirators for Prevention of Respiratory Infections: A State of the Science Review. *Clin. Microbiol. Rev.* **2024**, *37*, e0012324. [CrossRef]

Disclaimer/Publisher's Note: The statements, opinions and data contained in all publications are solely those of the individual author(s) and contributor(s) and not of MDPI and/or the editor(s). MDPI and/or the editor(s) disclaim responsibility for any injury to people or property resulting from any ideas, methods, instructions or products referred to in the content.

MDPI AG
Grosspeteranlage 5
4052 Basel
Switzerland
Tel.: +41 61 683 77 34

Journal of Clinical Medicine Editorial Office
E-mail: jcm@mdpi.com
www.mdpi.com/journal/jcm

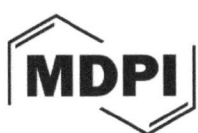

Disclaimer/Publisher's Note: The title and front matter of this reprint are at the discretion of the Guest Editor. The publisher is not responsible for their content or any associated concerns. The statements, opinions and data contained in all individual articles are solely those of the individual Editor and contributors and not of MDPI. MDPI disclaims responsibility for any injury to people or property resulting from any ideas, methods, instructions or products referred to in the content.

www.ingramcontent.com/pod-product-compliance
Lightning Source LLC
LaVergne TN
LVHW070000100526
838202LV00019B/2596